Nutrition Therapy for Chronic Kidney Disease

Nutrition Therapy for Chronic Kidney Disease

Edited by **Lynn K. Thomas**
Jennifer Bohnstadt Othersen

CRC Press
Taylor & Francis Group
Boca Raton London New York

CRC Press is an imprint of the
Taylor & Francis Group, an **informa** business

CRC Press
Taylor & Francis Group
6000 Broken Sound Parkway NW, Suite 300
Boca Raton, FL 33487-2742

Version Date: 20120215

International Standard Book Number: 978-1-4398-4949-1 (Hardback)

Library of Congress Cataloging-in-Publication Data

Nutrition therapy for chronic kidney disease / editors, Lynn K. Thomas, Jennifer Bohnstadt Othersen.
p. cm.
Summary: "This book presents variations in nutritional therapy through the five stages of chronic kidney disease. Chapters cover history of renal disease management and pathophysiology; electrolyte and acid-based disorders; acute renal disease; dialysis techniques; children/adolescents with chronic kidney disease; pregnancy with chronic kidney disease; bone and mineral disorders management; drug-nutrient/drug supplements; endocrine and lipid management; anemia management; enteral and parenteral support; nutrition post transplant; and establishing quality of life improvement parameters. The text links clinical applications to the Kidney Foundation Outcome Quality Initiative resources and provides dietary and supplement recommendations"-- Provided by publisher.
Includes bibliographical references and index.
ISBN 978-1-4398-4949-1 (hardback)
1. Kidneys--Diseases--Nutritional aspects. 2. Kidneys--Diseases--Diet therapy. I. Thomas, Lynn K. II. Bohnstadt Othersen, Jennifer.

RC903.N878 2012
616.6'1--dc23 2011052594

Visit the Taylor & Francis Web site at
http://www.taylorandfrancis.com

and the CRC Press Web site at
http://www.crcpress.com

To the many terrific dietitians that I have worked with and learned from over the years: Thank you.

Lynn K. Thomas

To Biemann for your patience and support,
to my amazing children who inspire me,
and to the patients whom I have had the privilege to treat.

Jennifer Othersen

Contents

Preface

Kidney disease is a global health concern. It has been classified into many stages and affects people of all ages and races. It can be acute or chronic. The National Kidney Foundation Disease Outcomes Quality Initiative (NKF KDOQI)™ and the Kidney Disease: Improving Global Outcomes (KDIGO)™ Foundation have done an outstanding job of outlining the many facets of the disease and describing the parameters for adequate care of patients with kidney disease. This book builds on those guidelines in the area of nutrition therapy.

Nutrition Therapy for Chronic Kidney Disease begins with a chapter on the history of the disease, which documents some of the early treatments for kidney disease. The next several chapters cover physiology, imbalance of electrolytes, acute kidney injury, and the techniques of dialysis. There are additional chapters on special populations and the unique concerns associated with end-stage disease and chapters on quality improvement programs and counseling strategies. Most of all, this book provides an expansive discussion on optimal nutritional management, which can improve the quality of life of people with kidney disease.

This book would not have been possible without the contribution of experts from many different professions who devoted their time and effort freely to construct chapters that are timely and practical and also provided guidance regarding the stages of kidney disease and the accompanying dietary restrictions. We, the editors, are forever grateful for their contributions.

Lynn K. Thomas
University of South Carolina School of Medicine
Columbia, South Carolina

Jennifer Othersen
WJB Dorn VA Medical Center
Columbia, South Carolina

Editors

Dr. Lynn K. Thomas is the assistant dean for preclinical curriculum in the Office of Medical Education and a clinical associate professor in the Department of Family and Preventive Medicine, University of South Carolina School of Medicine. She also serves as the director of the Nutrition Vertical Curriculum for the School of Medicine. She holds an associate degree in secondary education from Shawnee State University; dual bachelors' degrees in English and Dietetics plus a master's degree in Home Economics/Nutrition from Marshall University; and a doctorate in Public Health with an emphasis on nutrition education, from the University of South Carolina. She is a registered dietitian, licensed in South Carolina, and a certified nutrition support clinician. Dr. Thomas has over 25 years of experience as a nutrition support and renal dietitian. She publishes in both the nutrition and the education fields. In addition, she is a member of numerous professional organizations including the American Dietetic Association, American Society of Parenteral and Enteral Nutrition, and the National Kidney Foundation Council on Renal Nutrition.

Dr. Jennifer Othersen is the chief of the Division of Nephrology at the WJB Dorn VA Medical Center in Columbia, South Carolina. She is also a DVAMC assistant professor of clinical internal medicine at the University of South Carolina. She earned a BS in biology at Francis Marion University followed by a second BS in chemistry at the University of South Carolina. She holds an MD from the Medical University of South Carolina where she also received her training in internal medicine and nephrology. She is board certified in internal medicine and nephrology. She is active in clinical research and is a principal investigator on several research studies currently being conducted at the WJB Dorn VA Medical Center.

Contributors

Nicole Armellino-Nitti
Loyola University Medical Center
Maywood, Illinois

Malcolm L. Buford
Department of Medicine
Division of Nephrology and Hypertension
School of Community Medicine
University of Oklahoma-Tulsa
Tulsa, Oklahoma

Tai-Gen Cui
Department of Nephrology
Beijing Chaoyang Hospital
Capital Medical University
Beijing, China

Taixing Cui
Department of Cell Biology and Anatomy
University of South Carolina School of Medicine
Columbia, South Carolina

Charles J. Foulks
Department of Medicine
Division of Nephrology and Hypertension
School of Community Medicine
University of Oklahoma-Tulsa
Tulsa, Oklahoma

Ann Grothe
DaVita Peninsula Dialysis
Newport News, Virginia

Joseph Janicki
Department of Cell Biology and Anatomy
University of South Carolina School of Medicine
Columbia, South Carolina

Tamara Karosanidze
University of Virginia Health System
Charlottesville, Virginia

Pranay Kathuria
Department of Medicine
Division of Nephrology and Hypertension
School of Community Medicine
University of Oklahoma-Tulsa
Tulsa, Oklahoma

Anand Khurana
Department of Medicine
Division of Nephrology and Hypertension
School of Community Medicine
University of Oklahoma-Tulsa
Tulsa, Oklahoma

Fran Kittell
American Family Children's Hospital
University of Wisconsin–Madison
Madison, Wisconsin

Jeannine C. Lawrence
College of Human Environmental Sciences
Department of Human Nutrition and Hospitality Management
University of Alabama
Tuscaloosa, Alabama

Emily Dill McDonald
WJB Dorn VA Medical Center
Columbia, South Carolina

Lesley McPhatter
Renal Nutrition Services
University of Virginia
Charlottesville, Virginia

Tanis Vye Mihalynuk
School of Nutrition and Dietetics
Acadia University
Wolfville, Nova Scotia, Canada

Claire Moise
WJB Dorn VA Medical Center
Columbia, South Carolina

Matthew Orr
Department of Family and Preventive Medicine
University of South Carolina School of Medicine
Columbia, South Carolina

Jennifer Othersen
Division of Nephrology
WJB Dorn VA Medical Center
and
Clinical Internal Medicine
University of South Carolina School of Medicine
Columbia, South Carolina

Beth Parris
Blue Cross Blue Shield of South Carolina
Columbia, South Carolina

C.J. Parris
Columbia Nephrology
Columbia, South Carolina

Peggy Solan
Clinical Nutrition Service
Division of Nephrology
Seattle Children's Hospital
Seattle, Washington

Kim S. Stote
Empire State College
State University of New York
Saratoga Springs, New York

Lynn K. Thomas
Office of Medical Education and Curricular Affairs
University of South Carolina School of Medicine
Columbia, South Carolina

Kyle Thompson
Department of Nutrition and Health Care Management
Appalachian State University
Boone, North Carolina

L. Britt Wilson
Department of Pharmacology, Physiology, and Neuroscience
University of South Carolina School of Medicine
Columbia, South Carolina

1 Brief History of Kidney Disease

Lynn K. Thomas
University of South Carolina School of Medicine

CONTENTS

1.1 THE PAST

In most prehistoric cultures, there was a shared basic belief that all diseases and pain are caused by external means. Man had no control on unfriendly spirits and demons. He knew of no way to ease his suffering. It was in the Neolithic era (9500–3000 BCE) that man first tried to change the course of illness. Shamans, priests, and medicine men provided magical cures and herbal potions for use against supernatural illnesses. During the "Golden Age of Babylonia," physicians placated angry gods in return for good health. Physicians at this time were religious and were closely associated with temples. Ancient Egyptian medical papyri, *circa* 2000 BCE, describe the use of concoctions empowered with magical spells. This was early medicine (Longrigg, 1993).

In the sixth century BCE, Babylonian physicians started documenting symptoms and naming disease states, such as discharge diseases, kidney stones, and strictures. They also developed an extensive collection of prescriptions and procedures. However, if the patient was incurable, they still deferred the patient to the local incantation priest. This Babylonian system of observing symptoms is very similar to the one noted in the *Hippocratic Corpus*, and it most likely contributed greatly to the advancement of Greek medicine (Geller and Cohen, 1995).

It was not until the Greek physician Hippocrates Asclepiades (460–377 BCE; Figure 1.1) started his medical school on the island of Kos that the treatment of disease became based on science instead of religion. During this time, Hippocrates truly shifted the cause of illness from the mystic to the natural (Dolan and Adams-Smith, 1978). He borrowed documentation methods from the Babylonians and pharmacopeia, medical practices, and surgical techniques from the early Egyptians (Figure 1.2; Greek Medicine, 2010).

The faculty and students of the Kos medical school explored many diverse diseases and documented various descriptions of signs and symptoms of diseases (Bloom, 1997). They established

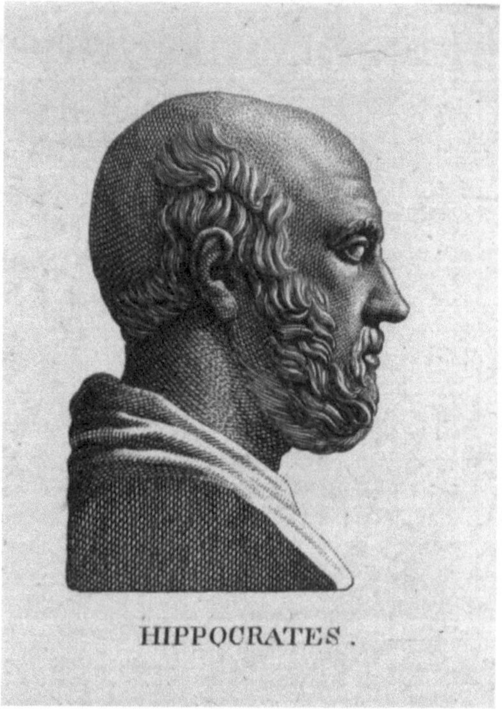

FIGURE 1.1 Hippocrates (460–377 BCE). (Courtesy of the National Library of Medicine.)

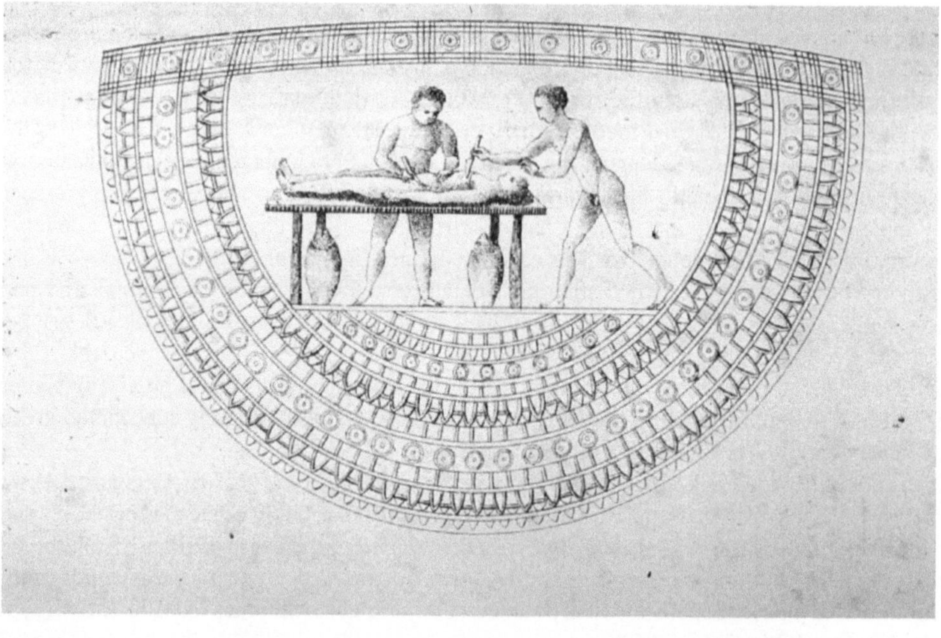

FIGURE 1.2 Early Greek medical practice. (Courtesy of the National Library of Medicine.)

TABLE 1.1
Humors

Characteristics	Empedocles's Elements	Hippocrates's Humors	Hippocrates's Seasons	Hippocrates's Organs
Bad temper	Fire	Yellow bile	Summer	Liver
Despondent	Earth	Black bile	Autumn	Brain/lungs
Calm	Water	Phlegm	Winter	Gall bladder
Hopeful	Air	Blood	Spring	Spleen

the belief that every living being contained certain mixtures of four humors (yellow bile, black bile, phlegm, and blood). This belief was based on another popular theory, *Essentialism*, postulated by Empedocles (495–435 BCE), which described four material elements (air, earth, water, and fire). The four material elements were controlled by forces called love and strife. The forces would continuously act on the elements, which would be either held together by love or driven apart by strife. The goal was to have both the elements and the forces in balance (Empedocles, 2010; Kirk et al., 1983).

Hippocrates associated his idea of "humoralism" with the four elements and the four seasons (Hippocratic Seasonal Diseases, 2010). He then related Empedocles's balance theory to the humors. A person in good health was considered "eucrasic." An ill person was someone with an imbalance of humors or "dyscrasic." Hippocrates also linked the humors to body organs (Table 1.1). The use of this system for diagnosis led the physicians to look for symptoms, or what is now known as "doing a clinical observation" (Hippocratic Method and the Four Humors in Medicine, 2010). An example is as follows: a fever was thought to be caused by too much blood in the body. This clinical observation led to the practice of "bleeding" the patient (Cataldi, 1998; Diamandopoulos et al., 2009; Figures 1.3 through 1.6).

Around the same time that Hippocrates was establishing scientific methods and describing diseases, the Medical School of Knidos, Asia Minor, was concerning itself with the classification of diseases by symptoms. In a book attributed to the school, *About Inner Sufferings*, four renal diseases were classified first. Two descriptions that are considered accurate even today include those of nephrolithiasis with renal colic and renal tuberculosis. The symptoms of the third disease resemble those of possible renal vein thrombosis or bilateral papillary necrosis. The fourth disease corresponds to chronic suppurative renal infection or sexually transmitted urethritis (Dardioti et al., 1997).

1.2 EARLY UNDERSTANDING OF KIDNEYS

Throughout antiquity, kidneys were not considered as important as the heart, liver, lungs, and intestines. One of the earliest references to the kidneys came from Aristotle Stagiritis (384–322 BCE). He wrote in his work *De Partibus Animalium* that "the human kidneys are of similar shape; being as it were made up of numerous small kidneys, and not presenting one unbroken surface …" Aristotle believed that the kidneys served two functions. One was to remove surplus liquid from the blood, and the other was to funnel this liquid through the ureter, bladder, and urethra. During this passage, the liquid would be filtered and transformed into "residuum" or urine.

Erasistratus of Ceos (304–250 BCE) was one of the early physicians to consider the kidneys as the source of urine (Twardowski, 2008). Another Greek physician, Claudius Galen (129–214 CE), in his book on functions of body parts, rejected the work of Aristotle and Erasistratus. He believed that the thin watery liquid in the blood was a vehicle for nutrients and that when the nutrients were depleted, the liquid would be extracted from the blood by the kidneys and directly passed to the ureters and then to the bladder. Galen (1968) rejected the possibility that

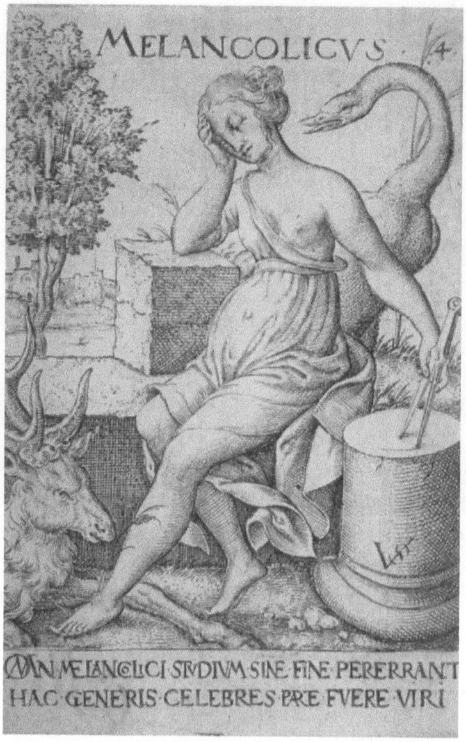

FIGURE 1.3 Black bile humor. (Courtesy of the National Library of Medicine.)

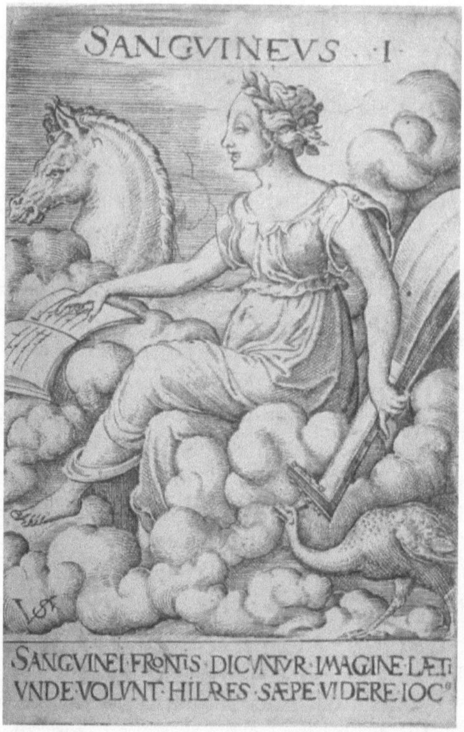

FIGURE 1.4 Blood humor. (Courtesy of the National Library of Medicine.)

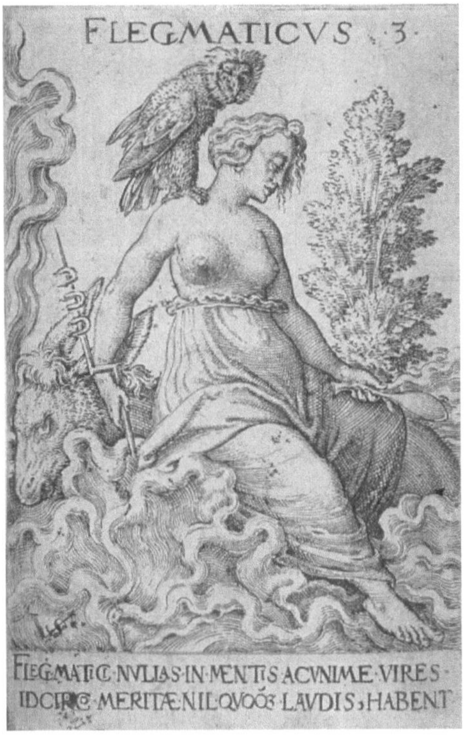

FIGURE 1.5 Phlegm humor. (Courtesy of the National Library of Medicine.)

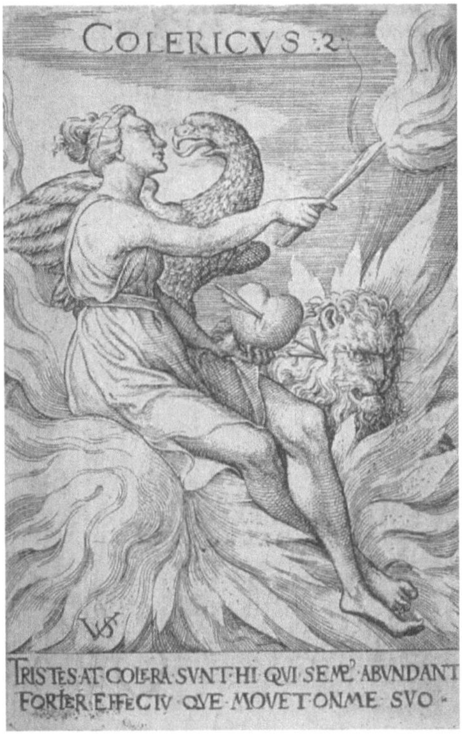

FIGURE 1.6 Yellow bile humor. (Courtesy of the National Library of Medicine.)

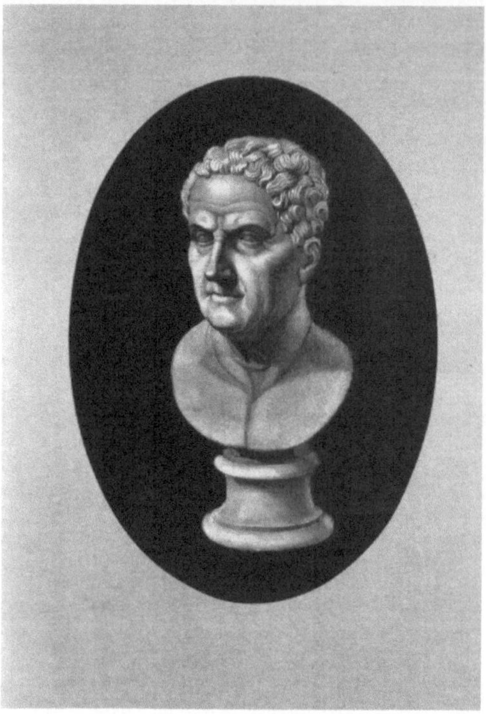

FIGURE 1.7 Claudius Galen (129–214 CE). (Courtesy of the National Library of Medicine.)

the kidneys filtered urine. He instead determined that the kidneys "attracted" the depleted liquid or urine (Galen, Translated by May, 1968; Figure 1.7).

For centuries, the gross anatomy of the kidneys was well documented. Leonardo da Vinci (1452–1519 CE) portrayed the anatomical features of the kidneys more accurately and artistically than anyone before him. Unfortunately, he did not provide any new knowledge about the urinary system. There continued to be little understanding of the functionality of the kidneys until the publication of *Opuscula Anatomica* (1564 CE) by Bartolomeo Eustachio (Figure 1.8). He illustrated the kidneys in 47 copper-plated engravings and first described renal collecting ducts. Eustachio proposed that the tiny ducts moved the urine from the kidney to the renal pelvis. He also described the adrenal glands and the differing locations of the left and the right kidney (Mezzogiorno, 1999).

In 1662, Lorenzo Bellini (1643–1704 CE) suggested that small, intertwined masses in the kidney were responsible for keeping urine separated from the blood. In 1666, at the University of Messina, Sicily, Marcello Malpighi, a professor of medicine and founder of microscopic anatomy discipline, was finally able to describe kidney histology and give physicians the first insight into the mechanism of urine formation. He described the actual structure of the kidney, including the glomerulus and the renal pyramids. Professor Malpighi utilized a microscope, made possible by the invention of the lens, and two different staining techniques to identify the tubular structures and the vascular tree (Andreucci, 1972; Eknoyan, 1996; Figure 1.9).

1.3 MORE DISCOVERIES

As medicine advanced, the documentation of the gross and microscopic anatomical description of the kidneys became more accurate. Frederich Henle (1809–1885) was a physician interested in the fine structure of organs and tissues. In 1862, he described the presence of perpendicular tubular loops imbedded on the kidney surface. He further described the tissue of the convoluted and straight cortical tubules found in the kidneys as epithelial in nature and declared that the same type of tissue

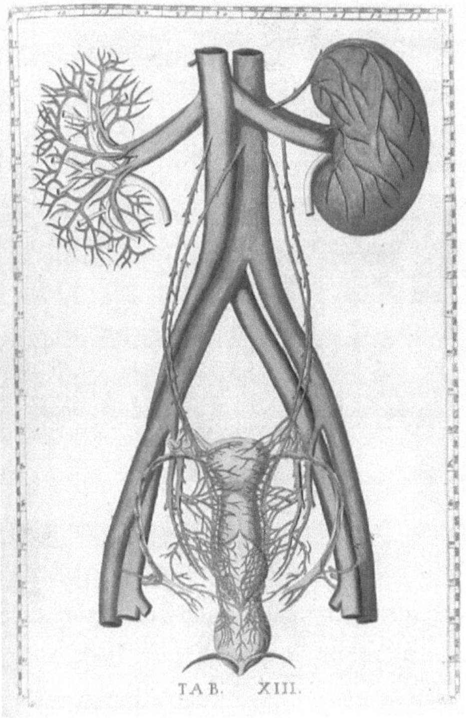

FIGURE 1.8 Depiction of urinary system in *Opuscula Anatomica* by Bartolomeo Eustachio. (Courtesy of the National Library of Medicine.)

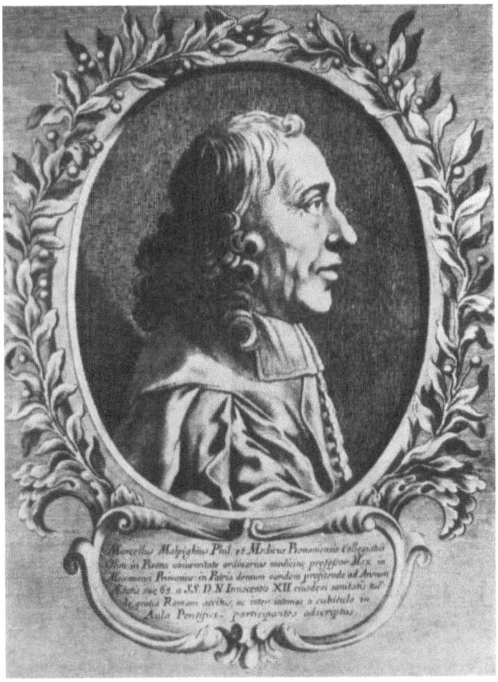

FIGURE 1.9 Marcello Malpighi. (Courtesy of the National Library of Medicine.)

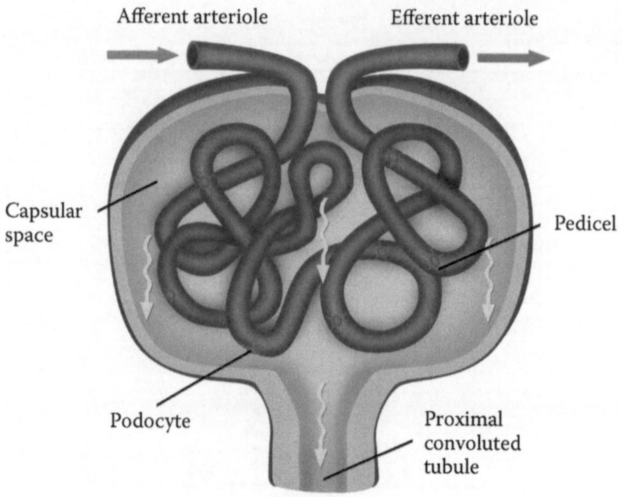

FIGURE 1.10 Bowman's capsule. (From Shaun Riffle, University of South Carolina School of Medicine, Columbia, SC. With permission.)

formed protective layers in the medullary and papillary collecting tubules and the duct of Bellini. Henle assigned no function to the structures. Urine-formation principles were the subject of intense debate during this period (Cataldi, 1998; Morel, 1999).

In 1842, William Bowman (1816–1892), a physiologist, investigated the relationship between the glomerulus and the renal tubules. He studied thin slices of kidneys using the high-power microscope of his days (300×) and described the glomerular capillary tuft and its relation to the afferent and efferent arterioles. He was the first to describe the basement membrane of the tubules and to demonstrate the function of the capsules. He concluded that the glomerular capsule functioned as a receptacle of filtrate separated from "blood in the capillaries" (Eknoyan, 1996; Todd and Bowman, 1856; Figure 1.10).

1.4 URINE

The work of Hippocrates in 400 BCE, *Corpus Hippocraticum*, contains approximately 400 aphorisms that refer to the practice of medicine. Several of these describe how the urine reflects different stages of renal disease.

When the urine is transparent and white, it is bad; it appears principally in cases of phrenitis.

Hippocrates (Section 4, Aphorsim 72 from Adams translation)

In those cases in which urine is thin at first, and the sediments become bilious, an acute disease is indicated.

Hippocrates (Section 7, Aphorism 32 from Adams translation)

Diseases about the kidneys and bladder are cured with difficulty in old men.

Hippocrates (Section 6, Aphorism 6 from Adams translation)

Early Babylonian medicine also looked at urine as the diagnostic tool for kidney disease. Markham Geller writes that the ancient physician consulted a list comprising statements such as *If his urine is like beer dregs, man suffers from discharge disease* (Geller and Cohen, 1995). Much later, Antoine François, comte de Fourcroy, a physician, and Louis Vauquelin, a pharmacist and chemist, in the early nineteenth century completed the analysis of urine and for the first time

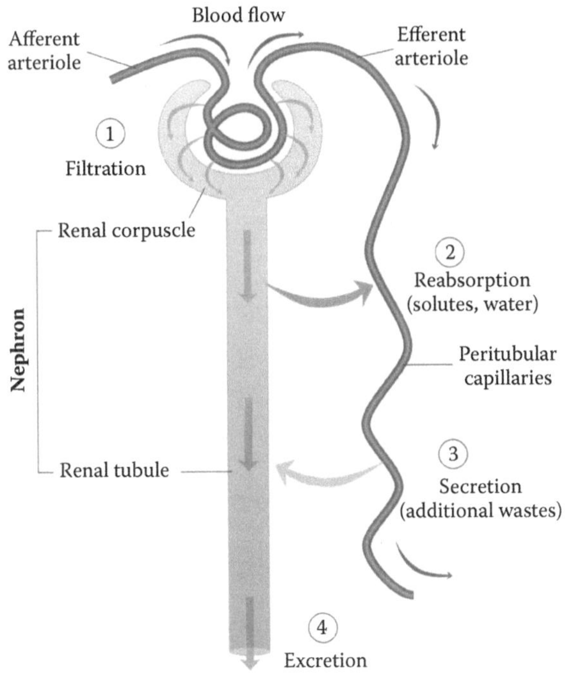

FIGURE 1.11 Urine formation. (From Alila07/Dreamstime.com, Dreamstime USA Headquarters, Brentwood, TN. With permission.)

noted the presence of nitrogen. They also were the first to surmise that urea overload could be capable of causing diseases, and that urea was a toxin. In the second half of the nineteenth century, further analytical studies concluded that potassium was the most toxic constituent of urine (Richet, 1999).

The mechanism of urine formation remained controversial from the time of William Bowman in 1856. Scientists supported either the "Filtration Theory" or the "Secretion Theory." Arthur Cushny (1866–1926) proposed a unified, modern theory in 1916 and reported that urine was formed by simple ultrafiltration in the glomeruli. By the mid-twentieth century, Alfred Richards (1876–1966) established the theory of salt and water reabsorption. He was one of the pioneers who established the true function of the kidneys (Morel, 1999; Figure 1.11).

1.5 DIALYSIS

Although nineteenth-century physicians and physiologists discerned the content and purpose of urine, Thomas Graham, a Scottish chemist (1805–1869), was the first scientist to separate colloids and crystalloids by using a "dialyzer." His dialysis technique involved the separation of a mixture of substances dissolved in a solution by passing the solution through semipermeable membranes (Figure 1.12).

"It may perhaps be allowed to me to apply the convenient term dialysis to the method of separation by the method of diffusion through a system of gelatinous matter" (Graham, 1854). The word "dialysis" was not new to Graham. It was derived from Greek and means "to part asunder." However, he did provide its new meaning, which is still in use. His research earned him the name "father of modern dialysis."

Thomas Graham constructed several simple devices during his study of diffusion and dialysis. His hoop dialyzer was made of gutta-percha and was closed on one end with parchment paper. The hoop floated on the water surface in a large basin. "Half a liter of urine, dialyzed for 24 hours, gave

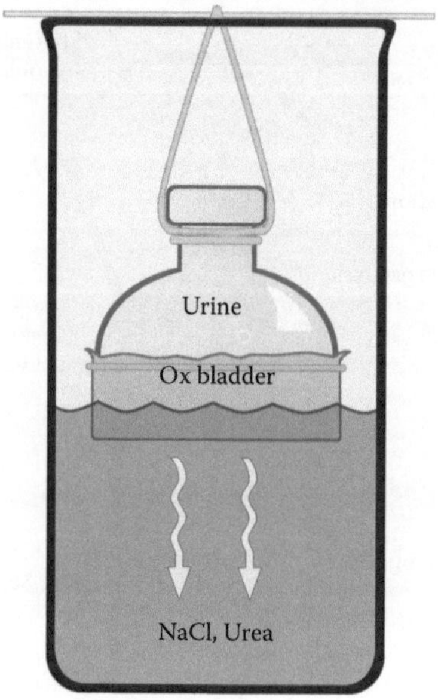

FIGURE 1.12 Depiction of the Graham dialyzer. (From Shaun Riffle, University of South Carolina School of Medicine, Columbia, SC. With permission.)

its crystalloid constituents to the external water. The latter, evaporated by a water bath yielded a white saline mass. From this mass, urea was extracted ..." Graham designed at least two other dialyzers, a water-jar type and a bulb type. He fitted these with a variety of membranes. He studied the effect of temperature and the efficacy of purification when using differing crystalloids. It was his work and later that of John Abel (Baltimore in 1913), who developed the first artificial kidney, which led to the current forms of hemodialysis treatment for kidney failure (Eknoyan, 2009; Graham, 1854; Gottschalk, 1998). Willem Kolff is considered the inventor of the first reliable artificial kidney. His rotating drum artificial kidney, in 1943, offered an effective method of dialysis. Dr. Kolff quickly put his artificial kidney into clinical use by successfully dialyzing a patient with acute kidney failure (AKF) (Kolff, 1965).

Georg Ganter performed the first human peritoneal dialysis in 1923 (Teschner et al., 2004). This type of dialysis was prone to complications and often failed secondary to peritoneum access issues.

Howard Frank, Arnold Seligman, and Jacob Fine at Boston's Beth-Israel Hospital established more successful peritoneal treatments for AKF in 1946. A new stylet catheter made access to the peritoneal cavity much easier and safer. Today, peritoneal dialysis, done at home, provides an alternative method to in-center hemodialysis.

Successful kidney transplants soon followed with the first successful transplant between identical twins in 1954 (Boston). In 1962, cadaver transplants and the first use of antirejection drugs began in Boston. The number of kidney transplants now exceeds 17,500 per year from both living related and cadaveric donors (National Institute of Diabetes and Digestive and Kidney Diseases, 2010).

1.6 NUTRITION

The link between diet and declining kidney function came to prominence in mid-1800s when Richard Bright suggested a milk diet to temporarily treat edema and proteinuria (Bright's disease) (Beebe, 1896). This type of extremely restricted diet was used well into the twentieth century (Fahnestock, 1896). Fritz Bischoff (1932) conducted one of the first scientific examinations to confirm the linkage between diet and kidney function. He used evidence from numerous studies on animals to conclude that nephrotoxic factors could be a result of dietary intake. Several decades later, studies on humans confirmed his hypothesis (Maschio et al., 1982; Rosman et al., 1984). In the interim, various practitioners proposed restricted diets to minimize uremic toxicity and delay the loss of kidney function (Addis, 1948). Patients with either acute or chronic kidney disease (CKD) were managed with a variety of diets that primarily limited sodium, protein, and fluids. These therapeutic diets extended the lives of patients in a time when treatment options were almost nonexistent (Addis et al., 1948).

1.6.1 Diet and AKF

Earlier diets for patients with AKF contained little, if any, protein, no salt, and a severely limited fluid allowance. For many years, they served as alternatives to dialysis. Professor J.G.G. Borst, Amsterdam 1948, formulated a gruel that provided approximately 1750 Cal/day to sustain patients with AKF. He also made butterballs from water (1.5 L), custard powder, sugar, and butter mixture (Table 1.2). Some amounts of protein were occasionally permitted in the diet. In 1955, Rose and Wixom established a minimal daily requirement for essential amino acids, and in 1963, Giordano established a ranking system so that high-biological value protein foods would be the preferred items in a protein-restricted diet. Today, the diet for patients with AKF is still very restricted until the kidney function is normal. Protein is now an essential part of the diet and is carefully calculated to ensure adequacy for the patient (Borst, 1948; Giordano, 1963; Rose and Wixom, 1955).

1.6.2 Diet and Stage 4 CKD

In 1934, the famous Rice Diet was developed by Walther Kempner, a doctor at Duke Hospital in Durham, NC, as a no-salt dietary treatment for patients with malignant hypertension and CKD. Besides restricting sodium, the diet limited calories and protein. Dr. Kempner named the diet after the bowl of white rice eaten at every meal. Today, this diet is generally regarded as a low-sodium, low-fat, low-calorie diet for weight reduction. White rice has been replaced with the healthier brown rice (Rice Diet Program, 2010).

Very low protein diets, first advocated in the 1960s, can be used to delay the start of dialysis. Protein is limited to 18–20 g/day of essential amino acids, ketoanalogs, or proteins of high biological value (eggs, soy, and whey). Special low-protein starches are also used to make breads and pastas. These diets help to reduce urea production. Symptomatic improvement is widely documented in those patients who are able to follow the very low protein diet, which requires many restrictions and special foods. The very low protein diet is also advocated as a way to completely avoid the start of dialysis in the elderly who do not wish to be treated or who have only a short time to live (Robson, 1969).

Typically, a 60-g protein, 2-g sodium, and 2-g potassium diet with adequate calories is prescribed for patients with CKD. Fluid restriction usually of 500–800 mL plus an amount equal to daily urine output of the patient is also recommended as kidney failure progresses. Currently, this diet is in use for patients with CKD who are considered for predialysis.

TABLE 1.2
Borst Soup and Butterballs

Borst Soup	Butterballs
Ingredients: Sugar 3/4 cup or ~150 g	Ingredients: Powdered sugar 1/2 cup or 100 g
Unsalted butter 2/3 cup or ~150 g	Unsalted butter 1/3 cup or ~80 g
Flour 1–2 tablespoons or ~20 g	Vanilla extract 3/4 teaspoon
Water 11/4 cups or ~ 300 g	Peppermint, lemon, or other flavorings (3–4 drops)
Mix all ingredients and heat slowly. Do not boil. Serve as soup. Divide into three servings	Combine sugar and butter; add peppermint (optional). Divide the mixture into 10 balls. Roll in powdered sugar. Store in a freezer until use. ~100 kcal/ball. Low protein
~590 calories per serving with <1 g of protein	

1.6.3 Diet and Stage 5 CKD

1.6.3.1 Hemodialysis

Once dialysis starts, protein restriction is lifted. Increased protein intake helps correct or prevent malnutrition. Sodium and potassium are generally limited to 2–3 g/day. Phosphorus restriction in the diet is based on the amount of protein intake. A limit of 10 mg of phosphorus in 1 g of protein is generally used. Fluids are also restricted to 800–1000 mL plus an amount equal to the urine output of the patient. Other restrictions are imposed as needed for management of comorbidities such as diabetes and cardiovascular disease.

1.6.3.2 Peritoneal Dialysis

Continuous ambulatory peritoneal dialysis was introduced in the 1970s. In the beginning, most patients were placed on an unrestricted diet since they received daily peritoneal exchange treatments. Now increased amounts of protein are recommended (1.2–1.3 g/kg) to offset protein losses due to dialysis. Additional dietary changes include modest restrictions on the intake of sodium and phosphorus. The intake allowance of potassium is liberalized to 4 g/day and fluid restrictions are minimal.

1.7 SOCIALIZED MEDICINE

In the 1960s, dialysis treatments became a standard of care for stage 5 CKD. Countries with socialized medicine started building local dialysis centers and increased the number of persons able to receive dialysis. The opportunity for dialysis in the United States during the same time was decided by patients' ability to pay and their social worth. Only one in seven patients considered suitable for treatment actually obtained it.

In 1967, a congressional committee, the Gottschalk Committee, stated that federal assistance was mandatory to defray the high cost of dialysis or transplant surgery for patients with CKD. The committee set up a national program that would ensure that 100% of candidates suitable for dialysis would be treated by 1973 (Kerr, 1973). The role of the renal dietitian expanded at that time, and the availability of dialysis brought a new approach to dietary management.

Approximately 10,000 Americans were eligible for the new program in 1973 (Nissenson and Rettig, 1999). Twenty-four years later (2007 data), the number of Americans receiving treatment for end-stage renal disease (ESRD) had grown to 368,544 (National Institute of Diabetes and Digestive and Kidney Diseases, 2010). Other countries have also seen large increases in the number of persons eligible for dialysis. This is accounted for by the increase in the number of patients with diabetes and hypertension, which are the primary causes of kidney failure, and by the increase in the number of elderly (65 years or older) who are now dialyzed. The cost of the ESRD program in the United States in 2007 was $35.32 billion in public and private spending or an annual average cost of $68,253 for every patient on hemodialysis and $56,807 for each patient on peritoneal dialysis.

1.8 SUMMARY

Future research holds the possibility of eliminating kidney disease. Until then, efforts would remain focused on the prevention and/or control of illnesses that contribute to the decline of kidney function. Dialysis techniques and equipment continue to be refined. Dialysis is becoming more "portable" with new peritoneal techniques. Nutritional therapy, for now, is the key stone that can prevent and control chronic renal diseases and make current dialysis techniques more effective.

REFERENCES

Adams, F., Translator. 1849. Hippocrates: Aphorisms. Online: http://classics.mit.edu/Hippocrates/aphorisms.html (accessed July 29, 2010).

Addis, T. 1948. Mechanism of proteinuria. *Science* 108(2816):680.

Addis, T., Gray, H., Barrett, E. 1948. Food protein consumption in glomerulonephritis: Effect on proteinuria and concentration of serum protein. *J Exp Med.* 87(4):353–368.

Andreucci, V. 1972. About the glomerulus. *Kidney Int.* 2: 349–351.

Beebe, H. 1896. Bright's disease. In Fisher, C., ed., *Medical Century, Volume IV.* New York: Medical Century Company, 17–19.

Bischoff, F. 1932. The influence of diet on renal and blood vessel changes. *J Nutr.* 5:431–450.

Bloom, D. 1997. Hippocrates and urology: The first surgical subspecialty. *Urology.* 50:157–159.

Borst, J. 1948. Protein katabolism in uraemia: Effects of protein free diet, infection, and blood transfusions. *Lancet.* 1:824–828.

Cataldi, L. 1998. The kidney through the ages. Proceeding of the 8th International Workshop of Neonatal Nephrology. Rome, Italy.

Dardioti, V., Angelopoulos, N., Hajiconstantiou, V. 1997. Renal diseases in the Hippocratic era. *Am J Nephrol.* 17:214–216.

Diamandopoulos, A., Goudas, P., Oreopoulous, D. 2009. Thirty-six Hippocratic aphorisms of nephrologic interest. *Am J Kidney Dis.* 54:143–153.

Dolan, J. and Adams-Smith, W. 1978. *Health and Society: A Documentary History of Medicine.* New York: The Seabury Press.

Eknoyan, G. 1996. Sir William Bowman: His contributions to physiology and nephrology. *Kidney Int.* 50:2120–2128.

Eknoyan, G. 2009. The wonderful apparatus of John Jacob Abel called the "artificial kidney." *Semin Dial.* 22:287–296.

Empedocles. Online: http://plato.stanford.edu/entries/empedocles (accessed July 29, 2010).

Fahnestock, J. 1896. Hints on the general management and homeopathic treatment of chronic Bright's disease. In Fisher, C., ed., *Medical Century, Volume IV.* New York: Medical Century Company, 14–17.

Galen, C. 1968. *On the Usefulness of the Parts of the Body.* Translated by Margaret Tallmadge May. Cornell University Press. Google online books (accessed October 11, 2010).

Geller, M. and Cohen, S. 1995. Kidney and urinary tract disease in ancient Babylonia, with translations of the cuneiform sources. *Kidney Int.* 47:1811–1815.

Giordano, C. 1963. Use of exogenous and endogenous urea for protein synthesis in normal and uremic subjects. *J Lab Clin Med.* 62:231–246.

Gottschalk, C. 1998. Thomas Graham, 1805–1869. *Nephrology.* 4:211–216.

Graham, T. 1854. The Bakerian lecture on osmotic force. *Philos Trans R Soc London.* 144:177–228.

Greek Medicine. Online: http://www.nlm.nih.gov/hmd/greek/greek_rationality.html (accessed July 24, 2010).

Hippocratic Method and the Four Humors in Medicine. Online: http://ancienthistory.about.com/cs/hippocrates/a/hippocraticmeds.htm (accessed June 16, 2010).

Hippocratic Seasonal Diseases. Online: http://ancienthistory.about.com/od/greekmedicine/tp/062709HippocraticSeasonalDiseases.htm (accessed June 18, 2010).

Kerr, D. 1973. Provision of services to patients with chronic uremia. *Kidney Int.* 3:197–204.

Kirk, G., Raven, J., and Schofield, M. 1983. *The Presoratic Philosophers*, 2nd edition. Cambridge: Cambridge Press.

Kolff, W. 1965. First clinical experience with the artificial kidney. *Ann Intern Med.* 62:608–619.

Longrigg, J. 1993. *Greek Rational Medicine.* London and New York: Routledge.

Maschio, G., Oldrizzi, L., Tessitore, N., et al. 1982. Effects of dietary protein and phosphorus restriction on the progression of early renal failure. *Kidney Int.* 22:371–376.

Mezzogiorno, A. 1999. Bartolomeo Eustachio: A pioneer in the morphological studies of the kidney. *Am J Nephrol.* 19:193–198.

Morel, F. 1999. The loop of Henle, a turning point in the history of kidney physiology. *Nephrol Dial Transpl.* 14:2510–2515.

National Institute of Diabetes and Digestive and Kidney Diseases (NIDDK). 2010. Kidney and Urologic Diseases Statistics for the United States. Online: http://Kidney.niddk.nih.gov/Kudiseases/pubs/kustats (accessed August 16, 2010).

Nissenson, A. and Rettig, R. 1999. *Medicare's End Stage Renal Disease Program: Current Status and Future Prospects.* People to People Health Foundation. Online: http://content.healthaffairs.org/cgi/reprint/18/1/161.full.pdf+html (accessed August 16, 2010).

Rice Diet Program. Online: http://www.ricedietprogram.com (accessed August 3, 2010).

Richet, G. 1999. The contribution of French-speaking scientists to the origins of renal physiology and pathophysiology (1790–1910). *Am J Nephrol.* 19(2):274.

Robson, J. 1969. Advances in the treatment of renal disease. *Practitioner* 203(216):483–493.

Rose, W. and Wixom, W. 1955. The amino acid requirement of man. *J Biol Chem*. 17:997–1004.
Rosman, J., Ter Wee, P., Meijer, S. 1984. Prospective randomized trial of early dietary protein restriction in chronic renal failure. *Lancet*. 2:1291–1296.
Teschner, M., Heidland, A., Klassen, A., et al. 2004. Georg Ganter—A pioneer of peritoneal dialysis and his tragic academic demise at the hand of the Nazi regime. *J Nephrol*. 17(3):457–460.
Todd, R. and Bowman, W. 1856. *The Physiological Anatomy and Physiology of Man*, Volume II. London, England: Parker.
Twardowski, Z. 2008. History of hemodialyzers. *Hemodial Int*. 12:173–210.

2 Renal Physiology

L. Britt Wilson
University of South Carolina School of Medicine

CONTENTS

2.1 OVERVIEW OF FUNCTION OF KIDNEYS

Kidneys are remarkable organs, and they play a pivotal role in whole-body homeostasis. In short, the kidneys regulate the extracellular environment, specifically extracellular water and electrolytes. In addition, they eliminate nitrogenous products from protein metabolism (urea) and creatinine, which is released from skeletal muscle. Mostly everyone, laypersons and professionals alike, recognizes the importance of the elimination function of the kidneys and the fact that the failure of the kidneys to eliminate urea (uremia or azotemia) does indeed cause profound pathologic disturbances. However, the ability of the kidneys to maintain extracellular water and electrolytes within an acceptable range has a profound influence on all the organs of the body because all cells reside in the extracellular environment. Retaining extracellular volume, for example, can result in hypertension, and disturbance in kidney function is one known cause of this disease (Dibona, 2002; Ganong, 2006; Kotchen, 2008). In fact, the use of diuretic therapy to treat hypertension illustrates the connection between the kidneys and blood-pressure regulation (Hoffman, 2006). Failure of the kidneys to eliminate or retain hydrogen and/or bicarbonate can result in acid–base disturbances, which of course affects the function of other organs of the body (Rose and Post, 2001). Extracellular potassium must be maintained within a narrow range; otherwise, fatal arrhythmias can result. In this chapter, we review some of the basic physiological processes of the kidneys, thus providing a foundation for understanding how alterations in these processes result in pathologic changes that occur in patients with renal disease. Understanding this underlying physiology also aids in making therapeutic and nutritional choices in treating patients with kidney disease.

The body is divided into two compartments (Figure 2.1): (1) intracellular and (2) extracellular. About two-thirds of the total body water is distributed in the intracellular compartment, whereas about one-third remains in the extracellular. The cell membrane divides these two compartments, and its fundamental function is to serve as a barrier. Although it acts as a barrier to some solutes, it does not act as a barrier to water because of water channels known as aquaporins (Barrett et al., 2010; Eaton and Pooler, 2009; Koeppen and Stanton, 2007). Thus, water moves easily between the

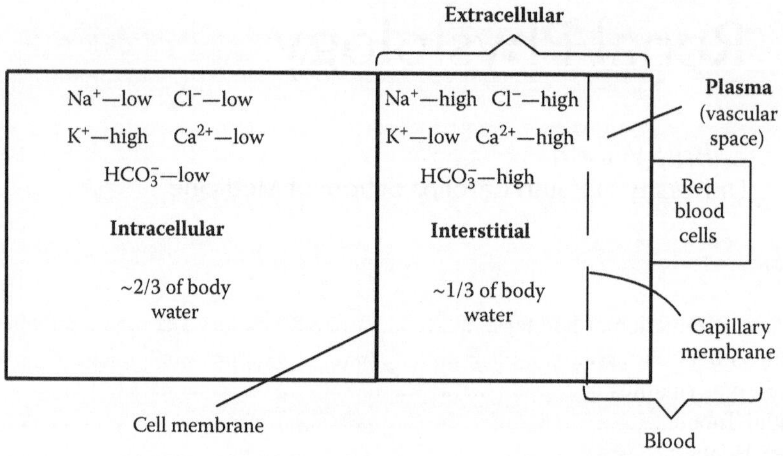

FIGURE 2.1 Schematic illustrating the major compartments of the body, relative distribution of water, and relative concentrations of the more prominent electrolytes. Although the distribution of water and electrolytes has been described for the interstitial compartment, the description applies to the extracellular compartment as well because the capillary membrane does not act as a barrier to water or the ions. See text for more details.

two major compartments via osmosis. Ions, on the other hand, do not easily penetrate cells, and thus a concentration gradient exists for the major ions. Of the more prevalent ions, the concentration of free sodium (Na^+), chloride (Cl^-), bicarbonate, and calcium (Ca^{2+})* is greater in the extracellular compartment, whereas the concentration of free K^+ is greater in the intracellular compartment. Na^+ is the most abundant ion in the extracellular space, and its relatively poor permeability into the cell means that it is the most abundant osmole of the extracellular compartment (Koeppen and Stanton, 2007; Rose and Post, 2001). The extracellular compartment is further subdivided into an interstitial compartment and a vascular compartment, the latter comprising plasma and red cells (erythrocytes). These are separated by the capillary membrane, which serves as a barrier for large molecular weight solutes (proteins, the most abundant in plasma being albumin) but does not exclude ions or water (Koeppen and Stanton, 2007).

As mentioned above, the kidneys regulate extracellular volume and the extracellular electrolytes. The fascinating aspect is how they achieve this. Although more details are provided below, in general, the kidneys achieve this in two basic ways. First, they regulate the extracellular volume by regulating Na^+. As is often said, where Na^+ goes, water follows. Although not precise, this is a good general rule of thumb to go by. Second, the kidneys regulate extracellular osmolality, and thus the concentration of electrolytes, by regulating water. Recall that water affects the concentration of solutes. Thus, by regulating water, the kidneys, at least in part, regulate extracellular electrolytes. Although this is an oversimplification, if one keeps these two basic constructs in mind, it can greatly facilitate one's ability to understand renal physiology.

2.2 STRUCTURE/FUNCTION

The nephron is the basic functional unit of the kidney, and Figure 2.2 is a schematic depicting the basic anatomy of the nephron. It is essential to know this basic anatomy along with the nomenclature to understand renal physiology and pathophysiology. Blood enters the kidney via the renal arteries (not depicted) and ultimately arrives at the glomerular capillaries (GC) via the afferent

* The Ca^{2+} difference here refers to free concentration. This does not take into account the intracellular stores of Ca^{2+}.

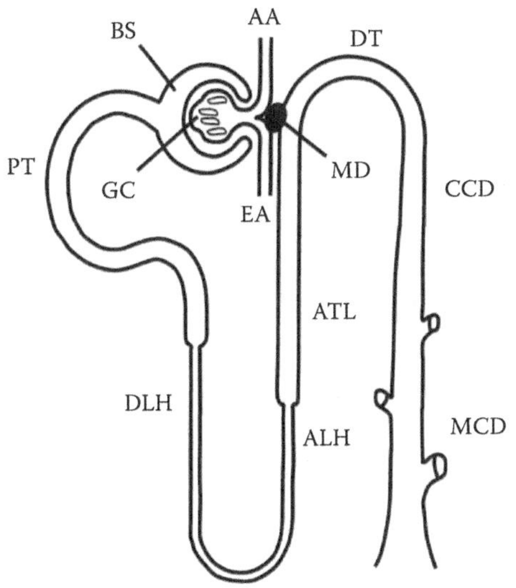

FIGURE 2.2 Basic drawing showing the fundamental anatomy of a nephron. Abbreviations are as follows: AA, afferent arteriole; EA, efferent arteriole; GC, glomerular capillary; BS, Bowman's space; PT, proximal tubule; DLH, descending loop of Henle; ALH, ascending loop of Henle; ATL, ascending thick limb (of loop of Henle); MD, macula densa; DT, distal tubule; CCD, cortical collecting duct; MCD, medullary collecting duct.

arteriole (AA). Some of the plasma then filters into Bowman's space (BS). The blood exits the GC via the efferent arteriole (EA) continuing into the peritubular or vasa recta capillary network (not illustrated for clarity). Vasa recta are limited to the juxtamedullary nephrons, which comprise about 10% of the total number of nephrons (Eaton and Pooler, 2009; Koeppen and Stanton, 2007). The venous drainage from these two capillary networks ultimately feeds into the renal vein and then into the inferior vena cava. The AA and EA represent resistors in series, and changes in their tone affect pressure in the GC, which in turn affects filtration. Filtration is the flux of fluid from the GC into the BS. Granular cells of the AA synthesize and release renin and are part of the juxtaglomerular apparatus. The macula densa (Figure 2.2) along with extraglomerular mesangial cells complete the structural components of the juxtaglomerular apparatus.

The GC is "leaky," meaning that it does not serve as a significant barrier to water and most of the other constituents of the plasma. Electron microscopy shows large spaces (fenestrae) between endothelial cells of the capillary endothelium, providing the anatomical basis for such leakiness (see Figure 2.3). However, the GC is remarkably adept at excluding proteins from the BS, and an electrostatic repulsion from the proteins lining the barrier is thought to be the mechanism for this exclusion of plasma proteins (Eaton and Pooler, 2009; Koeppen and Stanton, 2007; Rose and Post, 2001). Appreciating this architecture is important for understanding renal pathology because alterations in it form the basis for both nephritic and nephrotic syndromes (see Chapter 5). Minimal change disease is one form of nephrotic syndrome in which extravasation of proteins occurs, but there are no significant changes in the architecture of the GC or the Bowman's capsule (Alpers, 2005; Ix and Lingappa, 2006).

As described many years ago by Starling, fluid flux across the capillary is primarily caused by the hydrostatic and osmotic forces on both sides of the capillary (Eaton and Pooler, 2009; Koeppen and Stanton, 2007; Rose and Post, 2001). For the kidneys, the forces in the GC and the BS are relevant for filtration. Hydrostatic forces "push" the fluid away, and thus hydrostatic pressure in the GC (P_{GC}) promotes filtration. In contrast, hydrostatic pressure in the BS (P_{BS}) impedes filtration. Thus, the difference in the two plays an important role in determining the direction of fluid flux. Under normal circumstances, P_{GC} is much higher than P_{BS}, hence fluid filters into BS. However, this

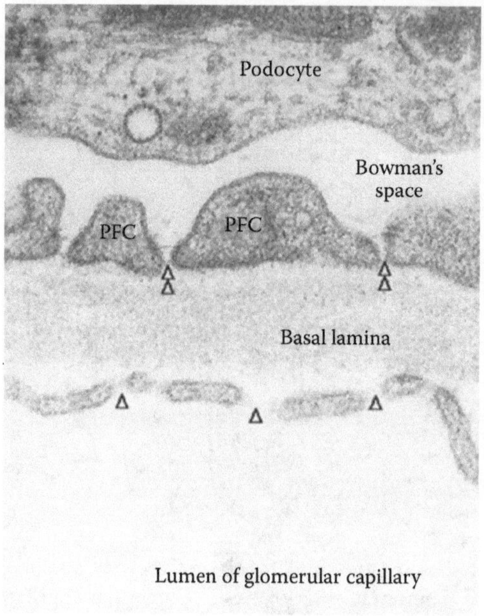

FIGURE 2.3 Electron micrograph showing the glomerular capillaries–Bowman's space (GC–BS) interface. Note the fenestrae or pores depicted by the arrows, creating a rather porous connection between the GC and the BS. Podocyte foot processes (PFC) provide support for the basal lamina of the basement membrane and contribute to the selective filtration of small solutes and water, but not plasma proteins. (Reproduced from Marshall, S. *Postgrad Med J.*, 80, 624–633, 2004. With permission from BMJ Publishing Group Ltd.)

filtration can be reduced if P_{BS} is elevated, as occurs in patients with kidney stones, pyelonephritis, and polycystic kidney disease. Albumin is the key component for oncotic forces in the capillary, and oncotic pressure in the GC (π_{GC}) retards filtration. Since proteins do not accumulate in the BS to any significant degree, the oncotic force that would result is ignored. Thus, P_{GC} is the driving force for fluid filtration across the GC, whereas P_{BS} and π_{GC} work against it. Under normal circumstances, P_{GC} exceeds the sum of P_{BS} and π_{GC}, thus fluid filters through the GC into BS. However, as indicated in the previous paragraph, alterations in the GC/BS junction (nephritic or nephrotic syndrome) can markedly alter this fluid flux (Alpers, 2005; Ix and Lingappa, 2006).

The rate at which fluid filters into the BS is called glomerular filtration rate (GFR). In essence, GFR represents the flow of protein-free fluid into BS and is an important marker of renal function. The kidneys must filter blood to perform their function; hence, determining or estimating GFR is considered an important first step in assessing the patient with suspected renal dysfunction. Classically, GFR is measured using inulin, but there are formulas that one can use to estimate it based, in part, on plasma creatinine, the rationale of which is as discussed below. Filtration, or GFR, represents one of the four basic mechanisms (see Figure 2.4) utilized by the kidney. The other three are reabsorption, which means the movement of water or solute from the tubule of the nephron back into the peritubular or vasa recta capillaries; secretion, which is defined as movement of solute from the capillary network surrounding the nephron into the tubule (note: this means that the solute was not filtered); and excretion, defined as loss of water or solute from the body via the urine.

2.3 RENAL HEMODYNAMICS

Because P_{GC} drives GFR, it is important to understand the basic hemodynamics of the renal microvasculature. As stated, the AA and EA represent two resistors in series, and Figure 2.5 is a

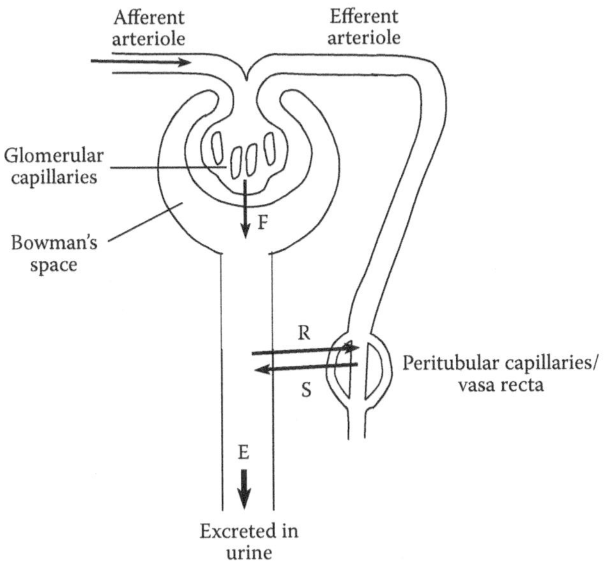

FIGURE 2.4 Schematic illustrating the four fundamental processes of the kidney. These are as follows: F = filtration, R = reabsorption, S = secretion, and E = excretion. See text for details.

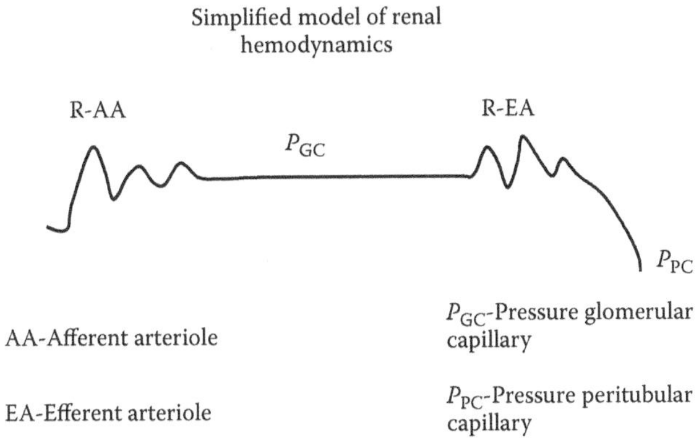

FIGURE 2.5 Simplified model showing the microcirculation of the nephron has two resistors and two capillary beds in series. Note that the glomerular capillary is between the two resistors, that is, it is downstream from the AA, but upstream of the EA.

simplified schematic depicting this. As a reminder, increasing resistance tends to decrease blood flow, increase pressure upstream, and decrease pressure downstream. Decreasing resistance has the opposite effect for all three. For example, if the AA vasoconstricts, then renal blood flow will tend to fall and pressure upstream from the AA increases, whereas pressure downstream from the AA decreases. Note that the GC is situated between the AA and the EA. Thus, constricting the AA decreases P_{GC}, whereas constricting the EA increases P_{GC}, yet renal blood flow falls regardless of which one is constricted. Since P_{GC} drives GFR, it decreases when the resistance upstream increases, but GFR increases if resistance downstream (EA) increases. Understanding these principles has many clinical implications. For instance, stenosis of the renal artery will compromise blood flow to the GC, and since the site of the stenosis is upstream from these capillaries, P_{GC} and GFR fall. Sympathetic stimulation can markedly constrict the AA (constricts EA also, but not as much), which will decrease P_{GC} and thus GFR. On the other hand, angiotensin II (AII) is considered to preferentially constrict the EA (Jackson, 2006b; Rose and Post, 2001). Constriction of the EA causes P_{GC} to increase, with a resultant rise in GFR despite a fall in renal blood flow. Clinical data also suggest that this is the case (Jackson, 2006b). If a patient, diabetic for example, has protein loss in the urine, one way to reduce this protein excretion would be to reduce P_{GC}. Angiotensin-converting enzyme (ACE) inhibitors can often stop or reduce protein loss in the urine, because reducing AII relaxes the EA, thereby dropping P_{GC} (Marshall, 2004). However, one must recognize that GFR will fall because of this drop in P_{GC}.

The kidney is considered a "good autoregulator." Autoregulation is the maintenance of a relatively constant blood flow despite changes in driving pressure. Intrinsic myogenic mechanisms participate as does tubular glomerular feedback (TGF). Delivery of sodium chloride to the macula densa is thought to be the signal driving TGF. The theory is that the macula densa "senses" the delivery of sodium chloride, and adenosine is released in proportion to the load of sodium chloride delivered (Eaton and Pooler, 2009; Koeppen and Stanton, 2007). Adenosine is a potent vasoconstrictor of the AA. Thus, increased delivery of sodium to the macula densa, such as would occur if flow through the nephron increases, causes vasoconstriction of the AA with the resultant fall in P_{GC} and GFR. This ability to autoregulate blood flow allows the kidneys to autoregulate, in large part, GFR. Although the kidneys do autoregulate well, renal blood flow can be compromised by stimulation of the sympathetic nervous system. Strong sympathetic activation can markedly reduce renal blood flow. Prostaglandins can also influence renal hemodynamics, but their role is subtle (Eaton and Pooler, 2009; Koeppen and Stanton, 2007). There is very little evidence that prostaglandins are important in the nonstressed state. However, vasodilator prostaglandins are released when renal blood flow is reduced, for example, during elevated sympathetic activity. For this reason, blocking prostaglandin production in stress states such as hemorrhage is often contraindicated. As mentioned above, AII can influence renal hemodynamics, and the kidneys can synthesize AII locally (Koeppen and Stanton, 2007).

2.4 PROXIMAL TUBULE

The proximal tubule does the "bulk" of reabsorptive work for the kidney (Eaton and Pooler, 2009; Koeppen and Stanton, 2007; Rose and Post, 2001). Since the GC is leaky to nonprotein solutes and water, the concentration of these solutes in the BS is the same as that in the plasma. As the fluid flows down the proximal tubule, about 67% of the filtered Na^+ is reabsorbed. This is primarily driven by the Na^+–K^+ ATPase on the basolateral membrane of the luminal epithelial cell (Figure 2.6). This ATPase keeps the intracellular concentration of Na^+ low, thereby maintaining a concentration gradient for Na^+ to enter the cell. In addition, the stoichiometry is three Na^+ out and two K^+ in, which creates a negative potential inside the cell, in turn aiding Na^+ movement into the cell. The proximal tubule is relatively permeable to water, so as solute gets reabsorbed, so does water. In turn, this movement of Na^+ and water causes ions such as Ca^{2+}, K^+, and Cl^- to follow. Although Cl^- lags a bit in its reabsorption, there is still significant reabsorption of this electrolyte. Many solutes, glucose and amino acids being the most relevant, are cotransported with Na^+, and under normal circumstances, all of the filtered glucose and amino acids are reabsorbed in the proximal tubule. However, the transporters are limited and can be saturated [follow transport maximum (T_M) kinetics] if the filtered load (GFR times plasma concentration) of these solutes is too great. For example, if plasma glucose becomes elevated in a diabetic, these transporters for Na^+–glucose cotransport cannot "capture" all of the filtered glucose and glucose remains in the lumen. These Na^+–glucose transporters are limited to the proximal tubule, and if all the glucose cannot be reabsorbed in the proximal tubule, then it is spilled into the urine. An important concept to bring in at this point is to remember that the solutes are osmoles. Thus, if a solute that is normally reabsorbed fails to be reabsorbed, then

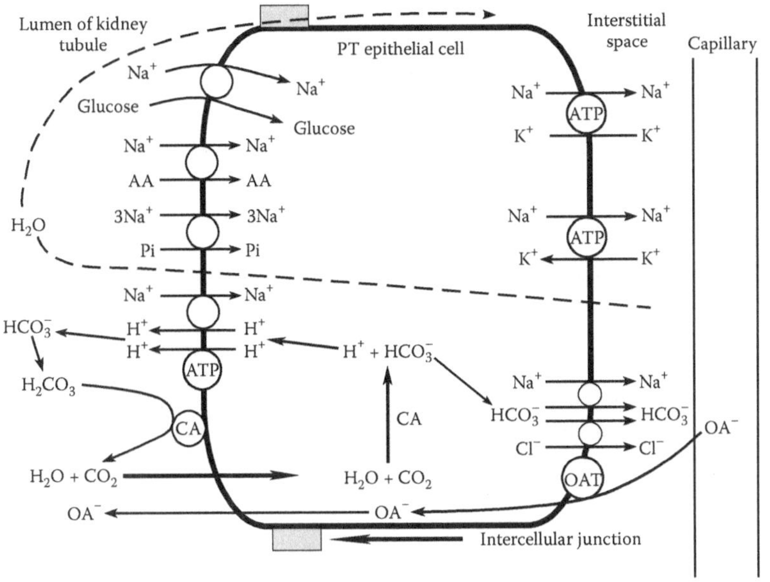

FIGURE 2.6 Details of the major transport processes in the proximal tubule. See text for a more complete description. The dashed line for water indicates its reabsorption follows the osmotic forces created by the reabsorption of other solutes, primarily sodium.

water follows the solute, which results in diuresis. For this reason, uncontrolled diabetes can result in significant diuresis since glucose is not reabsorbed completely. Mannitol is another example. It is freely filtered, but not reabsorbed. Thus, this solute stays in the lumen of the nephron, so water follows and diuresis results.

Phosphate (Pi) is another important solute that is cotransported with Na^+ (Figure 2.6), and it follows T_M kinetics similar to glucose transport. About 80% of the filtered Pi is reabsorbed via this transport mechanism. Parathyroid hormone (PTH) lowers the T_M, which thus reduces Pi reabsorption in the proximal tubule (Eaton and Pooler, 2009; Koeppen and Stanton, 2007; Rose and Post, 2001). Patients with renal failure retain phosphate despite often having elevated levels of PTH (Rose and Post, 2001). This likely reflects the loss of functioning nephrons rather than the inability of PTH to effectively diminish the activity of this transporter. Regardless, plasma Pi levels represent an important marker in patients with renal failure.

Bicarbonate is the most abundant base in the body, and approximately 80% of the filtered bicarbonate is reabsorbed in the proximal tubule (Eaton and Pooler, 2009; Koeppen and Stanton, 2007; Rose and Post, 2001). However, note that bicarbonate is reabsorbed across the luminal membrane as CO_2 (Figure 2.6). Thus, the filtered bicarbonate combines with H^+ to form CO_2, and this reaction is catalyzed by the carbonic anhydrase enzyme that exists on the luminal surface of the proximal tubular epithelium. Inside the cell, the bicarbonate is reformed from the CO_2 and exists on the basolateral membrane to return to the blood. Given this, one should see that bicarbonate reabsorption is coupled to H^+ availability and thus to H^+ secretion by the proximal tubule cell. The cellular concentration of H^+ is thought to be the primary factor driving H^+ secretion. Acidosis of the tubular epithelial cells, therefore, increases H^+ secretion and thus bicarbonate reabsorption. Reabsorbing bicarbonate is adaptive in an acidotic condition since it is a base. On the other hand, alkalosis of these cells decreases H^+ secretion and bicarbonate reabsorption. Again, this is adaptive because base is being eliminated from the body, thereby correcting alkalosis. This interplay illustrates one mechanism by which the kidneys regulate bicarbonate and H^+. Carbonic anhydrase inhibitors block the luminal carbonic anhydrase, thereby reducing bicarbonate reabsorption. This results in diuresis (failure to reabsorb the osmole) and elimination of base from the body, hence the treatment for respiratory alkalosis that occurs at high altitude. Finally, Fanconi syndrome is a genetic disorder in which many of the transport processes in the proximal tubule are deficient (Koeppen and Stanton, 2007). One deficit is the ability of the proximal tubule to reabsorb bicarbonate. As a result of excess loss of bicarbonate, the patient develops acidosis (type II renal tubular acidosis).

The other clinically relevant transport process in the proximal tubule involves organic acids and bases, particularly organic acids (Eaton and Pooler, 2009; Koeppen and Stanton, 2007; Rose and Post, 2001). The details of this transport are beyond the scope of this book, but in short, many organic acids are reabsorbed in the proximal tubule. However, the basolateral membrane contains transporters for organic acids, which are collectively called organic acid transporters (OATs). These OATs secrete organic acids into the proximal tubule, and in turn, these organic acids are secreted into the lumen of the nephron and eliminated via the urine. An important characteristic of these OATs is that they are relatively nonselective. Thus, a variety of organic acids are secreted via OATs, and therefore they compete for these transporters. This becomes particularly relevant for pharmacotherapy because the administration of two drugs that are organic acids may alter the pharmacokinetic profile of each drug, compared to the case when each was given in isolation. Further, furosemide is an organic acid that requires OAT function to be delivered to its site of action (El-Sheikh et al., 2008; Srimaroeng et al., 2008).

Uric acid is a particularly germane organic acid because of its role in gout. The renal handling of uric acid is actually quite complex, and the details are beyond the scope of this book. In short, about 90% of the filtered uric acid is reabsorbed in the proximal tubule; OATs play a role in this, although their precise role is controversial. Probenecid works on the kidney to increase the elimination of uric acid (Burke et al., 2006).

Organic base transporters also exist in the proximal tubule of the nephron (Eaton and Pooler, 2009; Koeppen and Stanton, 2007; Rose and Post, 2001). The important physiological organic base is creatinine. Creatinine is freely filtered but is not reabsorbed. Thus, what gets filtered gets eliminated, and the clearance of creatinine is the primary route of elimination for creatinine. Because of this, a fall in GFR causes a reduction in creatinine elimination and thus a rise in plasma creatinine. Therefore, plasma creatinine provides a rough marker for patients' GFR and thus their overall kidney function. However, the relationship between GFR and plasma creatinine is not linear. In addition, the number of functioning nephrons declines with age. Further, the amount of muscle mass and its breakdown can vary considerably from patient to patient. Thus, as indicated above, the estimation of plasma creatinine is often plugged into a formula that takes into account patients' age, size, and gender. Finally, the proximal tubule secretes creatinine, and about 10% of the elimination is tied to this secretion. Alterations in this protein-mediated transport could, at least in theory, alter the level of plasma creatinine.

2.5 LOOP OF HENLE

From the proximal tubule, the nephron bends toward the medulla and then loops back up toward the cortex, forming the loop of Henle (Figure 2.2). The descending limb of this loop is permeable to water but not solutes. By contrast, solutes are pumped out of the ascending limb but not water. This loop creates a countercurrent of luminal fluid flow, and the capillaries follow this loop and act as a multiplier for this countercurrent flow. Briefly, because of the differential characteristics of the descending and ascending limbs, the interstitium of medulla has an increasingly higher osmolality. The interstitium in the cortex of the kidney approximates blood osmolality (about 300 mOsm/kg), whereas the interstitium of the inner medulla may be as great as 1200 mOsm/kg. Functionally, this is pivotal for kidney function because the collecting ducts travel through the medulla. About half the osmolality of the medullary interstitium is due to NaCl, while urea contributes the other half (Eaton and Pooler, 2009; Koeppen and Stanton, 2007; Rose and Post, 2001). It is not imperative to understand the precise mechanism resulting in higher osmolality in the medullary interstitium, but appreciation of the fact that higher osmolality exists here is indeed important.

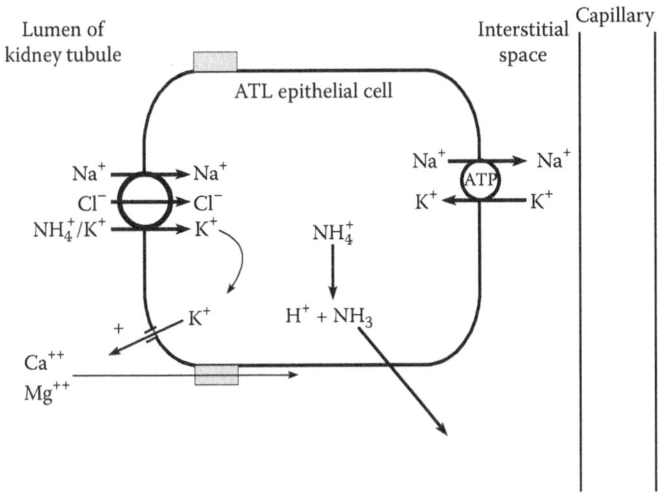

FIGURE 2.7 Schematic illustrating the Na^+–K^+–$2Cl^-$ transporter in the ascending thick limb (ATL) of the loop of Henle. See text for more details.

The critical transport process in the loop of Henle resides in the ascending thick limb (ATL), a Na^+–K^+–$2Cl^-$ transporter (Figure 2.7). Approximately, one-quarter of the filtered Na^+ gets reabsorbed via this transporter (Eaton and Pooler, 2009; Koeppen and Stanton, 2007; Rose and Post, 2001). This transport is electroneutral since two Cl^- ions move to balance the charge of the two cations. However, the luminal membrane of these cells is relatively permeable to K^+. As a result, K^+ can diffuse from the cell back into the lumen, thereby creating a lumen positive potential. This potential helps drive Ca^{2+} and Mg^{2+} reabsorption in the ATL via a paracellular (between cells) pathway. About 25% of filtered Ca^{2+} is reabsorbed in the ATL. In addition, ammonium (NH_4^+) can substitute for K^+ and move from the lumen into the epithelial cell. Although not described in detail in this chapter, this ammonium can dissociate into ammonia (NH_3) and H^+, and this ammonia in turn serves as the source that diffuses into the collecting duct (see below).

The Na^+–K^+–$2Cl^-$ transporter is the target for the loop diuretics (Eaton and Pooler, 2009; Koeppen and Stanton, 2007; Rose and Post, 2001). Blocking this transporter reduces the reabsorption of not only these three ions but also Ca^{2+} and Mg^{2+} because of reduced back diffusion of K^+ described above. Since several electrolytes are affected, loop diuretics can cause significant diuresis. Bartter's syndrome is a rare genetic disorder, which has several variants (Eaton and Pooler, 2009; Koeppen and Stanton, 2007; Rose and Post, 2001). However, in general, the syndrome is associated with a diminished function of the Na^+–K^+–$2Cl^-$ transporter in the ATL. As one might predict, patients with this syndrome typically present with low to normal blood pressure. As will be described later, they also exhibit hypokalemia and alkalosis, which is most likely the result of elevated aldosterone (ALDO).

2.6 DISTAL TUBULE

Epithelial cells of the distal tubule (DT) express a Na^+–Cl^- transporter (Figure 2.8). This electroneutral transport causes Na^+ and Cl^- reabsorption, and this is the site of action of the thiazide diuretics (Eaton and Pooler, 2009; Koeppen and Stanton, 2007; Rose and Post, 2001). The DT, similar to the ascending limb of the loop of Henle, is relatively impermeable to water. At first, this creates a quandary as to why thiazide diuretics do in fact cause diuresis. However, blocking NaCl transport increases the overall load of these ions, which exceeds the capacity of the remainder of the nephron to reabsorb them. Thus, osmoles remain in the lumen, keeping water with them. Another rare genetic condition

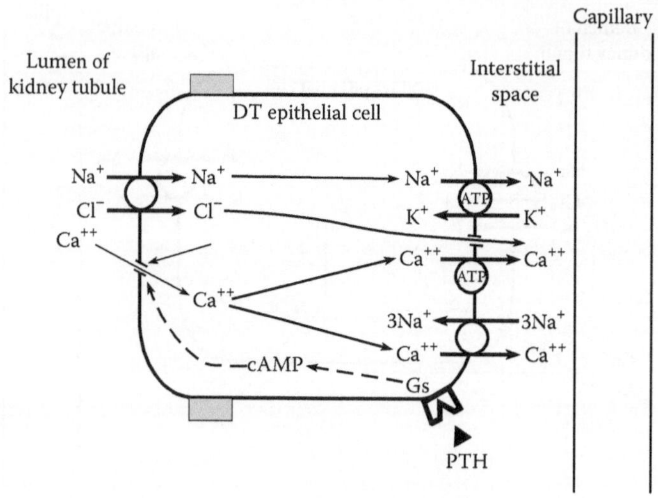

FIGURE 2.8 The cells of the distal tubule (DT) contain a Na^+–Cl^- symporter and calcium channels. See text for more details.

affecting renal transporters is Gitelman's syndrome. In this condition, there is a genetic deficit in the DT Na^+–Cl^- transporter. Similar to patients with Bartter's syndrome, these patients exhibit hypokalemia and alkalosis, which is most likely the result of hyperaldosterone. However, unlike the patients with Bartter's syndrome, patients with Giltelman's syndrome have low urine Ca^{2+} (see below).

DT epithelial cells also express Ca^{2+} channels (Figure 2.8). Ca^{2+} follows its electrochemical gradient into the epithelial cell via these channels, where Ca^{2+} is then shuttled back into the blood via a basolateral Ca^{2+}–ATPase and a Na^+–Ca^{2+} antiporter. These channels are regulated by intracellular cyclic adenosine monophosphate (cAMP), which is the second messenger for PTH. Thus, PTH enhances Ca^{2+} reabsorption in the DT (Eaton and Pooler, 2009; Koeppen and Stanton, 2007; Rose and Post, 2001). In addition, 1,25 dihdyroxycholecalciferol (active form of vitamin D) has a "permissive" action on the renal reabsorption of Ca^{2+}. Vitamin D induces the synthesis of calbindin, a Ca^{2+}-binding protein in the epithelial cells of the DT, which in turn binds intracellular free Ca^{2+} (Eaton and Pooler, 2009; Koeppen and Stanton, 2007; Rose and Post, 2001). This reduces the free concentration of cytosolic Ca^{2+}, thereby maintaining the concentration gradient needed for Ca^{2+} to diffuse from the lumen into the cell, in turn, increasing Ca^{2+} reabsorption. This is a minor site of action for vitamin D, with the cells of the duodenum being the main site.

The Na^+–Ca^{2+} antiporter may explain why thiazide diuretics often cause hypercalcemia (elevated blood calcium). This transporter moves three Na^+ in and one Ca^{2+} out (Figure 2.8). If Na^+ uptake via the Na^+–Cl^- transporter is reduced (mechanism of action for thiazide diuretic), this will reduce intracellular Na^+, which may in turn enhance the extrusion of Ca^{2+} from the cell since the Na^+ gradient is enhanced. Likewise, this may be the mechanism by which patients with Gitelman's syndrome have such low urine Ca^{2+}.

2.7 COLLECTING DUCTS

The collecting ducts form the final common pathway for tubular fluid, ultimately dumping this fluid into the renal pelvis. Beyond the collecting duct, the tubular fluid is no longer modified and is thus urine. Therefore, the final modifications and "fine tuning" of the urine occur here. Two cell types exist in the collecting duct (1) principal cells, called such because they constitute the majority of cells, and (2) intercalated cells (Eaton and Pooler, 2009; Koeppen and Stanton, 2007; Rose and Post, 2001). Although two subtypes of intercalated cells exist (alpha and beta), we will not delve into the differences.

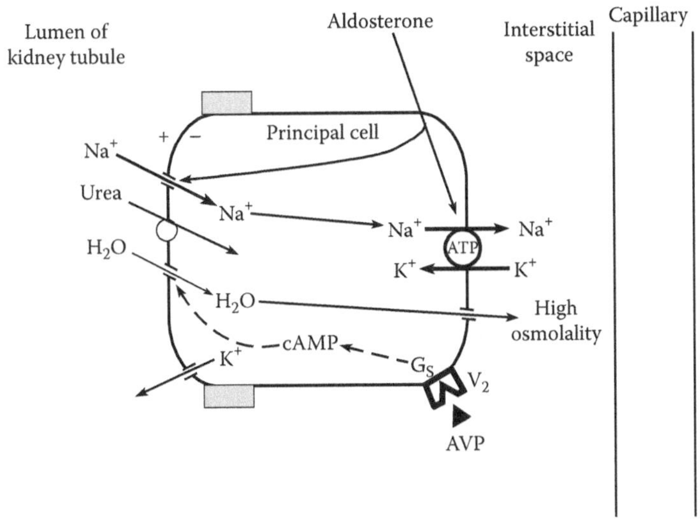

FIGURE 2.9 The principal cells of the collecting duct reabsorb sodium via epithelial sodium channels (ENaCs). Aldosterone exerts its primary effect on the principal cells, stimulating sodium reabsorption, which in turn causes potassium secretion. The principal cells also contain aquaporins that allow water reabsorption in the presence of AVP. Urea reabsorption is coupled to the reabsorption of water.

Principal cells are the target site for two of the three major hormones that target the kidney. Specifically, these cells express receptors for ALDO and arginine vasopressin (AVP) [also called antidiuretic hormone (ADH)]. The luminal membrane of the principal cells contains epithelial sodium channels (ENaCs) (Figure 2.9). These channels are blocked by amiloride and are also referred to as amiloride-sensitive sodium channels (Jackson, 2006a). Through these channels, Na^+ follows its electrochemical gradient into the cell, where it is then pumped into the interstitium by the Na^+–K^+ ATPase. The amount of Na^+ reabsorption is directly related to the Na^+ gradient, as would be predicted since Na^+ reabsorption into the cell is via a channel. Thus, if the luminal concentration of Na^+ is elevated, then the reabsorption is elevated. However, this is a time-dependent phenomenon, so if luminal flow is high, the overall percentage of Na^+ reabsorption will be reduced.

Reabsorption of the cation Na^+ causes K^+ to leave the cell and enter into the lumen (Figure 2.9). The concentration gradient favors K^+ secretion into the lumen (K^+ high inside cell vs. luminal concentration), and the addition of the cation Na^+ into the cells promotes K^+ secretion by electrostatic forces. In short, the salient feature to remember is that Na^+ reabsorption drives K^+ secretion. As indicated, ENaC can be blocked by amiloride (Jackson, 2006a). This results in diuresis but K^+ loss is minimized because its secretion by the principal cells is coupled to Na^+ reabsorption, and hence amiloride and amiloride-like drugs are K^+-sparing diuretics. ALDO also plays a pivotal role in Na^+ reabsorption in the principal cells. ALDO, a steroid hormone, increases the number of luminal ENaCs and enhances the activity of the basolateral Na^+–K^+ ATPase (Eaton and Pooler, 2009; Koeppen and Stanton, 2007; Rose and Post, 2001). Together, this can markedly increase Na^+ reabsorption, which in turn increases K^+ secretion. ALDO secretion is stimulated by plasma AII and K^+, the latter constituting a classic negative feedback pathway where hyperkalemia increases ALDO, which increases renal K^+ secretion, thereby reducing plasma K^+. ALDO receptor blockers, such as spironolactone, also serve as K^+-sparing diuretics (Jackson, 2006a). Liddle's syndrome is another rare genetic alteration affecting the kidneys (Ix and Lingappa, 2006; Koeppen and Stanton, 2007; Rose and Post, 2001). In this condition, genetic mutation of the ENaC results in enhanced Na^+ reabsorption. Because Na^+ reabsorption in the principal cells is markedly enhanced, these patients present with hyperaldosterone symptoms such as hypertension and hypokalemia. However, renin and, consequently, ALDO are markedly reduced.

The principal cells also express aquaporins, which are regulated by intracellular cAMP. AVP, via the V_2 receptor, stimulates adenylate cyclase, thereby increasing cAMP and allowing water to pass through the luminal channels. Recall that the medullary interstitium has a high osmolality (see Section 2.5). Thus, an osmotic gradient exists for water to move from the lumen into the interstitium. Under normal conditions, this osmotic gradient always exists; thus, whether or not water is reabsorbed is linked to circulating AVP levels. Not surprisingly, an important stimulus for AVP is plasma osmolality, and AVP secretion is directly related to it. Thus, if plasma osmolality increases, AVP increases, and water is reabsorbed by the kidney to reduce extracellular osmolality. If plasma osmolality falls, AVP is inhibited, and water is excreted by the kidneys to bring osmolality back up. In this way, the kidneys regulate extracellular osmolality.

Urea is also reabsorbed by the principal cells, and its reabsorption is linked to water (Eaton and Pooler, 2009; Koeppen and Stanton, 2007; Rose and Post, 2001). When AVP is high, and hence water reabsorption is high, the principal cells reabsorb urea with water. This reabsorption of urea is likely the result of the increased luminal concentration of urea that occurs as water leaves the lumen. As indicated above, urea constitutes about half the osmoles of the medullary interstitium, thus the reabsorption of this solute by the principal cells is the source of medullary urea. Urea then "cycles" within the medullary interstitium, being secreted into the ascending loop of Henle and then reabsorbed by the principal cells. This cycling provides the urea pool for the concentrated medullary interstitium. Although urea cycles in this manner, it should not be interpreted that all of the urea load to the collecting duct gets reabsorbed and cycled. In fact, about half the filtered load of urea is excreted, and this elimination of urea is an important function of the kidneys. As has been well described, renal failure causes urea retention; excess urea is toxic to the body, hence the term uremic poisoning.

Intercalated cells are the other cell type found in the collecting ducts. In short, intercalated cells play an important role in acid–base regulation (Eaton and Pooler, 2009; Koeppen and Stanton, 2007; Rose and Post, 2001). The luminal membrane of intercalated cells (technically alpha-intercalated cells) contains H^+–ATPase and a H^+–K^+ antiporter (Figure 2.10). Although not illustrated in the figure, the secreted H^+ can combine with bicarbonate to form CO_2 in the same manner as in the proximal tubule (see Section 2.4 and Figure 2.6). Thus, any bicarbonate remaining in the tubule (although not described, ATL does reabsorb some bicarbonate) is typically reabsorbed in the collecting duct. For those consuming a typical western diet, far more H^+ is generated than can be excreted as H^+. Recall that pH is measure of free H^+, and the luminal pH can only go so low before it begins to damage tissues. Thus, the excess H^+ must be excreted coupled to other compounds. The two most important compounds are Pi (predominant titratable acid) and ammonia. As depicted in Figure 2.10, H^+ in the lumen can combine with Pi to form diprotonated Pi, which is excreted. The secreted H^+ can also combine with ammonia forming ammonium, which is not reabsorbed and is thus excreted. The loss of H^+ via ammonium accounts for the bulk of H^+ excretion (about two-thirds), and the kidneys synthesize ammonia in proximal tubule cells. Acidosis will stimulate this renal synthesis of ammonia, which is quite adaptive. Note that for every H^+ lost via diprotonated Pi or ammonium, a "new" bicarbonate ion is added to body stores (Figure 2.10). ALDO also affects intercalated cells. This hormone stimulates H^+ secretion into the lumen, although the precise mechanism has not been well defined. Regardless, ALDO promotes H^+ loss from the body.

The preceding paragraph illustrates that the kidneys are long-term regulators of H^+ and bicarbonate and thus are pivotal in acid–base regulation. The kidneys play a crucial role in compensating for acid–base disturbances, and given the description above, one should be able to understand how this is accomplished. For example, acidosis increases H^+ secretion. This will enhance bicarbonate reabsorption, thereby preserving the major base in the body. In addition, acidosis stimulates ammonia synthesis, and the elevated H^+ can be eliminated in greater quantities via its binding to ammonia. Each H^+ lost via ammonium creates new bicarbonate, thereby increasing base within the body. On the flip side, renal dysfunction can cause acid–base disturbances. As mentioned, the kidneys must excrete significant quantities of H^+. Thus, chronic renal failure is one cause of acidosis. As mentioned above, failure to reabsorb bicarbonate in the proximal tubule results in type II renal

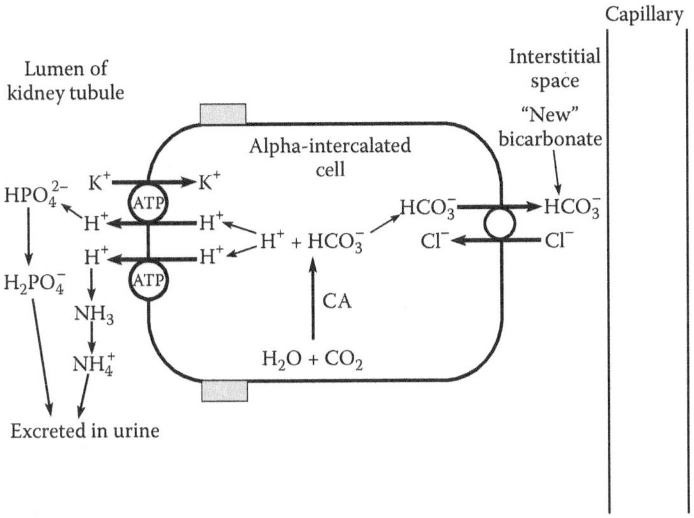

FIGURE 2.10 Role of alpha-intercalated cells of the collecting duct in acid–base regulation. See text for details.

tubular acidosis (e.g., Fanconi syndrome). Damage to the distal nephron (DT and collecting ducts), by ischemia, for example, can impair the ability of the kidneys to excrete H^+, resulting in type I renal tubular acidosis. Type IV renal tubular acidosis is the result of inadequate ALDO (Ix and Lingappa, 2006; Rose and Post, 2001).

2.8 K^+ DYNAMICS

Although the bulk of the body stores of K^+ reside within the intracellular compartment, extracellular K^+ is kept within a very narrow range. Excitable tissue, particularly the heart, can be markedly altered by changes in plasma K^+, and fatal arrhythmias can result if K^+ is not tightly regulated (Rose and Post, 2001). The kidneys play a pivotal role in this tight regulation of K^+. A thorough description of whole-body K^+ regulation is beyond the scope of this book. Instead, we describe the four fundamental factors that affect K^+ secretion by the principal cells. These are as follows: (1) *ALDO*: As described above, ALDO stimulates Na^+ reabsorption, which in turn causes K^+ secretion. Thus, there is a direct relationship between ALDO and K^+ secretion. This constitutes a negative feedback regulation because plasma K^+ concentration is one stimulus for ALDO. (2) *Tubular flow*: There is a direct relationship between tubular flow and K^+ secretion. As tubular flow increases, the concentration gradient for K^+ between the principal cells and the tubular lumen remains high; that is, there is not adequate time for K^+ to accumulate in the lumen, and thus more K^+ moves from the cell into the lumen. This likely explains why diuresis typically causes K^+ loss. (3) *Plasma* K^+: There is a direct relationship between the concentration of extracellular K^+ and its secretion. First, higher extracellular K^+ is thought to directly increase the K^+ concentration in the principal cells and thus increase its secretion. Second, elevated plasma K^+ stimulates ALDO release, which also increases K^+ secretion. (4) *Acid–base disturbances*: In general, alkalosis increases K^+ secretion, typically resulting in hypokalemia, whereas acidosis decreases (at least initially) K^+ secretion, resulting in hyperkalemia. There is evidence that H^+ directly inhibits the Na^+–K^+ ATPase (Eaton and Pooler, 2009; Koeppen and Stanton, 2007). If so, then it follows that K^+ secretion would fall in acidosis and rise in alkalosis (see Figure 2.9) because the basolateral Na^+–K^+ ATPase affects not only K^+ concentration inside the principal cells but also Na^+ reabsorption. As indicated, this is a generalization and an oversimplification since acid–base disturbances do not affect only the principal cells of the body. Thus, it should be appreciated that the clinical presentation for K^+ in acid–base disturbances can be quite varied from patient to patient.

2.9 INTEGRATION AND PATHOPHYSIOLOGY

As indicated at the beginning of this chapter, the kidneys regulate the extracellular volume by regulating Na^+. The principal cells provide the final fine-tuning of Na^+, and the reabsorption of this ion is greatly influenced by the hormone ALDO. In addition to being stimulated by plasma K^+, AII stimulates ALDO, and the rate-controlling step for AII production is catalyzed by renin, an agent released from the kidneys. This renin–angiotensin–ALDO system (RAAS) is a key element in the regulation of all production. There are three stimuli for renin secretion, the first step in the process of regulation of the extracellular volume (Eaton and Pooler, 2009; Koeppen and Stanton, 2007; Rose and Post, 2001). These are (1) reduced perfusion pressure to the kidney, (2) sympathetic stimulation of the kidney (beta-1 receptor), and (3) decreased delivery of Na^+ to the macula densa. If one examines these, one can find that, in general, they all go hand in hand. The first stimulus is a drop in arterial blood pressure (perfusion pressure to the kidney). If arterial blood pressure drops, sympathetic nerves are stimulated via the baroreflex. Further, if pressure drops, then GFR may drop (assuming incomplete autoregulation), which in turn would reduce Na^+ delivery to the macula densa. Even if the kidneys adequately autoregulate to compensate for the fall in arterial pressure, and thus GFR remains unchanged, the other two stimuli cause renin secretion. Regardless, the fall in pressure signals the kidneys to activate RAAS, and the rise in ALDO increases Na^+ reabsorption. This rise in Na^+ reabsorption causes water to follow the osmole and leads to expansion of the extracellular compartment because Na^+ is the most abundant osmole of the extracellular compartment. Sodium is the osmole and water follows. Thus, RAAS regulates the extracellular volume by regulating the osmole. This extracellular volume plays a pivotal role in determining arterial blood pressure. Thus, a drop in arterial blood pressure signals the kidneys to activate RAAS to bring arterial blood pressure back to its original level.

Numerous clinical entities that underscore the importance of RAAS and blood-pressure regulation exist. Even a cursory glance at many of the therapeutics for treating hypertension illustrates the importance of the kidneys and RAAS. Diuretics, ACE inhibitors, AII antagonists, and ALDO receptor blockers (often classified as diuretics) are frequently prescribed for treating hypertension (Hoffman, 2006). Congestive heart failure is another example of the role of RAAS in expanding extracellular volume (Rose and Post, 2001). Arterial blood pressure falls because of the inadequate cardiac output, which in turn activates RAAS and increases the extracellular volume. This continues as the heart fails more and more, hence the rationale for the term "congestive." Congestive heart failure is an example of secondary hyperaldosteronism—secondary because the hyperaldosterone is secondary to the fall in cardiac output. Interestingly, this degree of volume expansion is not seen in primary hyperaldosteronism (Conn's disease). By an undefined mechanism, the kidneys undergo an "ALDO escape," which prevents excessive extracellular expansion (Rose and Post, 2001). Although this escape occurs, these patients are typically hypertensive and show hypokalemia (K^+ loss) and alkalosis (H^+ loss). However, they rarely show hypernatremia, further illustrating that Na^+ regulation is related to volume regulation. Similarly, patients with renal artery stenosis often exhibit hypertension even though they do not exhibit the edema common for congestive heart failure. Renal artery stenosis increases RAAS because the stenosis causes a reduced perfusion pressure to the kidney (pressure downstream from the resistor falls; see Section 2.3).

AVP is the second hormone targeting the principal cells. As indicated, AVP causes water reabsorption in these cells. From a whole-body perspective, this subserves two functions, both of which can be predicted based upon the factors stimulating AVP. These are increased plasma osmolality and decreased blood pressure/volume (Abboud and Thames, 1983; Bishop et al., 1983; Eaton and Pooler, 2009; Koeppen and Stanton, 2007; Rose and Post, 2001). Considering osmolality first, increasing water reabsorption in response to increased plasma osmolality provides negative feedback regulation of extracellular osmolality, which in turn helps control the intracellular volume. Recall that water moves via osmosis and that changes in extracellular osmolality alters the intracellular volume. For example, inadequate water intake will increase extracellular osmolality, causing water to shift from the intracellular compartment to the extracellular. Cells will shrink in response.

The rise in extracellular osmolality stimulates AVP, which in turn causes the kidneys to conserve water. Diabetes insipidus is the pathologic correlate of this condition (Else et al., 2006; Rose and Post, 2001). In this condition, there is a lack of functional AVP because either AVP is not secreted (central diabetes insipidus) or the kidneys fail to respond to the circulating levels of AVP (nephrogenic diabetes insipidus). Regardless, the lack of AVP causes the kidneys to excrete water in excess. This causes a rise in extracellular osmolality and a loss of water from cells (cellular dehydration). Lithium can also have the negative consequence of producing a diabetes insipidus-like condition. Lithium may alter the function of V_2 receptors, thus causing marked water loss. In addition, lithium can be nephrotoxic (Rose and Post, 2001). On the opposite end of the spectrum, one can consume too much water, a condition called primary polydipsia. In this case, extracellular osmolality falls, resulting in water moving into cells. To combat this, AVP levels fall, water reabsorption in the kidney decreases, and the excess water is eliminated in an attempt to correct the reduced extracellular osmolality. This process occurs even if there is no pathologic consumption of water, that is, simply drinking water. The AVP pathology correlate is a syndrome of inappropriate ADH (SIADH). In SIADH, there is excess AVP (Else et al., 2006; Rose and Post, 2001). This causes a pathologic increase in water reabsorption with a concomitant fall in extracellular osmolality, causing water to move intracellularly.

The second factor regulating AVP is blood pressure/volume. Both cardiopulmonary and arterial baroreceptor stimulation inhibit AVP release (Abboud and Thames, 1983; Bishop et al., 1983; Eaton and Pooler, 2009; Koeppen and Stanton, 2007; Rose and Post, 2001). Thus, a rise in arterial blood pressure and/or intravascular volume decreases AVP, thereby causing water excretion and a subsequent reduction in the extracellular volume. On the other hand, a drop in arterial blood pressure and/or intravascular volume stimulates AVP release, causing water retention. In this regard, AVP works in tandem with RAAS and thus plays some role in the overall regulation of the extracellular volume. However, when AVP is considered alone, the process is self-limiting. If intravascular volume falls, AVP increases, which in turn increases water reabsorption. Since this is water alone, extracellular osmolality falls, which has a negative effect on AVP secretion. The opposite occurs if arterial blood pressure and/or intravascular volume rises. Thus, significant and sustained increases in the extracellular volume must occur using osmoles, for example, Na^+ and thus RAAS. Nevertheless, one should appreciate that severe intravascular volume loss, for example, hemorrhage, can produce profound increases in AVP, which in turn can reduce overall osmolality.

2.10 SUMMARY

Understanding renal physiology is the backbone for understanding the clinical disturbances associated with renal dysfunction. The kidneys play a crucial role in regulating the extracellular compartment. In this chapter, we reviewed the various transport mechanisms that exist in the nephron to accomplish this feat. Via a countercurrent mechanism, a concentrated medullary interstitium of the kidneys is created, and it is this concentrated interstitium that provides the osmotic driving force for water reabsorption. In turn, AVP acts on the kidneys to regulate water reabsorption, thereby regulating overall extracellular osmolality. Not surprisingly, extracellular osmolality is an important regulator of AVP secretion. The kidneys also serve as the mode of elimination for urea, a breakdown product of protein metabolism, that exerts toxic effects on the body if it is not eliminated. In addition, the principal cells reabsorb Na^+, and this reabsorption is primarily under the influence of the hormone ALDO. Since Na^+ is the predominant osmole of the extracellular compartment, regulating this ion helps control the extracellular volume. Since the extracellular volume is an important component of arterial blood pressure, the kidneys play a crucial role in long-term regulation of blood pressure. One factor affecting ALDO release is plasma AII, and thus RAAS is a key player in blood pressure regulation. In addition, ALDO stimulates K^+ secretion, and plasma K^+ is the second stimulus for ALDO secretion. This forms a negative feedback loop to help tightly regulate extracellular K^+. Finally, the kidneys are long-term regulators of H^+ and bicarbonate, and thus they play a pivotal role in acid–base regulation of the body. Considering all this, it is not surprising that pathology of the kidney can evoke multiple problems for a variety of organs, which underscores the important role the kidneys play in whole-body homeostasis.

REFERENCES

Abboud, F. and Thames, M. 1983. Interaction of cardiovascular reflexes in circulatory control. In Shepherd, J.T. and Abboud, F.M., eds., *Handbook of Physiology*. Baltimore, MD: American Physiological Society, 675–753.

Alpers, C. 2005. The kidney. In Kumar, V., Abbas, A.K., and Fausto, N., eds., *Pathologic Basis of Disease*. Philadelphia, PA: Elsevier Inc., 955–1021.

Barrett, K., Barman, S., Boitano, S., et al. 2010. Renal physiology. In Barrett, K.E., Barman, S.M., Boitano, S. and Brooks, H.L., eds., *Ganong's Review of Medical Physiology*. New York: McGraw-Hill Companies, 639–686.

Bishop, V., Malliani, A., Thoren, P. 1983. Cardiac mechanoreceptors. In Shepherd, J.T. and Abboud, F.M., eds., *Handbook of Physiology*. Baltimore, MD: American Physiological Society, 675–753.

Burke, A., Smyth, E., FitzGerald, G. 2006. Analgesic–antipyretic and antiinflammatory agents: Pharmacotherapy of gout. In Brunton, L.L., ed., *Goodman and Gilman's the Pharmacological Basis of Therapeutics*. New York: McGraw-Hill Companies, 671–715.

Dibona, G. 2002. Sympathetic nervous system and the kidney in hypertension. *Curr Opin Nephrol Hypertens*. 11:197–200.

Eaton, D. and Pooler, J. 2009. *Vander's Renal Physiology*. New York: McGraw-Hill Companies.

El-Sheikh, A., Masereeuw, R., Russel, F. 2008. Mechanisms of renal anionic drug transport. *Eur J Pharmacol*. 585:245–255.

Else, T., Hammer, G., Lingappa, V. 2006. Disorder of the hypothalamus and pituitary gland. In McPhee, S.J. and Ganong, W.F., eds., *Pathophysiology of Disease: An Introduction to Clinical Medicine*. New York: McGraw-Hill Companies, 456–481.

Hoffman, B. 2006. Therapy of hypertension. In Brunton, L.L., ed., *Goodman and Gilman's the Pharmacological Basis of Therapeutics*. New York: McGraw-Hill Companies, 845–868.

Jackson, E. 2006a. Diuretics. In Brunton, L.L., ed., *Goodman and Gilman's the Pharmacological Basis of Therapeutics*. New York: McGraw-Hill Companies, 737–770.

Jackson, E. 2006b. Renin and angiotensin. In Brunton, L.L., ed., *Goodman and Gilman's the Pharmacological Basis of Therapeutics*. New York: McGraw-Hill Companies, 789–822.

Ix, J. and Lingappa, V. 2006. Renal disease. In McPhee, S.J. and Ganong, W.F., eds., *Pathophysiology of Disease: An Introduction to Clinical Medicine*. New York: McGraw-Hill Companies, 456–481.

Ganong, W. 2006. Cardiovascular disorders: Vascular disease. In McPhee, S.J. and Ganong, W.F., eds. *Pathophysiology of Disease: An Introduction to Clinical Medicine*. New York: McGraw-Hill Companies, 300–326.

Koeppen, B. and Stanton, B. 2007. *Renal Physiology*. Philadelphia, PA: Mosby Inc.

Kotchen, T. 2008. Hypertensive vascular disease. In Fauci, A.S., Braunwald, E., Kasper, D.L., Hauser, S.L., Longo, D.L., Jameson, J.L. and Loscalzo, J., eds. *Harrison's Principles of Internal Medicine*. New York: McGraw-Hill Companies, 1549–1562.

Marshall, S. 2004. Recent advances in diabetic nephropathy. *Postgrad Med J*. 80:624–633.

Rose, B. and Post, T. 2001. *Clinical Physiology of Acid–Base and Electrolyte Disorders*. New York: McGraw-Hill Companies.

Srimaroeng, C., Perry, J., Pritchard, J. 2008. Physiology, structure, and regulation of the cloned organic anion transporters. *Xenobiotica* 38:889–935.

3 Electrolyte and Acid–Base Disorders

Malcolm L. Buford and Charles J. Foulks
The University of Oklahoma-Tulsa

CONTENTS

3.1 FLUID AND ELECTROLYTES INTRODUCTION

Chronic kidney disease (CKD) affects more than 25 million Americans, including more than 350,000 persons on dialysis, at a current cost of $17 billion annually (Fox et al., 2010; Ikizler, 2009). Renal disease is very frequently accompanied by electrolyte abnormalities, which must be recognized and managed. In modern medicine, it is impossible to have a comprehensive discussion on the spectrum of disease, goals of treatment, and prognostic factors that determine patient outcomes without including nutrition and electrolytes, which influence the management of these issues. This chapter provides the reader with information about electrolytes from a systemic and pathophysiologic perspective.

3.1.1 Sodium

Sodium (Na^+) is ubiquitous in nature and second to potassium in its distribution in the human body. The average human body contains 9 oz (250 g) of sodium (Harvard, 2010). The roles of sodium in the health of the individual are numerous and include maintaining normal plasma osmolality and normal blood pressure, and nerve conduction (central, peripheral, and cardiac). In the kidney, sodium also acts as a cotransporter for various elements, namely, potassium and phosphorus. Increased Na^+ intake is a leading contributor to hypertension, second only to obesity. The average American diet contains 3.4 g/d ("d" denotes "day") of dietary sodium (roughly 1.5 teaspoons), and in other countries, dietary sodium intake is even higher (e.g., Finland has ranges of 7–11.2 g/d in men) (Charlton et al., 2007). Due to the morbidity and mortality associated with chronic disease states such as hypertension and atherosclerosis, in order to decrease the contribution to these diseases by dietary discretion, the World Health Organization recommends limiting intake to <7 g/d in men and 6 g/d in women, with the ideal intake being 4 g/d (Harvard, 2010). In United States, the Recommended Daily Allowance (RDA) for sodium is 2.3 g/d if there is no associated medical illness and 1.5 g/d in the presence of hypertension, CKD, or in persons of African American descent. To better define actual dietary intake in hypertension that may be "refractory" to therapy utilizing 3+ agents, there should be further evaluation by measuring 24-h urine collection for sodium excretion. Numerous studies have shown a discrepancy between a patient's reported dietary intake and actual urinary quantitative excretion. This 24-h urine may be used to determine the actual dietary sodium or reveal the presence of insidious sources of salt intake and help facilitate patient education.

There are several disease states in which sodium levels may rise or fall or where changes in sodium levels may be a component of a larger disease process. As with all plasma electrolytes, sodium levels are maintained within narrow limits, and the variation is divided into two groups, "hyper" or elevated levels, "hypo" or depressed levels. *Hypernatremia*, defined as a serum $Na^+ > 145$ mmol/L and *hyponatremia,* defined as serum $Na^+ < 135$ mmol/L. The fluctuation of serum Na^+ in most cases actually reflects changes in volume status. It is imperative to note that serum Na^+ levels reflect free-water concentrations rather than an absolute abundance or deficit of total body sodium content. Invariably, dietary Na^+ is considered the culprit; however, this is rarely, if ever, the case. Table 3.1 depicts the typical differential of elevated Na^+ levels, and Table 3.2 does the same for depressed levels. In hyponatremia, it is customary to consider perceived volume status on examination of the patient in addition to urinary Na^+ concentration to help establish the source of the aberration.

3.1.1.1 Hyponatremia

Patients presenting with hyponatremia should first be evaluated by assessing their effective intravascular volume. This is done by history and physical examination, obtaining vital signs such as orthostatic blood pressures, and by laboratory evaluations such as for the fractional excretion of sodium

TABLE 3.1
Hypernatremia—Associated Disease States

High volume

- Iatrogenic (hyperalimentation, hyperosmolar fluids)
- Early diabetes insipidus

Low to normal volume

- Dehydration (insensible loss, gastrointestinal, burns)
- Late diabetes insipidus (nephrogenic or central)

TABLE 3.2
Hyponatremia—Associated Disease States

Low volume states
- Dehydration
- Diuretic-induced (particularly thiazide diuretics, spironolactone)
- Adrenocortical deficiency
- Medication induced
- Nausea/emesis prior to replacement fluids

Euvolemia (normal volume state)
- Depression
- Syndrome of inappropriate antidiuretic hormone (SIADH)
- Acute kidney injury without volume overload
- Fever
- Pain
- Acute psychosis
- Pseudo hyponatremia
- Pancreatitis
- Nausea/emesis after inappropriate repletion

Excess volume states
- Acute kidney injury
- Chronic kidney disease
- Congestive heart failure
- Liver disease

(FeNa) and serum uric acid levels. In prerenal or underperfusing disease states, the FeNa will be <1% unless there are compounding issues regarding kidney function or in patients on diuretics. The serum uric acid level can provide clues to intravascular volume and renal perfusion. Hypovolemia can result in elevated levels of antidiuretic hormone (ADH), which increases permeability of the distal tubule to free water, resulting in dilution of measured serum Na^+. Patients with decreased oral intake, nausea, or emesis may show such findings. In this scenario, volume resuscitation with isotonic electrolyte repletion would be appropriate. Hyponatremia with volume excess can also be present. Congestive heart failure, liver disease or cirrhosis, and chronic renal disease are such scenarios. Patients may have decreased peripheral perfusion pressures, thus increasing ADH and causing retention of free water. This may occur despite the use of salt restriction and diuretics. A newer class of medications, aquaporin channel inhibitors, are available and capable of indirect inhibition of the normal function of vasopressin in the distal kidney and may be used to prevent the pathologic lowering of sodium in the aforementioned disease states. There is currently no survival benefit for patients, and their availability is still limited. Free-water restriction is typically recommended, as well as attempts to provide adequate kidney perfusion pressure. A difficult situation arises when the patient is euvolemic without an identifiable cause of low Na^+. These patients should raise suspicion of the syndrome of inappropriate antidiuretic hormone release (SIADH) after testing rules out other causes listed in Table 3.2. Because of its association with malignant conditions, hyponatremia thought to be due to SIADH should prompt exhaustive testing to find a source. In evaluating the patient with an unidentified source for hyponatremia, a thorough medication history should be obtained, including over-the-counter medications and holistic/ritualistic medications as patients may omit these agents believing them to be innocuous though the substances may be the causative agent.

Low-serum uric acid in patients with hyponatremia suggests volume excess with adequate distal delivery and may serve to help differentiate SIADH from other causes of hyponatremia. Though SIADH is placed in the "euvolemic volume" category, it is in fact a mildly volume-expanded disease state. *Pseudohyponatremia* is a laboratory phenomenon in which unmeasured osmoles such as triglycerides and mannitol may expand the volume being measured by instruments and cause falsely low levels of sodium due to dilution.

3.1.1.2 Hypernatremia

Hypernatremia has a more limited differential. In this particular disease state, the elevation in Na^+ content results from a deficit of serum-free water. Hypernatremia is usually found in patients with impaired access to free water (either due to dementia or bed-bound physical states or iatrogenic) or who have an impaired thirst mechanism. Hypernatremia may be due to a lack of access to free water with an inability to reabsorb appropriate levels in the kidney, so-called diabetes insipidus (DI). This particular disease state can be both central (originating in the posterior pituitary where ADH, also called *arginine vasopressin*, is stored after being formed in hypothalamic nuclei along its carrier protein, neurophysin) or as a result of intrinsic kidney disease (making the disease state "nephrogenic"). There are many potential causes of either one of these disease states, with central etiologies most often secondary to stroke, infiltrative disease (such as sarcoid), or Sheehan's disease, and nephrogenic etiologies often caused by medications such as lithium, orlistat, amphotericin B, and foscarnet or may be the result of excess amounts of calcium. Correction of the underlying cause either with supplemental ADH in the case of central DI or with supraphysiologic doses in the case of nephrogenic DI can usually afford some regulation to residual sodium/free-water control, though, if possible, treatment of the underlying cause or withdrawal of the offending agents is always the initial treatment.

3.1.2 Potassium

Potassium (K^+), the second element in our discussion, is a monovalent element similar to sodium and is often found in the body working in conjunction with sodium. It is the most abundant cation in the human body, with 2% in the extracellular compartment and 98% of body stores in the intracellular areas. Typical serum concentrations of potassium are 3.5–5 mmol/L, and intracellular concentrations are 125–135 mmol/L (Rastergar et al., 2001; Wang et al., 1997). Typical daily intake of potassium is 80–120 mmol/d, and yet the body filters 700–800 mmol/d in the urine, with the majority being reabsorbed proximally in the kidney or in the limb of Henle. The majority of potassium loss from the kidney occurs distally under the influence of aldosterone and sodium absorption at the epithelial sodium channel. Potassium functions mainly in the maintenance of action potential gradients because of its marked distribution difference and the ratio of that difference (Ki/Ke) (Rastergar et al., 2001; Tang et al., 2004). Intracellular K^+ is maintained by plasma Na–K ATPase channels that are phosphorylated to allow the exit of three molecules of sodium from the cell and then hydrolyzed to allow the entry, via conformational change, of two molecules of potassium. Potassium contributes to lacrimation, mucus in the lung, or surfactant elaboration and gastrointestinal (GI) peptide secretion. In acute hypoxic events, K^+ channels are inhibited resulting in large calcium influx into cells, particularly carotid body chemoreceptors, inducing dopamine release, intense muscle cell contraction, and vasoconstriction of responsive vessels (Tang et al., 2004; Wang et al., 1997; Weir and Rolfe, 2010).

Disorders of potassium are quite frequent, with *hyperkalemia*, defined as a serum K^+ >5.5 mmol/L found in 5%–10% of all patients with end-stage renal disease (ESRD), contributing to 2%–5% of all deaths in patients on dialysis. Hyperkalemia causes 1.4% of all hospitalizations, with levels >6.0 mmol/L being particularly dangerous because it is at this level that cardiovascular conduction issues begin to be clinically relevant. *Hypokalemia*, defined as a serum concentration <3.5 mmol/L, is also associated with worsening hypertension, and in one study, K^+ levels <4.0 mmol/L were associated with increased mortality.

Signs and symptoms of clinical K^+ irregularity are fairly similar in both elevated and suppressed levels of potassium. Muscle weakness and potential paralysis are shared between the two extreme levels. With hyperkalemia, there is usually a continuous spectrum of findings on electrocardiogram, from initial peaked T waves with a normal to mildly prolonged PR interval to a finally widened

QRS with prolonged duration and eventual sine-wave "conduction" with eventual failure and death. These changes are not truly reflective of a particular level and can occur suddenly because of the nature of potassium handling. See Tables 3.3 and 3.4.

Dietary recommendations for potassium in persons without risk for symptomatic hyperkalemia are 4 g/d. This is roughly twice of what self-reporting instrument studies suggest persons in the United States consume. Multiple sources of potassium are known, some of the more abundant ones being legumes, fruits, and dairy products. Increasing K^+ intake has shown to improve mortality, lower blood pressure, and suppress progressive cardiovascular disease (CVD) and interstitial fibrosis in the kidney. However, patients with CKD are typically at high risk for developing hyperkalemia because of the kidney's important role in potassium handling (Naito et al., 2010; Unwin et al., 2011).

3.1.3 Calcium

Calcium (Ca^{2+}) is the fifth most abundant element in the body. In man, calcium in combination with phosphorus helps to make up the mineralizing strength of the bone, where >99% of body calcium is found (Peacock, 2010). Bone is composed of 70% mineral, 8% water, and 22% protein (in the form of type I collagen) (Dawson-Hughes, 2003). Calcium is bound to plasma proteins such as albumin and is free extracellularly in an ionized, physiologically active form to facilitate neurologic function and muscular contraction. Intracellular systems utilize Ca^{2+}, either free or bound to a protein called *calmodulin*, to allow for hormonal signaling. Ca^{2+} is only available to humans through dietary gain, although various mechanisms maintain physiologic ranges. The recommended intake for calcium is 1000–1500 mg per day, of which 30% of the ingested amount is absorbed. This goal, however, is rarely met, and numerous studies have been done or are currently underway with the goal of both maximizing the education of the public about the importance of adequate dietary Ca^{2+} and encouraging more fortification by the food industry.

The homeostatic mechanisms to maintain ideal ranges of calcium in the body (8.5–10 mg/dl) are complex, and disturbances in them have the potential to cause disease in various organ systems. Three mechanisms maintain normal levels of calcium: intestinal absorption from dietary

TABLE 3.3
Causes of Hypokalemia

Renal losses
- Medication
- Renal tubular acidosis type I and II
- Osmotic diuresis
- Hyperaldosteronism
- Liddle's syndrome

Malnutrition

GI losses
- Diarrhea
- Laxative abuse

Consumptive loss
- Malignancy
- Refeeding

Transcellular shift[a]
- Acid/base
- Insulin administration
- β-receptor agonists

[a] Transient decrease.

TABLE 3.4
Causes of Hyperkalemia

Renal disease
- Renal tubular acidosis type IV
- Chronic interstitial disease
- Decreased glomerular filtration rate
- Gordon's syndrome
- Addison's disease (hypoaldosteronism)

Marked volume depletion

Tissue damage
- Rhabdomyolysis
- Chemotherapy with aggressive tumor

Medication
- Nonsteroidal anti-inflammatory drugs
- Potassium supplementation
- Angiotensin-converting enzyme inhibitors
- Angiotensin receptor blockers
- β-receptor blockers
- Heparin

Transcellular shift[a]
- Systemic acidosis
- Hyperglycemia

[a] Transient.

intake, renal reabsorption, and bone turnover. To understand the balance of these systems, one must look to the parathyroid hormone (PTH) and vitamin D metabolism. Beginning in the gut, dietary Ca^{2+} absorption is facilitated by activated $1,25(OH)_2$ vitamin D, which when present increases intestinal absorption and when absent decreases intestinal absorption. The absorption of dietary Ca^{2+} is also affected by other ingested items such as oxalic acid or the presence of phosphate, both of which form insoluble salts in the gut and result in the Ca^{2+} being excreted in the feces (Taylor and Curhan, 2009). This can be minimized by diet planning if desired. Increased absorption can be facilitated by supplementing the dietary Ca^{2+} with calcium supplements. Historically, aluminum was utilized to bind phosphorus, but that has since fallen out of favor, particularly in patients with severe kidney disease because of the risks of causing relatively refractory anemia. After gut absorption, Ca^{2+} metabolism is also controlled by PTH. In the presence of increased PTH, the renal reabsorption of Ca^{2+} is increased in the proximal tubule cells, and the hormone stimulates osteoclastic activity, increasing the liberation of Ca^{2+} from bony stores. Interestingly, the latter would concomitantly liberate phosphorus (P), but PTH's actions in the proximal kidney counteract the accumulation of serum P in the presence of intact kidney function by causing a P-wasting state. Recent evidence also shows that fibroblast growth factor 23 has a significant role in the functioning of vitamin D and renal handling of P, which can indirectly also affect Ca^{2+} handling (Taylor and Curhan, 2009).

Numerous disease states affect calcium and its metabolism. In renal disease, the usual Ca^{2+} abnormality is hypocalcemia (serum levels < 8.5 mg/dL). This is typically due to diminished dietary intake coupled with impaired 25-OH vitamin D activation with decreased 1a-hydroxylase activity. Exogenous Ca^{2+} and vitamin D supplementation can be introduced to treat this hypocalcemia; if hypocalcemia is not treated, adaptive mechanisms in the body will lead to decreased bone density (*renal osteodystrophy*) as well as elevated PTH levels, resulting in secondary hyperparathyroidism syndrome. This is important because the known association between elevated PTH levels and accelerated atherosclerosis may explain the higher incidence of heart disease and peripheral arterial disease in patients with CKD. The two most common forms of hypercalcemia are not renal in etiology: primary parathyroid adenoma in the outpatient setting and malignancy when previously undiagnosed patients present to the hospital. See Tables 3.5 and 3.6.

3.1.4 Phosphorus

Phosphorus (P) is a multivalent element in the nitrogen family, which has great utility for normal physiologic function. In nature, P is rather reactive and is never found as a lone element, but it is always adjoined chemically in a compound, usually with oxygen. P has many different roles both inside and outside the body. P is commonly found in fertilizers, detergents, and pesticides (Isakova and Wolf, 2010). From a nutritional perspective, P is mainly found in dairy products, meats, and fish. The RDA allowance for P is 700–1250 mg/d depending on age and comorbidities such as pregnancy. In normal physiologic conditions, around 95% of dietary absorption is excreted in the kidneys to maintain the normal serum concentration. Phosphorus is critical in cellular membrane stability and generation of ATP within the Krebs' cycle, and it plays significant roles in intracellular hormonal action and tissue oxygenation via 2,3-BPG with hemoglobin. The majority of P (~85%) is stored in bone alongside Ca^{2+} as a salt called *hydroxyapatite*. P is also typically found in food additives, consumption of which may play a rather significant role in generating potentially harmful imbalances in most people.

TABLE 3.5
Causes of Hypocalcemia

Medications
- Loop diuretics
- Carbonic anhydrase inhibitors
- Antiepileptics

Aggressive blood transfusion
Bartter's syndrome
Malnutrition and refeeding syndrome
Secondary hyperparathyroidism
Vitamin D deficiency
Familial hypocalcaemia hypercalciuria
Post parathyroidectomy syndrome

TABLE 3.6
Causes of Hypercalcemia

Volume depletion
Malignancy
- Multiple myeloma
- Prostate cancer with lytic lesions
- Parathyroid carcinoma

Medications
- Thiazide diuretics

Gitelman's syndrome
Primary and tertiary hyperparathyroidism

Phosphorus homeostasis is maintained both by dietary intake and the feedback mechanisms in the body that control vitamin D and PTH (Kalantar-Zadeh et al., 2010). In fact, aside from dietary intake, the strict range of serum P in patients without clinical kidney dysfunction (2.5–4.5 mg/dl) is mostly mitigated through changes in how PTH affects P distribution. Upon ingestion of food, the absorption of P averages between 40% and 80%, greatly influenced by PTH levels and the presence of associated "binders" in the diet. For example, available Ca^{2+} and other phosphate-adherent molecules decrease systemic P absorption to the degree that has clinical utility. From a pathophysiologic perspective, concerns about systemic P stem from several studies that have linked serum P levels to advancing or accelerated atherosclerosis and CVD (Isakova and Wolf, 2010). Limiting phosphorous intake has been shown to delay or decrease the rate of progressive atherosclerosis, particularly in patients with chronic kidney disease. The challenge is maintaining healthy nitrogen/protein balance in a diet while trying to minimize phosphorous ingestion. The K/DOQI guidelines (National Kidney Foundation, 2003) recommend 1.2 g/kg/d dietary intake, and Shinaberger et al. found in follow-up reanalysis of their patients that a slightly higher goal of 1.4–1.5 g/kg/d showed improved long-term survival for patients on maintenance dialysis (Boaz and Smetana, 1996). The challenge stems from the fact that the vast majority of easily available foodstuffs are laden with either high P/protein ratios or are associated with inorganic P, which is more readily available for absorption from the gut and hence systemically. Boaz and Smetana showed that dietary P was in fact an independent risk factor for accelerated renal-function decline. Other authors have shown a measurable atherogenic potential of these higher levels. The challenge therefore for patients and health care providers is education that can help them make dietary choices that reflect our current understanding of P and its impact, at least in renal disease, on CVD and long-term risk (Ix et al., 2009).

Several things may affect serum P levels (see Table 3.7). Aside from dietary change and the above-mentioned roles of vitamin D, PTH, and calcium ingestion, other disease states may have transient effects and must be kept in mind when approaching the patient with P levels outside of the normal range, though with presumably normal kidney function. Assessment of the patient's condition should help to identify complicating factors that may influence treatment decisions.

3.1.5 Magnesium

Magnesium (Mg) is the fourth most common cation found in humans, and it is abundant in the environment. Fifty-two percent of the total body Mg is contained within bone, 27% in muscle, and 19% in soft tissues. Less than 1% of total body magnesium is present in the extracellular space. Magnesium is required for many metabolic and enzymatic processes, including the synthesis of nucleic acids and proteins, and in intermediary metabolism (Swaminathan, 2003). Hypomagnesemia is much more common than hypermagnesemia, which is generally only seen in patients with kidney dysfunction

TABLE 3.7
Disease States Associated with Aberrant Phosphorus

Rhabdomyolysis
Burns
Acute or chronic renal failure
Hyperparathyroidism (PTH elevated in all)
• Primary (low with elevated Ca^{2+})
• Secondary (normal to high with low Ca^{2+})
• Tertiary (high with elevated Ca^{2+})
Anorexia
Malignancy
Granulomatous disease

or those receiving a massive intake of Mg, generally given intravenously (e.g., the eclamptic patient receiving magnesium sulfate). Magnesium is contained in food and water, and the daily intake is dependent upon the Mg concentrations in these sources. Chlorophyll is magnesium rich, and green leafy vegetables are excellent dietary sources. Magnesium is also found in nuts, legumes, and grains. Other vegetables, fruits, meats, fish, and chocolates are not as Mg-rich, and dairy products are Mg-poor. The Mg content of drinking water varies widely, and the Mg content of hard water can be high. As long as dietary energy intake is not primarily obtained from sugar and alcohol, the Mg intake roughly parallels the intake of energy. The Mg content of foods can be markedly reduced (>85% loss) by boiling and refining or industrial processing of foods (Fawcett et al., 1999). The current RDA for Mg is 4.5 mg/kg/d and is higher in pregnancy and lactation.

Many consuming a Western diet have an inadequate intake of Mg. About half of the Mg contained in bone is exchangeable, and this acts as an Mg pool that can stabilize the serum Mg. The normal range for serum Mg concentration is very narrow and is not affected by acid–base status. Magnesium balance is a function of intake (absorption from food or medicine or intravenous administration) and GI or renal conservation or loss. In persons who are exposed to a Mg-deficient diet, renal excretion and GI excretion fall to 0.5–1.0 mEq/d each. Although the extracellular space contains little Mg, with 1/4 of the content within the intravascular space, the filtered load of Mg in the kidney is high. A 2.0 mEq/L serum Mg concentration in a person with a GFR of 120 mL/min (173 L/d) will have a 24-h Mg-filtered load of 346 mEq/d. The total body Mg of a 70-kg adult is about 2000 mEq. It is clear that any impairment of renal conservation mechanisms can have rapid and potentially devastating effects. Thirty percent of the serum Mg is protein bound and 70% is ultrafiltered by the glomerulus. Over 95% of the filtered Mg is reabsorbed; of this, 20% is reabsorbed in the proximal tubule; 70%, in the thick ascending limb of Henle; and the remainder is reabsorbed distally. Absorption in the thick ascending limb is directly related to sodium chloride reabsorption and is inversely related to the rate of urine flow. Diuretics increase urinary Na and urinary flow rate thereby increasing urinary Mg losses and may lead to hypomagnesemia (Dai et al., 2001; Quamme, 1997).

GI absorption is inversely related to intake, and the majority of Mg is reabsorbed in the ileum and cecum. PTH may be important in regulating Mg absorption, but the roles of vitamin D and $1,25(OH)_2D$ are unclear. Dietary phytates bind Mg, but the low levels found in the usual diet are not believed to impair absorption. Oxalate, phosphate, proteins, zinc, and potassium may affect absorption. The regulation of intracellular Mg is poorly understood. Less than 5% of intracellular Mg is ionized; the remainder is bound to anionic compounds such as ATP, ADP, citrate, RNA, DNA, and other proteins as well as being sequestered within the mitochondria and endoplasmic reticulum. Different rates of Mg transport occur, with the highest transport rates being found in the heart, liver, and kidney (Fawcett et al., 1999; Saris et al., 2000). Serum Mg is poorly reflective of the total body Mg content (Rude, 1993). Although many measures of Mg exist, they are of no real clinical use. The serum Mg remains the best measure available. When the serum Mg is low, intracellular Mg tends to be low as well. Unfortunately, when the serum Mg is normal, the intracellular Mg may be low (Fox et al., 2002; Whang et al., 1994). Patients with acute kidney injury (AKI) are unable to properly secrete or reabsorb Mg secondary to primary renal damage to secretory and absorptive sites. Patients with CKD have impaired Mg reabsorption due to tubular damage from diseases such as obstructive uropathy, tubulointerstitial diseases, renal transplantation, tubular dysfunction caused by electrolyte disorders (prolonged hypokalemia) or mineral disorders (hypercalcemia), or inherited disorders such as Bartter's or Gitelman's syndromes. Certain drugs are known to cause renal Mg wasting, for example, aminoglycosides and amphotericin, especially when used in prolonged courses of therapy or in the presence of malignancies. Antineoplastic agents such as cisplatin are also associated with renal Mg wasting as are some immunosuppressive agents such as cyclosporine (Lewis, 2009).

3.1.5.1 Hypomagnesemia and Hypermagnesemia

Hypomagnesemia symptoms and signs are similar to those of many disorders: anorexia, vomiting, lethargy, profound weakness, spontaneous carpopedal spasm, muscle fasiculations, and tremor. Carpopedal spasm in hypomagnesemia is generally seen when the patient has concomitant hypocalcemia and hypokalemia. Generalized tonic-clonic seizures can be seen in young children (Lewis, 2009). Mg concentrations < 1.0 mEq/L should be treated and intravenous Mg considered. Magnesium can be replaced orally or intravenously. Unfortunately, the oral intake of high Mg-containing medications can result in diarrhea caused by the Mg load. Intravenous Mg is well tolerated but can result in hypermagnesemia, especially when there is any degree of CKD. If intravenous Mg is given, it must be closely monitored. Mg salts should, in general, be avoided in patients with CKD, especially in CKD Stages 3–5. However, magnesium carbonate has been used as a phosphate-binding agent, with 4% of the studied population developing diarrhea and 4% developing hypermagnesemia (Tzanakis et al., 2008). Hypermagnesemia is characterized by muscle weakness, respiratory depression, and cardiac dysrhythmias, especially Toursade de Pointes. Although hypermagnesemia is defined as Mg > 2.1 mEq/L, these signs are not generally seen unless the Mg is 2×–3× normal. Intravenous calcium and volume expansion with NaCl solution with a loop diuretic are treatments that can be used for severe or serious hypermagnesemia. In the presence of AKI, CKD, or impaired urine output, hemodialysis (HD) may be required (Lewis, 2009).

3.1.5.2 Recommendations

Since most adult patients have multiple medical and surgical disorders and take multiple medications, serum Mg should be measured in any adult patient admitted to the hospital and should be routinely followed in the outpatient clinic in patients who have diseases or who take medications known to be associated with hypomagnesemia. Serum Mg should also be measured in all patients with CKD Stages 3–5 since these patients may take many nonprescription drugs and supplements, and nonrenal physicians sometime prescribe Mg-containing medications. Disorders of Mg should be considered in patients who have altered or inadequate food intake, impaired absorption, renal or GI losses, disorders associated with intercompartmental shifts, and in all patients who present or develop hypokalemia.

Malnutrition is seen in many clinical circumstances and intracellular Mg deficiency must be considered. Examples include patients with alcoholism; the homeless; the elderly; patients taking multiple drugs; and patients with anorexia, severe depression, organic brain syndrome, decreased mobility, inadequate resources to obtain or prepare foods, and unbalanced or nutritionally deficient diets. Malnutrition is also caused by any disorder that interferes with intake, swallowing, digestion, absorption, or processing and metabolism. Losses may occur in diarrheal illnesses and in renal losses. Patients who have marginal total body Mg stores are at particular risk of developing severe Mg deficiency when stressed by catabolic illnesses. Starved or malnourished patients when fed may develop the refeeding syndrome and severe Mg deficiency can be seen. Mg-shifting occurs in diabetes mellitus, the refeeding syndrome, correction of acidosis, administration of sympathomimetic amines, the hungry bone syndrome following parathyroidectomy, and in massive blood transfusion. Renal Mg wasting can be caused by drugs such as aminoglycosides, amphotericin, and cisplatin as well as being caused by Bartter's or Gitelman's syndromes (Swaminathan, 2003).

Hypermagnesemia is seen in patients with AKI or CKD who have been given or who have ingested Mg-containing medications. It can also be seen in patients who have been given large intravenous doses of Mg. Treatment involves the use of intravenous calcium, NaCl volume expansion and loop diuretics, or emergency HD.

3.2 TRACE ELEMENTS INTRODUCTION

Trace elements (TE) are a subset of micronutrients that are essential for the optimal functioning of metabolic pathways and that are found in minute quantities in humans, such as zinc (Zn), selenium, (Se), manganese (Mn), chromium (Cr), cadmium (Cd), fluoride (F), iodine (I), molybdenum (Mo), arsenic (As), aluminum (Al), lithium (Li), tin (Sn), lead (Pb), and mercury (Hg). Some of these elements such as Al, Li, and Pb accumulate in the body as glomerular filtration rate (GFR) falls, leading to increased tissue burdens that cause disease. Even with a normal GFR, Li and Pb can accumulate in persons exposed to high amounts, such as those living close to a lead smelter. Other elements, such as As and Hg, are toxic and lead to serious and often fatal disorders. The importance of Mo in the activity of xanthine oxidase, sulfite oxidase, and aldehyde oxidase is known, but deficiency is exceedingly rare and toxicity nearly nonexistent (Johnson, 2008c). Although there are no data on the use of weight-reduction diets in patients with CKD or ESRD, it is concerning that a recent publication has shown that each of four popular weight-loss diets was insufficient in the minimum Reference Daily Intake (RDI) for 27 micronutrients. Six micronutrients were consistently low in all diets: vitamin B7, vitamin D, vitamin E, Cr, I, and Mo (Calton, 2010). The impact of using these diets for weight loss in obese adults with CKD should cause concern and clinicians should monitor the use of these diets closely. In this chapter, we will focus on the metabolism of Zn, Se, Cu, F, Cr, and Al.

3.2.1 Zinc

3.2.1.1 Zinc Metabolism

Zinc (Zn) is an essential TE that is involved in numerous aspects of cellular metabolism. Zn supports normal growth and development, is active in immune function, protein synthesis, and wound healing (Fabris and Mocchegiani, 1995; Heyneman, 1996; Institute of Medicine, 2001; Maret and Sandstead, 2006; Prasad, 1995; Simmer and Thompson, 1985; Solomons, 1998). Zn is also required for proper sense of taste and smell (Prasad et al., 1997). Zn is necessary for the proper transcriptional control of specific genes associated with cellular proliferation and differentiation as well as intracellular signaling (Cousins, 1996). Zn is primarily found in teeth, hair, skin, bones, liver, muscles, leucocytes, and the testes, and over 80% of blood Zn is found in carbonic anhydrase, essential in acid–base balance (Linder, 1991).

A daily intake of Zn is required to maintain a steady state because the body has no specialized Zn storage system. Whole grains and milk products are good sources of Zn, and many ready-to-eat breakfast cereals are fortified with Zn. Oysters, red meat, and poultry are excellent sources of Zn, as are baked beans, chickpeas, and nuts (such as cashews and almonds) (Office of Dietary Supplements, 2009). Phytates (whole-grain breads, cereals, legumes, primarily) bind Zn and inhibit its absorption (Sandstrom, 1997; Solomons, 1998; Wise, 1995). Thus, the bioavailability of Zn from grains and plant foods is lower than that from animal foods, although many grain- and plant-based foods are still good sources of Zn.

Zn deficiency in the United States is seen only when there is insufficient intake, increased loss, or an increased requirement (Hambidge, 1989; Institute of Medicine, 2001; King and Cousins, 2005; Prasad, 1996). Insufficient intake is seen in those with marginal diets such as the elderly, the homeless, or those with alcoholism (Institute of Medicine, 2001; Menzano and Carlen, 1994; Navarro et al., 1994). Vegetarians are at particular risk of inadequate Zn intake not only because meat is higher in Zn than nonmeat foods but also because the vegetarian diet is high in legume and grain intake. Vegetarians can overcome some of the phytate binding by soaking or dialyzing the grains or legumes in water for several hours prior to intake and by using grains in leavened products since the leavening process breaks down phytates (American Dietetic Association, Dietitians of Canada, 2003; Hunt, 2003). Other persons at risk of Zn deficiency include those with GI diseases such as malabsorption syndromes, inflammatory bowel disease, and short bowel syndromes in which there is an increased GI loss, or renal wasting of Zn such as patients with AKI or CKD and persons who may have increased requirements for Zn (Hambidge, 1989; Solomons, 1998; Valberg et al., 1986). Decreased Zn can also be seen in patients with chronic liver disease, CKD, diabetes mellitus, sickle cell disease, in women who are pregnant or lactating, and in older infants who are exclusively breast-fed (Caulfield et al., 1998; Krebs, 1998; Solomons, 1998).

Symptoms of Zn deficiency include anosmia, impaired taste, impotence, gonadal dysfunction, impaired wound healing, depression and mood lability, impaired cell-mediated immunity, and skin lesions (parakeratosis) (Cousins, 1996; Linder, 1991). Acrodermatitis enteropathica, an autosomal recessive disorder characterized by an impairment of Zn absorption, leads to diarrhea, dermatitis (especially perioral and perianal), poor growth, and impaired immune function (Prasad, 1985). It is readily treated with Zn supplementation that has to be continued indefinitely.

Zn deficiency has been associated with impotence (testicular atrophy), growth retardation, immune system dysfunction, dysgeusia, anorexia, and anosmia in CKD patients (Antoniou et al., 1997; Mahajan et al., 1982a, 1989). Patients on maintenance HD have been found to be in negative Zn balance secondary to augmented fecal Zn excretion. It is not clear whether decreased secretion or enhanced secretion by the GI tract or both contribute to the negative balance (Mahajan et al., 1982). Patients on HD and continuous ambulatory peritoneal dialysis have been found to have Zn levels that were normal or low (Danielson et al., 1986; Hosokawa et al., 1990a, 1990b; Hosokawa and Yoshida, 1993, 1995; Lin et al., 1996; Muirhead et al., 1986; Richard et al., 1991; Van Renterghem et al., 1992; Wallaeys et al., 1986). The majority of Zn in a human is in erythrocytes, and correction of anemia and a decrease in the protein catabolic rate result in an increase in serum Zn levels (Hosokawa and Yoshida, 1993, 1995). Low Zn concentrations are more likely to be seen in CKD patients treated conservatively prior to the initiation of dialysis. The conservative diet is lower in protein and dairy products and legumes, and whole grains are limited. In CKD Stage 4 and 5, patients may have anorexia due to medications, the effects of CKD, and underlying and acute illnesses. Vascular and peritoneal access surgeries increase catabolism, and increased Zn is needed for wound healing. Intercurrent infections are frequent, and the majority of patients have diabetes mellitus or long-standing hypertension with a high incidence of vascular disease. Interventions to treat peripheral vascular, cardiovascular, and cerebrovascular disease are frequent. Hospitalizations are common, and oral intake is generally depressed in the hospitalized patient who may have been put on a restricted diet or have meals withheld for testing or in preparation for surgery. The typical dialysis patient is older (the average age of a dialysis patient is >62 years) and therefore more comorbid diseases are present, many of which can be associated with decreased Zn intake or absorption, increased loss, or increased need for wound healing or response to infections. A recent meta-analysis has demonstrated that patients on HD have lower levels of Zn compared to the general population (Tonelli et al., 2009).

In hypogeusic patients, Zn supplementation has been found to increase serum and erythrocyte Zn levels with either no change or an improvement in taste (Eggert et al., 1982; Watson et al., 1983). Improved nerve conduction velocity, increased serum testosterone and sperm counts, improved libido and potency, and increased frequency of intercourse, as well as a fall in serum luteinizing hormone and follicle-stimulating hormone have been associated with Zn supplementation (Mahajan et al., 1982b). However, other studies have not corroborated these findings (Antoniou et al., 1997; Joven et al., 1985; Rodger et al., 1989).

Uremic patients with low Zn levels have depressed immune function and impaired granulocyte motility (Antoniou and Shalhoub, 1985; Briggs et al., 1982; Kouw et al., 1991; Prasad and McDonald, 1982). Zn has also been shown to stimulate the production of IL-1, IL-1 beta, tumor necrosis factor, and calcitriol function (Briggs et al., 1982). It is possible that Zn supplementation might improve or restore impaired cell-mediated immunity and lymphocyte function (Antoniou and Shalhoub, 1985; Grekas et al., 1985). Normalization of Zn levels in dialyzed patients has shown increases in the helper/suppressor T-cell ratio and in tetanus antibody titers, as well as increased delayed hypersensitivity (Brodersen et al., 1994; Holtkamp et al., 1991). However, Zn supplementation has not been shown to influence immunoglobulin or complement levels; nor is there an increase in anti-HBs antibodies in response to revaccination. Influenza antibody response to vaccination is not enhanced by Zn supplementation (Brodersen et al., 1994; Grekas et al., 1992; Kouw et al., 1991; Migneco et al., 1990).

3.2.1.2 Recommendations

Patients with CKD who are on restricted diets or being treated with conservative therapy should have their Zn levels determined on whole blood samples if there is a concern that malnourishment is present or may develop. Whole-blood Zn should be measured in patients with CKD with GI diseases that affect food intake or proper absorption lasting more than 1–2 weeks. If the patient is already malnourished, Zn levels should be measured. If the Zn level is low, short-term Zn supplementation should be considered until the patient has returned to an acceptable and stable clinical status.

Zn levels should be measured in patients on dialysis who develop malnutrition or anorexia, and if the disorder is prolonged over 1–2 weeks, Zn supplementation should be considered. Patients who are malnourished when they begin dialysis should have their Zn measured if the malnutrition does not improve after 1 month of adequate dialysis. Patients with CKD who have dysgeusia that is not due to medications, inadequate dialysis, or readily reversible illness (e.g., sinusitis) should have their Zn checked, and they should be treated for 4–6 weeks to determine if there is a clinical response. Zn supplementation should be considered in malnourished patients with CKD or on dialysis who are hospitalized, especially if they have a prolonged illness that interferes with food intake or absorption or if the patient's catabolic rate is high. Hospitalized patients with CKD or ESRD who are receiving total parenteral nutrition (TPN) or peripheral parenteral nutrition (PPN) should have TE added to the TPN; however, the amount needed is unknown. It is generally thought that TE solution should be given 2–3 times weekly. It may be better to also follow the whole blood Zn level and to add supplemental Zn to the TPN or PPN solution. TE solution for TPN can also be used to provide TE to patients receiving enteral feedings who are TE deficient.

3.2.2 Selenium

3.2.2.1 Selenium Metabolism

Selenium (Se) in the diet comes from two Se-containing amino acids: selenocysteine and selenomethionine (Burk and Levander, 1999). Dietary sources of these two amino acids are various seafoods, kidney, liver, and meat. Grains may also contain appreciable amounts of Se, although this depends on the Se content of the soil (10th Edition of the RDAs, 1989b). Dietary Se is highly bioavailable. Se is active in glutathione peroxidase, which metabolizes hydroperoxides formed from polyunsaturated fatty acids, and it is also active in enzymes that deiodinate thyroid hormones (Johnson, 2008d).

The methionine absorptive pathways in the small intestines are responsible for Se absorption (Burk and Levander, 1999) Inorganic Se (dietary supplements) is passively absorbed in the duodenum, and Se absorption appears to be unregulated (Thomas and Robinson, 1993). There is no storage pool for Se; however, the incorporation of Se-methionine into amino acids serves the same purpose. Se-cysteine is absorbed directly from foodstuffs and is also metabolized from Se-methionine (Thomas and Robinson, 1993). It can also be synthesized from Se replacement of oxygen residue on serine while serine is bound to a specific tRNA (Burk and Levander, 1996). Se is released when Se-cysteine and Se-methionine are catabolized. Se is excreted in the urine.

The typical Se intake in the United States is 100–250 mcg/d; whereas in Finland and New Zealand, it is 30–50 mcg/d. Despite this broad range of intake, Se deficiency is rare (Johnson, 2008d). Muscle weakness and cardiomyopathy, impaired immune function, macrocytosis, and white nail beds are associated with and seen in Se deficiency (Hawkes et al., 1996; Rayman, 2000). In certain areas of China, where Se intake can be as low as 10 mcg/d, an endemic cardiomyopathy that affects children and women of childbearing age can been seen, which improves with Se supplementation. Se supplementation can prevent Keshan Disease (cardiomyopathy caused by Se deficiency) (Johnson, 2008d). High intakes of Se can be toxic, causing hair loss, the formation of abnormal fingernails and toenails, dermatitis, peripheral neuropathy, nausea, diarrhea, fatigue, irritability, or halitosis (imparting a garlic odor to the breath). However, there is no good definition of toxic Se blood levels (Johnson, 2008d).

Se levels are lower in HD patients than in the general population (Tonelli et al., 2009). Plasma Se concentrations and erythrocyte glutathione peroxidase activity are strongly correlated, and glutathione peroxidase activity increases with Se supplementation (Koenig et al., 1997; Saint-Georges et al., 1989). There is greater decrease in serum and platelet Se in dialyzed patients with CVD than in those without (Girelli et al., 1993). However, Se supplementation in patients with low Se concentrations did not improve echocardiographical parameters of left ventricular function or morphology (Maher et al., 1987). Low Se levels and abnormal thyroid function abnormalities are frequently seen in dialyzed patients (Napolitano et al., 1996). Uremic patients who received selenium supplementation demonstrated increased T-cell response to phytohemagglutinin and increased delayed-type hypersensitivity (Bonomini et al., 1995).

3.2.2.2 Recommendations

The manifestations of Se deficiency mimic the findings in patients with advanced CKD and patients with ESRD who are receiving dialysis therapy. It is impossible to distinguish between disorders caused by CKD or other comorbid conditions and those potentially caused by Se. Since Se deficiency syndromes do not occur in the United States in patients who have access to food, they should not be considered unless the patient has a reason to have inadequate intake of food or normal absorption of food. Since we do not know how long it takes for Se-cysteine and Se-methionine stores to become depleted, we do not know how long it takes to become Se deficient in the face of inadequate Se intake. It seems reasonable to follow the Clinical Guidelines of the American Society for Parenteral and Enteral Nutrition: Nutritional Support in Adult Acute and Chronic Renal Failure (ASPEN, 2011). Se intoxication is extremely rare and should only be considered in patients who are receiving Se supplementation.

3.2.3 Copper

3.2.3.1 Metabolism

Virtually all copper (Cu) in the human is bound to body proteins, since free or unbound Cu is highly toxic. Cu metabolism is highly controlled both by genetic mechanisms that regulate the incorporation of Cu into apoproteins and by processes that prevent toxic Cu accumulation. As long as the genetic mechanisms that control Cu metabolism are normal, Cu deficiency rarely occurs. It is seen in severe, long-standing Kwashiorkor; persistent infantile diarrhea, typically in a child whose diet is limited to milk; severe malabsorption syndromes, and excessive Zn intake (Johnson, 2008b).

Cu is abundant in vegetable products, grains, legumes, seeds, and meat, in that order. Of all foods, liver contains the highest concentration of Cu (Johnson and Kays, 1990). After being absorbed in the proximal small intestine, Cu is bound to albumin and amino acids. Transcuprin, a specific Cu transporter may be involved. The majority of the Cu is taken up by the liver on the first pass. Once in the liver, Cu is incorporated into ceruloplasmin, a protein that acts as the transfer agent for moving Cu from the liver to the peripheral tissues. Ceruloplasmin also plays a role in Fe metabolism, serving as a plasma ferroxidase. Methionone may act as a Cu storage protein (Chan and Rennert, 1980; Harris, 1995). All Cu excretion occurs through the GI tract, with bile excretion accounting for half. The exception is the loss of ceruloplasmin in the urine in nephritic syndrome, causing a decrease in serum Cu levels (Stec et al., 1990).

Biological roles for Cu include incorporation into several important Cu-containing enzymes including Zn–Cu superoxide dismutase (antioxidant defense), dopamine mono-oxygenase (neurotransmitter synthesis), lysyl oxidase (collagen cross-linking, bone formation), ceruloplasmin (Cu transport and ferroxidase), cytochrome c oxidase (electron transport), factor V (hemostasis), and tyrosinase (melatonin production) (Danks, 1988; Lutsenko, 2010).

Cu deficiency is unusual in the absence of genetic disorders and is mostly seen in premature babies receiving milk formulas, patients with chronic diarrhea (or malabsorption syndromes), gastrectomy, Roux-en-Y gastric bypass surgery, patients receiving chronic parenteral nutrition without TE supplementation, patients on prolonged oral Zn supplementation or patients who have ingested Zn-containing coin(s) (Zn and Cu are competitively absorbed in the jejunum), and patients on chronic peritoneal dialysis. Cu deficiency is marked by skin depigmentation, fragile and kinky hair, weakness, edema, hepatosplenomegaly, osteoporosis, and neurological abnormalities such as ataxia, neuropathy, and cognitive defects that closely mimic vitamin B12 deficiency (Fleming, 1989; Griffith et al., 2009; Juhasz-Pocsine et al., 2007; Kumar et al., 2004; Shaw, 1992; Tan et al., 2006). Menkes disease is a congenital x-linked genetic disorder that is caused by a mutation in the intestinal transport protein for Cu. The severe Cu deficiency leads to profound neurological deterioration and death in early childhood. The involved gene is closely linked to the gene responsible for Wilson's disease (Danks, 1988).

Wilson's disease is an autosomal recessive disorder characterized by excessive Cu accumulation. It is caused by a mutation in a Cu-ATPase enzyme that is closely related to the gene defect in Menkes disease. Many tissues are involved in Cu overload deposition leading to cardiac dysfunction (congestive heart failure, rhythm disturbances), hepatic cirrhosis, diabetes mellitus, renal failure, and malignancies (Harris, 2000; Linder, 1996). Wilson's disease is treated with a low-Cu diet and the use of a Cu chelating agent. Oral Zn may be used early in the course of the disease since it is a competitor ofGI absorption.

Cu levels (plasma and serum) have been reported to be normal to high in patients with renal failure, but levels have been reported to be low in patients treated with HD or PD (Borner et al., 1984; Hasanoğlu et al., 1994; Hosokawa et al., 1985; Picchota et al., 1983; Thomson et al., 1983). The increased Cu found in some patients is not accompanied by an increase in plasma ceruloplasmin. The cause of the delinking of this relationship is unknown (Sondheimer et al., 1988). Hemo- and peritoneal dialysates do not represent sources of Cu. However, it is important that the plumbing within the water pathway leading to the water preparation area for hemodialysate does not have any copper piping. This is an especially important consideration when reviewing the home situations for patients who will be hemodialyzed at home using their tap water to generate dialysate in a proportioning dialysis system. This is of much less concern now because home HD machines that have a premixed dialysis solution are available. Cu contamination of water supplies in devastated areas would be unlikely to cause Cu overload and toxicity as long as the untreated water is used for only 2–3 dialysis sessions or a dialysis sorbent system is used.

3.2.3.2 Recommendations

It is highly unlikely that Cu deficiency will be seen in the United States. The clinical scenario in which Cu deficiency is likely to be seen is severe malnutrition with little to no intake of food or severe malabsorption. Milk-fed babies are at risk, as are patients with a previous gastrectomy or gastric bypass surgery with a Roux-en-Y diversion, and patients on long-term oral Zn supplementation. Since Cu deficiency mimics vitamin B12 deficiency, it should be considered when vitamin B12 deficiency is suspected. At-risk populations also include the homeless, alcoholics and drug addicts, and children or psychiatrically disturbed patients who swallow Zn-containing objects such as coins. Serum Cu levels should be measured; however, the utility of ceruloplasmin concentrations in diagnosing Cu deficiency in patients with CKD is unknown. Cu can be administered by increasing the patient's dietary intake of Cu-containing foods or by the oral or parenteral use of TE solutions.

3.2.4 Fluoride

3.2.4.1 Metabolism

Fluoride (F) is a ubiquitous mineral in the earth's crust, but its concentration in natural water supplies is quite variable. It is known to be important in preventing dental caries and has been added to the drinking water in most public water supplies in the United States for many years. It is a beneficial TE rather than an essential TE (10th Edition of the RDAs, 1989a). Other important sources of F are black tea, seafood with edible bones or shells (sardines, herring, soft-shell crabs), supplements, and fluoridated toothpaste and mouthwash. Dietary F is rapidly absorbed in the stomach and small intestines. Up to one-third of ingested F is deposited in calcified tissue; the rest is excreted by the kidney (Stamp, 1993). Fluoride displaces hydroxyapatite and produces fluorapatite or fluorhydroxyapatite. Over 99% of the total body F is contained within bones. F supplementation causes an increase in bone density, but there is no corresponding decrease in fractures; nonvertebral fractures may actually increase (Haguenauer et al., 2000).

Other than an increase in dental caries, there is no known disease caused by F deficiency. Fluoride toxicity is caused by ingestion of high amounts of F by water, use of F-containing medicaments (toothpaste, especially flavored toothpastes in children; F-containing mouthwash), F supplements, exposure to fluorine-containing insecticides, or in industrial exposure, for example, to hydrofluoric acid (HF) acid (Augenstein et al., 1991). Nonspecific GI complaints are the hallmark of acute fluoride toxicity, which may lead to kidney and cardiac failure, coma, and death. Exposure to small amounts of F in children (F-containing mouthwash or toothpaste ingestion) can cause acute F toxicity (Augenstein et al., 1991).

Chronic toxicity is generally caused by high F concentrations in drinking water and the use of F supplements or F-containing products such as mouthwash or pica for toothpaste in adults. Dental fluorosis, a cosmetic disorder with mottled teeth is caused by high-F intake. In more severe instances, there may be skeletal fluorosis, a condition in which radiologically, bone appears dense but is brittle and prone to fracture, and ligaments can calcify, leading to joint immobility (Stamp, 1993). Other than fluorosis, it is not evident that chronic F intoxication is seen more often in CKD patients compared to normal patients. Acute fluoride poisoning occurs in industrial accidents and in intentional overdoses. Acute dialysis may be effective in patients who receive medical attention (Bjornhagen et al., 2003). Bottled water that is produced by a process of reverse osmosis and replenished with minerals is low in F. Water used for the preparation of dialysate is treated by reverse osmosis, and the F content is well within Association for Advancement of Medical Instrumentation (AAMI) standards (<0.02 mg/L). It is unlikely that F toxicity would be seen in an adult CKD or ESRD population. The possibility of F toxicity in the pediatric population is always present.

3.2.5 Chromium

3.2.5.1 Metabolism

Less than 3% of ingested chromium (Cr) is absorbed, and plasma levels are therefore quite low (0.05–0.50 mcg/L) (Johnson, 2008a). Because Cr potentiates insulin activity, Cr deficiency has been associated with glucose intolerance. Low plasma Cr levels have been described in patients with glucose intolerance, diabetes mellitus, hypercholesterolemia, and in aged persons (Linder, 1991). Cr deficiency has also been described in patients receiving long-term TPN who exhibited weight loss, ataxia, and peripheral neuropathy; most responded when trivalent Cr was administered (Johnson, 2008a). Skin irritation occurs with high-dose trivalent Cr therapy, but lower doses are well tolerated. Industrial exposure to hexavalent Cr (CrO_3) is associated with lung and skin irritation, GI disturbances, nasal perforation, and lung cancer (Johnson, 2008a).

Dialyzed patients and renal transplant patients have increased whole-blood and serum Cr levels (Danielson et al., 1986; Granadillo et al., 1994; Wallaeys et al., 1986). Chromium-rich dialysate may be the source of the Cr since the Cr levels were increased in the dialyzed patients (Thomson et al., 1983). There is no known Cr toxicity in CKD or ESRD patients unless they have significant industrial exposure.

3.2.6 Aluminum

3.2.6.1 Metabolism

Aluminum (Al) is the most ubiquitous and abundant metal. It is found in natural waters, plants, animals, and the earth's crust (Jiang et al., 2008; Verstraeten et al., 2008). Al is trivalent and highly reactive and is only found bound with other elements. The amount of Al in the diet is exceedingly small and of no consequence unless there is renal impairment. Al is used in water purification systems, which remove organic compounds that can bind free Al, thereby increasing the amount of free Al in the water supply. Again, with normal renal function, this is of no consequence. Given the usual water intake in humans of 1–4 + L/d depending upon the climate, Al intoxication from the oral intake of treated municipal water does not occur. It is a totally different matter when a patient is hemodialyzed where the patient may be exposed to 270–720 L of water as dialysate per week. Clearly, dialysis water supplies must be Al-free.

Al does not appear to be a required TE for normal physiological functioning. Because of its atomic weight and electrical charge, it is a competitive inhibitor of several essential minerals (calcium, magnesium, and iron). Over 95% of ingested Al is bound to transferrin and albumin in the intravascular space. It is then eliminated through the kidneys. Al will only accumulate in the human when there is increased oral or intravenous intake of Al in patients with AKI, CKD, or ESRD. Association for Advancement of Medical Instrumentation (AAMI) (Brown et al., 2008; Mayor et al., 1981).

Patients with an impaired GFR are at risk of Al intoxication if they are treated with Al salts [$Al(OH)_3$] used as phosphate-binding agents in CKD, intravenously through contaminated dialysate or TPN, or through bladder irrigation with Al-containing solution. Lactate, citrate, and ascorbate all increase Al absorption from the GI tract. These compounds should not be taken by patients who are receiving oral aluminum products. The effects of Al cookware and Al-containing antiperspirants on Al levels in patients with an impaired GFR are not known. Excess Al is deposited in bone, brain, muscle, heart, liver, and spleen. Up to this time, no biological function has been attributed to this metal. More importantly, Al accumulation in the tissues and organs results in dysfunction and toxicity.

Acute Al intoxication is rare. The original reports described dialysis patients whose dialysate was made with untreated water who developed an osteomalacic form of renal osteodystrophy. This improved when the dialysate was prepared with deionized water (Ward et al., 1978). The dominant feature of this bone disease was a defect in mineralization of bone and excessive deposits of aluminum at the osteoid mineralization front where calcium should have been deposited. A dialysis encephalopathy was described that was thought to be due to Al deposition in the brain, and high Al levels were noted in patients receiving dialysis with high Al-containing dialysate (Alfrey et al., 1976).

The elimination half-life of Al in the brain is 7 years, which can lead to cumulative damage. Al has been suggested as an agent in the development of Alzheimer's disease and possibly autism spectrum disorders (Blaylock and Strunecka, 2009; Ferreira et al., 2008). Al acts as an excitotoxin, which can exacerbate a clinical disorder by increasing cell excitation and oxidative stress and by priming microglial cells to proliferate (Bihaqi Blaylock and Strunecka, 2009; Mailloux et al., 2009). Excitotoxicity describes the process of neuron damage and death that is caused by overactive receptors such as the N-methyl D-aspartate (NMDA) and α-amino-3-hydroxy-5-methyl-4-isoxazole propionic acid (AMPA) receptors for glutamate, an excitatory neurotransmitter. Excitotoxins bind to these receptors and in the presence of high intracellular glutamate allow high levels of calcium to enter the cell. This activates several enzymes that cause cell damage and death, including phospholipases, proteases, and endonucleases (Science Daily, 2011). Brain Al can cause these changes to occur (Blaylock, 2009). Al has a direct toxic effect on hematopoiesis and can cause a microcytic anemia very similar to that found in patients suffering from lead intoxication. Al intoxication results in decreased heme synthesis and may be related to increased hemolysis although the role of PTH as a cause of decreased RBC survival in ESRD patients is unclear (Foulks et al., 1989; Wu et al., 1998). Al also directly interferes with iron absorption and iron transport in addition to competitively replacing iron binding to transferrin (Drüeke et al., 1986). Anemia exacerbated by Al overload was commonly seen into the 1980s when toxic Al-containing phosphate-binding agents were gradually replaced by calcium-containing binding agents such as calcium carbonate, calcium acetate, and calcium lactate.

Aluminum may cause anemia through decreased heme synthesis, decreased globulin synthesis, and increased hemolysis. Aluminum may also have a direct effect on iron metabolism: it influences absorption of iron via the intestine; it hinders iron's transport in the serum; and it displaces iron's binding to transferrin. Patients with anemia from Al toxicity often have increased reticulocyte counts, decreased mean corpuscular volume, and mean corpuscular hemoglobin (Bernardo et al., 2010).

Considering the increasing prevalence of CKD in our society, it behooves us to review what is known about Al absorption from the diet and from the use of Al cookware and packaging. The best review is by Fimreite et al. (1997), who showed that cooking in an aluminum container, especially if the food being cooked was acidic, caused a significant increase in the Al content of the food. This was also seen in brewed tea. Significant Al accumulation has also been found in coffee brewed and reheated in aluminum percolators (Lione et al., 1984). The content of Al in various liquids boiled in an Al pot increased 10–945-fold depending upon the liquid (the lowest was coffee; the highest, 2% acetic acid). The Al content of various beverages ranged from 53 mcg/L for apple juice in an aluminum-foil-lined carton to 1800 mcg/L in tea with lemon. Coca-Cola™ had an Al concentration of 70 mcg/L (Nagy and Jobst, 1994). Clearly, dietary Al sources can present a large amount of Al to the GI tract. This poses no problem to those with normal kidney function but could be of consequence to those with advanced CKD who live for a long time. When CKD patients were studied while using aluminum kitchen utensils compared to the use of stainless steel kitchen utensils, serum aluminum levels and urinary excretion of aluminum were significantly higher among the patients using aluminum utensils. This suggests that patients with CKD should be concerned about the long-term use of aluminum cooking utensils (Lin et al., 1997).

3.2.6.2 Recommendations

At this time, Al-containing phosphate-binding agents should not be used for the chronic long-term management of hyperphosphatemia and secondary hyperparathyroidism. Many safer agents, such as calcium carbonate, calcium acetate, sevelamer, lanthanum, and others, are available. Rarely, $Al(OH)_3$ may be used as a phosphate-binding agent for a period not to exceed a week. This may come into play when the CKD or ESRD patient has extremely high phosphate levels (>15) and/or a very elevated CaXP product (>100). Al-salts should never be used in patients who are receiving citrate. Patients who have CKD and are presumed to have longevity should probably be cautioned about extensive use of Al-containing cookware and of large intake of beverages in Al-containing cans.

3.3 CONCLUSION

TE roles and disorders in CKD and ESRD patients are still poorly understood. Many of the methodological publications appeared at a time when dialysis adequacy was poorly understood and medical technologies were less advanced than they are today. We still have insufficient information about many TEs. The metabolism of even those TE that are known to be necessary such as Mo has not been fully explored in non-CKD patients, let alone in CKD and ESRD patients. Zn supplementation may be of use in clinical circumstances, but one should be careful about giving Zn to potential renal transplant patients because of the risk of stimulating a rejection episode, although the degree of this risk during our modern era of excellent antirejection drugs is unknown. Cu deficiency does occur but is rare, as is Cr deficiency. Se deficiency is likely unusual as well. Common to TE disorders are malnutrition, malabsorption syndromes, severe or chronic diarrhea, impaired GI transport, increased need due to illness, and genetic disorders. The clinical presentations of many of these deficiencies are very similar to the uremic state and to common complaints seen in CKD and ESRD patients, and it is difficult to separate them. As in most clinical situations, the wise clinician observes, correlates, and keeps an open mind.

REFERENCES

Alfrey, A., LeGendre, G., Kaehny, W. 1976. The dialysis encephalopathy syndrome. Possible aluminum intoxication. *N Engl J Med.* 294(4):184–188.
American Dietetic Association, Dietitians of Canada. 2003. Position of the American Dietetic Association and Dietitians of Canada: Vegetarian diets. *J Am Diet Assoc.* 103:748–765.
Antoniou, L. and Shalhoub, R. 1985. Zinc-induced enhancement of lymphocyte function and viability in chronic uremia. *Nephron* 40:14–21.
Antoniou, L., Sudhakar, T., Shalhoub, R., et al. 1997. Reversal of uraemic impotence by zinc. *Lancet* 350:895–898.
Augenstein, W., Spoerke, D., Kulig, K., et al. 1991. Fluoride ingestion in children: A review of 87 cases. *Pediatrics* 88(5):907–912.
Bernardo, J., Edwards, M., Barnett, B. 2010. Toxicity, Aluminum. http://emedicine.medscape.com/article/165315-overview
Bihaqi, S., Sharma, M., Singh, A., et al. 2009. Neuroprotective role of Convolvulus pluricaulis on aluminum induced neurotoxicity in rat brain. *J Ethnopharmacol.* 124(3):409–415.
Bjornhagen, V., Hojer, J., Karlson-Stiber, C., et al. 2003. Hydrofluoric acid-induced burns and life-threatening systemic poisoning-favorable outcome after hemodialysis. *J Toxicol Clin Toxicol.* 41(6):855–860.
Blaylock, R. 2009. A possible central mechanism in autism spectrum disorders, Part 3: The role of excitotoxin food additives and the synergistic effects of other environmental toxins. *Altern Ther Health Med.* 15(2):56–60.
Blaylock, R. and Strunecka, A. 2009. Immune-glutamatergic dysfunction as a central mechanism of the autism spectrum disorders. *Curr Med Chem.* 16(2):157–170.
Boaz, M. and Smetana, S. 1996. Regression equation predicts dietary phosphorus intake from estimate of dietary protein intake. *J Am Diet Assoc.* 96:1268–1270.
Bonomini, M., Forster, S., De Risio, F., et al. 1995. Effects of selenium supplementation on immune parameters in chronic uraemic patients on haemodialysis. *Nephrol Dial Transplant.* 10:1654–1661.
Borner, H., Mehnert, E., Falkenhagen, D., et al. 1984. Behavior of copper and manganese in serum in hemodialysis. *Urol Nephrol.* 77:483–487.
Briggs, W., Pedersen, M., Mahajan, S., et al. 1982. Lymphocyte and -granulocyte function in zinc-treated and zinc-deficient hemodialysis patients. *Kidney Int.* 21:827–832.
Brodersen, H., Holtkamp, W., Larbig, D. 1994. Zinc supplementation and cellular and humoral immune function in chronic haemodialysis patients. *Nephrol Dial Transplant.* 9:736–737.
Brown, R., Morgan, L., Bhattacharya, S., et al. 2008. Potential aluminum exposure from parenteral nutrition in patients with acute kidney injury. *Ann Pharmacother.* 42(10):1410–1415.
Burk, R.F, and O.A. Levander. 1999. Selenium. In M. Shils, J. Olson, M. Shike, and A. C. Ross, eds., Modern Nutrition in Health and Disease, 9th Edition. Baltimore, MD: Williams & Wilkins, 265–276.
Calton, J. 2010. Prevalence of micronutrient deficiency in popular diet plans. *J Int Soc Sports Nutr.* 7:24. http://www.ncbi.nlm.nih.gov/pubmed/20537171
Caulfield, L., Zavaleta, N., Shankar, A., et al. 1998. Potential contribution of maternal zinc supplementation during pregnancy to maternal and child survival. *Am J Clin Nutr.* 68(2 Suppl):499S–508S.
Chan, W. and Rennert, O. 1980. The role of copper in iron metabolism. *Ann Clin Lab Sci.* 10:338–344.
Charlton, K., Steyn, K., Levitt, N., et al. 2007. Development and validation of a short questionnaire to assess sodium intake. *Public Health Nutr.* 11(1):83–94.
Cousins, R. 1996. Zinc. In Zioegler, E. and Filer, I., eds. *Present Knowledge in Nutrition,* 7th ed. Washington: ILSI Press, 293–306.
Dai, L., Ritchio, G., Kerstan, D., et al. 2001. Magnesium transport in the renal distal convoluted tubule. *Physiol Rev.* 81:51–84.
Danielson, B., Fellstrom, B., Nilsson, P., et al. 1986. Trace element levels in patients with renal failure and after transplantation. *Acta Pharmacol Toxicol.* 59:438–441.
Danks, D. 1988. Copper deficiency in humans. *Annu Rev Nutr.* 8:235–257.
Dawson-Hughes, B. 2003. Calcium and protein in bone health. *P. Nutr. Soc.* 62:505–509.
Drüeke, T., Lacour, B., Touam, M., et al. 1986. Effect of aluminum on hematopoiesis. *Kidney Int Suppl.* 18:S45–S48.
Eggert, J., Siegler, R., Edomkesmalee, I. 1982. Zinc supplementation in chronic renal failure. *Int J Pediatr Nephrol.* 3:21–24.
Fabris, N. and Mocchegiani, E. 1995. Zinc, human diseases and aging. *Aging (Milano)* 7:77–93.
Fawcett, W., Haxby, E., Male, D. 1999. Magnesium: Physiology and pharmacology. *Br J Anaesth.* 83:302–320.

Ferreira, P., Piaikde, A., Takayangui, A., et al. 2008. Aluminum as a risk factor for Alzheimer's disease. *Rev Lat Am Enfermagem.* 16(1):151–157.

Fimreite, N., Hansen, O., Pettersen, H. 1997. Aluminum concentrations in selected foods prepared in aluminum cookware, and its implications for human health. *Bull Environ Contam Toxicol.* 58(1):1–7.

Fleming, C. 1989. Trace element metabolism in adult patients requiring total parenteral nutrition. *Am J Clin Nutr.* 49:573–579.

Foulks, C., Mills, G., Wright, L. 1989. Parathyroid hormone and anaemia—An erythrocyte osmotic fragility study in primary and secondary hyperparathyroidism. *Postgrad Med J.* 65:136–139.

Fox, C., Gona, P., Larson, M., et al. 2010. A multi-marker approach to predict incident CKD and microalbuminuria. *J Am Soc Nephrol.* 21:2143–2149.

Fox, C., Ramsoomair, D., Carte, C. 2002. Magnesium: Its proven and potential clinical significance. *South Med J.* 94:1195–1201. medscape.com/viewarticle/423568_print

Girelli, D., Olivieri, O., Stanzial, A., et al. 1993. Low platelet glutathione peroxidase activity and serum selenium concentration, in patients with chronic renal failure: Relations to dialysis treatments, diet and cardiovascular complications. *Clin Sci.* 84:611–617.

Granadillo, V., Parra de Machado, L., Romero, R. 1994. Determination of total chromium in whole blood, blood components, bone, and urine by fast furnace program electrothermal atomization AAS and using neither analyte isoformation nor background correction. *Anal Chem.* 66:3624–3631.

Grekas, D., Alivanis, P., Kotzadamis, N., et al. 1992. Influenza vaccination in chronic hemodialysis patients. The effect of zinc supplementation. *Ren Fail.* 14:575–578.

Grekas, D., Tsakalos, N., Giannopoulus, Z., et al. 1985. Effect of zinc treatment on cell mediated immunity of chronic renal failure patients. *Proc Eur Dial Transplant Assoc Eur Ren Assoc.* 21:825–829.

Griffith, D., Liff, D., Ziegler, T., et al. 2009. Acquired copper deficiency: A potentially serious and preventable complication following gastric bypass surgery. *Obesity* (Silver Spring). 17(4):827–831.

Haguenauer, D., Welch, V., Shea, B., et al. 2000. Fluoride for the treatment of postmenopausal osteoporotic fractures: A meta-analysis. *Osteoporos Int.* 11(9):727–738.

Hambidge, K. 1989. Mild zinc deficiency in human subjects. In Mills, C.F., ed. *Zinc in Human Biology.* New York: Springer-Verlag, 281–296.

Harris, E. 2000. Cellular copper transport and metabolism. *Annu Rev Nutr.* 20:291–310.

Harris, E.D. 1995. The iron-copper connection: The link to ceruloplasmin grows stronger. *Nutr Rev.* 53:170–173.

Harvard Medical School. 2010. Salt and your health series. The Sodium Connection. *Har Men's Health Watch* 15:3–4.

Hasanoğlu, E., Altan, N., Sindel, S., et al. 1994. The relationship between erythrocyte superoxide dismutase activity and plasma levels of some trace elements (Al, Cu, Zn) of dialysis patients. *Gen Pharmacol.* 25:107–110.

Hawkes, W. and Hornbostel, L. 1996. Effects of dietary selenium on mood in healthy men living in a metabolic research unit. *Biol Psychiatry.* 39:121–128.

Heyneman, C. 1996. Zinc deficiency and taste disorders. *Ann Pharmacother.* 30:186–187.

Holtkamp, W., Brodersen, H., Thiery, J., et al. 1991. Effect of zinc substitution on lymphocyte subsets and cellular immune function in hemodialysis. *Lkin Wochenschr.* 69:392–396.

Hosokawa, S., Nishitani, H., Tomita, K., et al. 1985. Serum copper concentration changes in chronic hemodialysis patients. *Uremia Invest.* 9:63–67.

Hosokawa, S., Nishitani, H., Umemura, K., et al. 1990a. Serum and corpuscular nickel and zinc in chronic hemodialysis patients. *Nephron.* 45:151–153.

Hosokawa, S., Oyamaguchi, A., Yoshida, O. 1990b. Trace elements and complications in patients undergoing chronic hemodialysis. *Nephron.* 55:375–379.

Hosokawa, S. and Yoshida, O. 1993. Effects of erythropoietin on trace elements in patients with chronic renal failure undergoing hemodialysis. *Nephron.* 65:414–417.

Hosokawa, S. and Yoshida, O. 1995. Effects of recombinant human erythropoietin (rHuEPO) on protein zinc (Zn), nickel (Ni) and manganese (Mn) in patients undergoing hemodialysis. *Int Urol Nephrol.* 27:207–214.

Hunt, J. 2003. Bioavailability of iron, zinc, and other trace minerals from vegetarian diets. *Am J Clin Nutr.* 78 (3 Suppl):633S–639S.

Ikizler, T. 2009. CKD classification: Time to move beyond KDOQI. *J Am Soc Nephrol.* 20:929–930.

Institute of Medicine, Food and Nutrition Board. 2001. *Dietary Reference Intakes for Vitamin A, Vitamin K, Arsenic, Boron, Chromium, Copper, Iodine, Iron, Manganese, Molybdenum, Nickel, Silicon, Vanadium, and Zinc.* Washington, DC: National Academy Press.

Isakova, T. and Wolf, M. 2010. FGF23 or PTH: Which comes first in CKD? *Kidney Int.* 78:947–949.

Ix, J., De Boer, I., Peralta, C., et al. 2009. Serum phosphorus concentrations and arterial stiffness among individuals with normal kidney function to moderate kidney disease in MESA. *Clin J Am Soc Nephrol.* 4:609–615.

Jiang, H., Chen, L., Zheng, J., et al. 2008. Aluminum-induced effects on Photosystem II photochemistry in citrus leaves assessed by the chlorophyll a fluorescence transient. *Tree Physiol.* 28(12):1863–1871.

Johnson, L. 2008a. Chromium. In *The Merck Manuals Online Medical Library.* www.merckmanuals.com.

Johnson, L. 2008b. Copper. In *The Merck Manuals Online Medical Library.* www.merckmanuals.com.

Johnson, L. 2008c. Molybdenum. In *The Merck Manuals Online Medical Library.* www.merckmanuals.com.

Johnson, L. 2008d. Selenium. In *The Merck Manuals Online Medical Library.* www.merckmanuals.com.

Johnson, M. and Kays, D. 1990. Copper: Its role in human nutrition. *Nutr Today.* 25:6.

Joven, J., Villabona, C., Rubies-Prat, J., et al. 1985. Hormonal profile and serum zinc levels in uraemic men with gonadal dysfunction undergoing hemodialysis. *Clin Chem Acta.* 148:239–245.

Juhasz-Pocsine, K., Rudnicki, S., Archer, R., et al. 2007. Neurologic complications of gastric bypass surgery for obesity. *Neurology.* 68:1843–1850.

Kalantar-Zadeh, K., Gutekunst, L., Mehrotra, R., et al. 2010. Understanding sources of dietary phosphorus in the treatment of patients with chronic kidney disease. *Clin J Am Soc Nephrol.* 5:519–530.

King, J. and Cousins, R. 2005. Zinc. In Shils, M., Shike, M., Ross, A., et al., eds. *Modern Nutrition in Health and Disease*, 10th ed. Baltimore, MD: Lippincott Williams & Wilkins, 271–285.

Koenig, J., Fischer, M., Bulant, E., et al. 1997. Antioxidant status in patients on chronic hemodialysis therapy: Impact of parenteral selenium supplementation. *Wein Klin Wochenschr.* 109:13–19.

Kouw, P., Konings, C., deVries, P.M, et al. 1991. Effects of zinc supplementation on zinc status and immunity in haemodialysis patients. *J Trace Elem Electrolytes Health Dis.* 5:115–119.

Krebs, F. 1998. Zinc supplementation during lactation. *Am J Clin Nutr* 68 (2 Suppl):509S–512S.

Kumar, N., Ahlskog, J., Gross, J. 2004. Acquired hypocupremia after gastric surgery. *Clin Gastroenteroal Hepatol.* 2:1074–1079.

Lewis, J. 2009. Disorders of magnesium metabolism. In *The Merck Manuals Online Medical Library.* http://www.merckmanuals.com/professional/sec12/ch156/ch156i.html#sec12-ch156-ch156i-956.

Lin, T., Chen, J., Liaw, J., et al. 1996. Free elements and lipid peroxidation in uremic patients on hemodialysis. *Biol Trace Elem Res.* 51:277–283.

Lin, J.L., Yang, Y.J., Yang, S.S., and Leu, M.L. November 1997. Aluminum utensils contribute to aluminum accumulation in patients with renal disease. *Am J Kidney Dis.*, 30(5):653–658.

Linder, M. 1991. Nutrition and metabolism of the trace elements. In Linder, M., ed. *Nutritional Biochemistry and Metabolism with Clinical Application*, 2nd ed. Englewood Cliffs: Prentice-Hall, 215–276.

Linder, M. 1996. Nutrition and metabolism of the trace elements. In Ziegler, E. and Filer, L., eds. *Present Knowledge in Nutrition.* Washington, DC: ISLI Press, 215–276.

Lione, A., Allen, P., Smith, J. 1984. Aluminum coffee percolators as a source of dietary aluminum. *Food Chem Toxicol.* 22(4):265–268.

Lutsenko, S. April 2010. Human copper homeostasis: a network of interconnected pathways. *Curr Opin Chem Biol.*, 14(2):211–217. Epub February 1, 2010.

Mahajan, S., Abbasi, A., Prasad, A., et al. 1982a. Effect of oral zinc therapy on gonadal function in hemodialysis patients. A double-blind study. *Ann Intern Med.* 97:357–361.

Mahajan, S., Bowersox, E., Rye, D., et al. 1989. Factors underlying abnormal zinc metabolism in uremia. *Kidney Int.* 36(suppl 27):269–273.

Mahajan, S., Prasad, A., Rabbani, P., et al. 1982b. Zinc deficiency: A reversible complication of uremia. *Am J Clin Nutr.* 36:1177–1183.

Maher, E., Sampson, B., Curtis, J. 1987. Is selenium deficiency the cause of uraemic cardiomyopathy? *Adv Exp Med Biol.* 223:221–230.

Mailloux, R., Puiseux-Dao, S., Appanna, V. 2009. Alpha-ketoglutarate abrogates the nuclear localization of HIF-1alpha in aluminum-exposed hepatocytes. *Biochimie.* 91(3):408–415.

Maret, W. and Sandstead H. 2006. Zinc requirements and the risks and benefits of zinc supplementation. *J Trace Elem Med Biol.* 20:3–18.

Mayor, G., Sprague, S., Sanchez, T. 1981. Determinants of tissue aluminum concentration. *Am J Kidney Dis.* 1(3):141–145.

Menzano, E. and Carlen, P. 1994. Zinc deficiency and corticosteroids in the pathogenesis of alcoholic brain dysfunction—A review. *Alcohol Clin Exp Res.* 18:895–901.

Migneco, C., Tripi, S., Navett, A., et al. 1990. Serum zinc concentration and antibody response to hepatitis B vaccine. *Minerva Med.* 81:19–21.

Muirhead, N., Kertesz, A., Flanagan, P., et al. 1986. Zinc metabolism in patients on maintenance hemodialysis. *Am J Nephrol.* 6:422–426.

Nagy, E. and Jobst, K. 1994. Aluminum dissolved from kitchen utensils. *Bull Environ Contam Toxicol.* 52:396–399.

Naito, S., Ohta, A., Sohara, E., et al. 2010. Regulation of WNK1 kinase by extracellular potassium. *Clin Exper Nephrol.* 12 September, 195–202. DOI 10.1007/s10157-010-0378-9

Napolitano, G., Bonomini, M., Bomba, G., et al. 1996. Thyroid function and plasma selenium in chronic uremic patients on hemodialysis treatment. *Biol Trace Elem Res.* 55:221–230.

National Kidney Foundation. 2003. K/DOQI clinical practice guidelines for bone metabolism and disease in chronic kidney disease. *Am J Kidney Dis.* 42(Suppl 3):S1–S201.

Navarro, S., Valderrama, R., To-Figueras, J., et al. 1994. Role of zinc in the process of pancreatic fibrosis in chronic alcoholic pancreatitis. *Pancreas.* 9:270–274.

Office of Dietary Supplements. 2009. NIH, Dietary Supplement Fact Sheet: Zinc. http://ods.od.nih.gov/FactSheets/Zinc/.

Peacock, M. 2010. Calcium metabolism in health and disease. *Clin J Am Soc Nephrol.* 5:S23–S30.

Picchota, W., Dobrucki, T., Symonowicz, N., et al. 1983. Zinc in patients with chronic renal failure. *Int Urol Nephrol.* 15:377–382.

Prasad, A. and McDonald, F. 1982. Lymphocyte and granulocyte function in zinc-treated and zinc-deficient hemodialysis patients. *Kidney Int.* 21:827–832.

Prasad, A. 1985. Clinical, endocrinological and biochemical effects of zinc deficiency. *Clin Endocrinol Metab.* 14:567.

Prasad, A. 1995. Zinc: An overview. *Nutrition* 11:93–99.

Prasad, A. 1996. Zinc deficiency in women, infants and children. *J Am Coll Nutr.* 15:113–120.

Prasad, A., Beck, F., Grabowski, S., et al. 1997. Zinc deficiency: Changes in cytokine production and T-cell subpopulations in patients with head and neck cancer and in noncancer subjects. *Proc Assoc Am Physicians.* 109:68–77.

Quamme, G.A. 1997. Renal magnesium handling: New insights in understanding old problems. *Kidney Int.*, 52(5):1180–1195.

Rastergar, A. and Soleimani, M. 2001. Hypokalaemia and hyperkalaemia. *Postgrad Med J.* 77:759–764.

Rayman, M.2000. The importance of selenium to human health. *Lancet.* 356:233–241.

Richard, M., Arnaud, J., Jurkovits, C., et al. 1991. Trace elements and lipid peroxidation abnormalities in patients with chronic renal failure. *Nephrol* 57:10–15.

Rodger, R., Sheldon, W., Watson, M., et al. 1989. Zinc deficiency and hyperprolactinemia are not reversible causes of sexual dysfunction in uraemia. *Nephrol Dial Transplant.* 4:888–892.

Rude, R. 1993. Magnesium metabolism and deficiency. *Endocrinol Clin North Am.* 22:377–390.

Saint-Georges, M., Bonnefont, D., Bourely, B., et al. 1989. Correction of selenium deficiency in hemodialyzed patient. *Kidney Int.* 27(suppl):274–277.

Sandstrom, B. 1997. Bioavailability of zinc. *Eur J Clin Nutr.* 51(1 Suppl):S17–S19.

Science Daily. 2011. Excitotoxicity and cell damage. http://www.sciencedaily.com/articles/e/excitotoxicity.htm

Shaw, J. 1992. Copper deficiency in term and preterm infants. In Fomon, S. and Zlotkin, S., eds. *Nutritional Anemias.* New York: Vevey/Raven Press, 105.

Saris, N., Mervaala, E., Karppanen, H., et al. 2000. Magnesium. An update on physiological, clinical, and analytical aspects. *Clin Chim Acta.* 291:1–46.

Simmer, K. and Thompson, R. 1985. Zinc in the fetus and newborn. *Acta Paediatr Scand Suppl.* 319:158–163.

Solomons, N. 1998. Mild human zinc deficiency produces an imbalance between cell-mediated and humoral immunity. *Nutr Rev.* 56:27–28.

Sondheimer, J., Mahaman, S., Rye, D., et al. 1988. Elevated plasma copper in chronic renal failure. *Am J Clin Nutr.* 47:896–899.

Stec, J., Podracha, L., Pavkovcekova, O. 1990. Zinc and copper metabolism in nephritic syndrome. *Nephron* 56(2):186–187.

Subcommittee on the Tenth Edition of the RDAs. 1989a. Fluoride. In *Recommended Dietary Allowances*, 10th ed. Washington, DC: National Academy Press.

Subcommittee on the Tenth Edition of the RDAs. 1989b. Selenium. In *Recommended Dietary Allowances*, 10th ed. Washington, DC: National Academy Press.

Swaminathan, R. 2003. Magnesium metabolism and its disorders. *Clin Biochem Rev.* 24(2):47–66.

Tan, J., Burns, D., Jones, H. 2006. Severe ataxia, myelopathy, and peripheral neuropathy due to acquired copper deficiency in a patient with a history of gastrectomy. *J Parenter Enteral Nutr.* 30:446–450.

Tang, X., Santarelli, L., Heinemann, S., et al. 2004. Metabolic regulation of potassium channels. *Annu Rev Physiol.* 66:131–159.

Taylor, E. and Curhan, G. 2009. Demographic, dietary, and urinary factors and 24-h urinary calcium excretion. *Clin J Am Soc Nephrol.* 4:1980–1987.

Thomas, C. and Robinson, M. 1993. Selenium. In Macrae, R., Robinson, R., Sadler, M., eds. *Encyclopedia of Food Science, Food Technology, and Nutrition.* London: Academic Press, 5117–5124.

Thomson, N., Stevens, B., Humphrey, T. 1983. Comparison of trace elements in peritoneal dialysis, hemodialysis and uremia. *Kidney Int.* 23:9–14.

Tonelli, M., Wiebe, N., Hemmelgarn, B., et al. 2009. Trace elements in hemodialysis patients: A systematic review and meta-analysis. *BMC Med.* 7:25, online publication.

Tzanakis, I., Papadaki, A., Mingxin, W., et al. 2008. Magnesium carbonate for phosphate control in patients on hemodialysis. A randomized controlled trial. *Int Urol Nephrol.* 40(1):193–201.

Unwin, R., Luft, F., Shirley, D. 2011. Pathophysiology and management of hypokalemia: A clinical perspective. *Nature Rev Nephrol.* 7:75–84.

Valberg, L., Flanagan, P., Kertesz, A., et al. 1986. Zinc absorption in inflammatory bowel disease. *Dig Dis Sci.* 31(7):724–731.

Van Renterghem, D., Cornelis, R., Mees, L., et al. 1992. The effect of adding Br or Zn supplements to the dialysate on the concentrations of Br and zinc in the blood of hemodialysis patients. *J Trace Elem Electrolytes Health Dis.* 6:105–109.

Verstraeten, S., Aimo, L., Oteiza, P. 2008. Aluminum and lead: Molecular mechanisms of brain toxicity. *Arch Toxicol.* 82(11):789–802.

Wallaeys, B., Cornelia, R., Mees, L., et al. 1986. Trace elements in serum, packed cells, and dialysate of CAPD patients. *Kidney Int.* 30:599–604.

Wang, W., Hebert, S., Giebisch, G., 1997. Renal K+ Channels: Structure and function. *Annu Rev Physiol.* 59:413–436.

Ward, M., Feest, T., Ellis, H., et al. 1978. Osteomalacic dialysis osteodystrophy: Evidence for a water-borne aetiological agent, probably aluminum. *Lancet.* 1(8069):841–845.

Watson, A., Stuart, A., Wells, F., et al. 1983. Zinc supplementation and its effect on taste acuity in children with chronic renal failure. *Hum Nutr Clin Nutr.* 37:219–225.

Weir, M. and Rolfe, M. 2010. Potassium homeostasis and renin-angiotensin-aldosterone system inhibitors. *Clin J Am Soc Nephrol.* 5:531–548.

Whang, R., Hampton, E.M., Whang, D.E.D. 1994. Magnesium homeostasis and clinical disorders of magnesium deficiency. *Ann Pharmacother.*28:220–225.

Wise, A. 1995. Phytate and zinc bioavailability. *Int J Food Sci Nutr.* 46:53–63.

Wu, S., Jeng, F., Wie, S. 1998. Red blood cell osmotic fragility in chronically hemodialyzed patients. *Nephron* 78:28–32.

4 Acute Kidney Injury

Pranay Kathuria and Anand Khurana
University of Oklahoma-Tulsa

CONTENTS

4.1 DEFINITION

Acute renal failure (ARF) is an abrupt decrease in the glomerular filtration rate (GFR) occurring over a period of hours to days, resulting in the failure of the kidney to excrete nitrogenous waste products and maintain fluid and electrolyte homeostasis. The retention of nitrogenous wastes is usually assessed by measuring blood urea nitrogen (BUN) and serum creatinine. However, immediately after a kidney injury, BUN or creatinine levels may be normal, and the only sign of a kidney injury may be decreased urine production.

The above definition is largely subjective, given that neither time nor the quantitative changes in kidney function are specified. In past medical literature, more than 35 different definitions of ARF have been used. This hampered our ability to characterize the true incidence of the disease, assess its impact, and make progress in clinical and scientific research. All these factors led to the realization that there needed to be a consensus definition of ARF. The term ARF was replaced by acute kidney injury (AKI). AKI encompasses the entire spectrum of the syndrome from minor changes in renal function to need for kidney replacement therapy. The initial definition of AKI was proposed by the Acute Dialysis Quality Initiative (ADQI) and subsequently modified by the Acute Kidney Injury Network (AKIN; Bellomo et al., 2004; Srisawat et al., 2010). AKI is defined as an abrupt (within 48 h) reduction in kidney function with an absolute increase in serum creatinine of more than or equal to 0.3 mg/dL, a percentage increase in serum creatinine of more than or equal to 50% (1.5-fold from baseline), or a reduction in urine output (documented oliguria of less than 0.5 mL/kg/h for more than 6 h; Srisawat et al., 2010). The stages of AKI are summarized in Table 4.1.

4.2 EPIDEMIOLOGY

The worldwide incidence of AKI is poorly known because of underreporting, regional disparities, and differences in definition and case mix. It is recognized that the epidemiology of AKI in developing countries differs from that of the developed world in many important ways. Whereas in developed regions elderly patients predominate, in developing countries, AKI is a disease of the young and children. In developing countries, the most common causes of AKI are frequently associated with volume-responsive "prerenal," obstetric, infectious or toxic mechanisms. In the developed world, AKI is seldom a community-acquired disease; the condition develops primarily in hospitalized patients. The common causes include sepsis, intravenous iodinated contrast and other nephrotoxins, postoperative and hypovolemia. In these regions, the incidence of hospital-acquired AKI exceeds that of community-acquired AKI by 5–10 times, having an estimated yearly incidence of 0.15%–7.2%. The incidence of AKI exceeds 20% in the critically ill patients (Cerda et al., 2008). Approximately 4%–5% of general intensive care unit patients will be treated with renal replacement therapy (RRT). Intensive care unit patients with AKI have a longer length of stay and therefore associated with greater costs. Patients with AKI have increased mortality, even after correction for

TABLE 4.1
Stages of Acute Kidney Injury (AKIN Classification)

AKI Stage	Creatinine Criteria	Urine Output Criteria
Stage I	Increase of serum creatinine by ≥0.3 mg/dL or increase to ≥150%–200% from baseline	Urine output < 0.5 mL/kg/h for >6 h
Stage II	Increase of serum creatinine to >200%–300% from baseline	Urine output < 0.5 mL/kg/h for >12 h
Stage III	Increase of serum creatinine to >300% from baseline or serum creatinine ≥4.0 mg/dL with an acute rise of at least 0.5 mg/dL or treatment with RRT	Urine output < 0.3 mL/kg/h for >24 h or an-uria for 12 h

covariates. Patients treated with RRT have a mortality rate of 50%–60%. Of surviving patients, 5%–20% remain dialysis dependent at hospital discharge (Hoste and Schurgers, 2008).

4.3 CAUSES OF AKI

The causes of AKI traditionally are divided into three categories: (1) prerenal AKI, (2) AKI caused by obstruction of the urinary-collecting system (postrenal AKI), and (3) AKI caused by acute intrinsic renal diseases. This longstanding, simple clinical classification of AKI remains useful because it provides a logical basis for the diagnosis and treatment of AKI. The most common causes of AKI are prerenal failure (>35% of cases) and acute tubular necrosis (ATN) (>50% of cases). Obstruction accounts for approximately 10% of cases, whereas intrinsic diseases of the kidney other than ATN account for the minority of cases (Thadhani et al., 1996).

4.3.1 Prerenal Azotemia

Prerenal azotemia is a reduction in GFR caused by reduced renal perfusion. It is not associated with any intrinsic renal parenchymal disease and resolves rapidly when the underlying causes of renal hypoperfusion are corrected.

Whenever there is a decrease in the effective arterial blood volume, or portion of the extracellular volume that effectively perfuses the tissues, normal homeostatic mechanisms attempt to preserve the GFR by causing afferent vasodilatation and efferent vasoconstriction. Prerenal ARF develops only when these adaptive mechanisms fail causing the GFR to fall. Those with proteinuria, preexisting kidney disease, and the elderly are more susceptible to AKI. Commonly used classes of drugs, nonsteroidal anti-inflammatory drugs (NSAIDs), angiotensin receptor blockers, and angiotensin-converting enzyme (ACE) inhibitors can cause prerenal azotemia by impairing renal autoregulation (Abernethy and Lieberthal, 2002).

The causes of prerenal azotemia are listed in Table 4.2. These causes can be broken down into three major categories: intravascular volume depletion, decreased effective circulating volume, and intrarenal hemodynamic changes. In the outpatient setting, gastrointestinal losses, fever, diuretics, and heart failure are the common causes. Among hospitalized patients, prerenal azotemia is often due to cardiac failure, liver dysfunction, or septic shock. Among surgical patients, anesthesia can cause redistribution of blood and consequent prerenal azotemia (Thadhani et al., 1996).

4.3.2 Postrenal Causes

AKI develops when both urinary tracts are obstructed or when one tract is obstructed in a patient with a single functioning kidney. The condition is most often due to obstruction of the lower urinary tract. Among children, obstruction of the ureteropelvic junction, urethral strictures, and posterior urethral valves are common. In the mature male, tumors of the prostate and benign prostatic hyperplasia, and in women, gynecological malignancies predominate as causes of obstructive uropathy. An extensive list of causes is presented in Table 4.3.

The presence of a urinary obstruction causes the pressure to rise within the ureters and renal pelvis leading to dilatation of these structures. The increased pressure inside the urinary space of the glomerulus causes a decline in the net hydrostatic pressure, reducing GFR. Vasodilatory hormones initially increase renal arterial flow and pressure in the glomerular capillary. However, as obstruction continues, the renal blood flow is markedly reduced because vasoconstrictor hormones are released, increasing the resistance of renal vasculature (Loo et al., 1988).

The potential for recovery of renal function is often inversely related to the duration of obstruction. Checking a postvoid residual volume in the bladder by either a bladder scan or catheterization

TABLE 4.2
Causes of Prerenal Azotemia

1. Intravascular Volume Depletion
   - Acute blood loss
   - Gastrointestinal fluid loss (vomiting, diarrhea, NG suction)
   - Kidney losses (diuretics, hypoaldosteronism, diabetes inspidus)
   - Dermatological losses (burns, hyperthermia)
   - Third-space fluid loss (pancreatitis, peritonitis, crush syndrome)
2. Decreased Effective Circulating Volume
   - Reduced cardiac output (congestive heart failure, valvular diseases, pericardial tamponade, pulmonary embolism, positive pressure ventilation)
   - Systemic vasodilatation (sepsis, anaphylaxis, cirrhosis, anesthetics)
   - Abdominal compartment syndrome
3. Intrarenal Hemodynamic Changes
   - Hepatorenal syndrome
   - Drugs: angiotensin-converting enzyme inhibitors, angiotensin receptor blockers, cyclosporine, radiocontrast media, nonsteroidal anti-inflammatory drugs
   - Hypercalcemia

TABLE 4.3
Causes of Postrenal Acute Kidney Injury

1. Ureteral Obstruction
   - Intraureteral: Obstruction: Stones, blood clots, cancer, sloughed papillae
   - Extraureteral: Malignancy, retroperitoneal fibrosis, trauma or accidental ligation of ureter, abdominal compartment syndrome
2. Bladder Neck: Neurogenic bladder, prostatic hyperplasia, calculi, blood clots, anticholinergic drugs, malignancies of bladder, prostate or cervix
3. Urethral: Urethral strictures, posterior urethral valves, phimosis

is an easy way to make a diagnosis of a bladder or urethral obstruction. A kidney ultrasound will detect obstructive uropathy with a very high sensitivity and specificity. False-negative ultrasound examinations can occur if the obstruction is very early or retroperitoneal fibrosis is present.

4.3.3 Intrinsic AKI

Intrinsic kidney diseases that result in AKI are categorized according to the primary site of injury: tubules, interstitium, vessels, or glomerulus (Table 4.4).

4.3.3.1 Acute Tubular Necrosis

Prerenal azotemia and ischemic tubular necrosis represent a continuum, with the former leading to the latter when blood flow is sufficiently compromised to result in the death of tubular cells. In its most extreme form, ischemia leads to bilateral renal cortical necrosis and irreversible renal failure.

Nephrotoxic ATN may result from either endogenous or exogenous toxins. The endogenous heme pigments hemoglobin and myoglobin cause ATN in the settings of massive intravascular

TABLE 4.4
Intrinsic Acute Kidney Injury

1. Tubular
   - Ischemic
   - Nephrotoxic
     - Pigment (rhabdomyolysis, intravascular hemolysis)
     - Toxins (aminoglycosides, lithium, amphotericin B, pentamidine, cisplatinum, ifosfamide, radiocontrast agents)
2. Interstitial
   - Allergic (penicillins, cephalosporins, quinolones, sulfonamides, nonsteroidal anti-inflammatory drugs, allopurinol, rifampin, mesalamine)
   - Infection (pyelonephritis, viral nephritides)
   - Systemic disease (Sjögren syndrome, sarcoidosis, lupus, lymphoma, leukemia, tubulonephritis with uveitis)
3. Glomerular
   - Antiglomerular basement membrane disease (Goodpasture syndrome)
   - Antineutrophil cytoplasmic antibody-associated glomerulonephritis (Wegener granulomatosis, Churg–Strauss syndrome, microscopic polyangiitis)
   - Immune complex glomerulonephritis (GN) (lupus, postinfectious, cryoglobulinemia, primary membranoproliferative glomerulonephritis)
4. Vascular (large and small vessel)
   - Renal artery obstruction (thrombosis, emboli, dissection, vasculitis)
   - Renal vein obstruction (thrombosis)
   - Microangiopathy (thrombotic thrombocytopenic purpura, hemolytic uremic syndrome, disseminated intravascular coagulation, malignant hypertension, scleroderma renal crisis)
   - Atheroembolic disease
5. Crystal Nephropathies
   - Endogenous (uric acid, light chains, oxalosis)
   - Exogenous (phosphate, methotrexate, calcium oxalate, acyclovir, indinavir)

hemolysis or rhabdomyolysis, respectively. Most cases of nephrotoxic ATN from exogenous toxins are associated with antimicrobial agents such as aminoglycosides and amphotericin B, radiocontrast media, and chemotherapeutic agents including cisplatinum and ifosfamide. From a clinical perspective, patients are often divided into oliguric and nonoliguric. Oliguria is defined as urine output less than 500 mL/day. Patients without oliguria typically have a better prognosis (Thadhani et al., 1996).

The pathogenesis of ischemic ATN can be divided into several phases. There usually is an initiation phase characterized by epithelial and endothelial cell injury. Cell injury is most often seen in the proximal tubule and the medullary portion of the thick ascending limb of the loop of Henle. These segments are very metabolically active and are located in the outer medulla, which has low oxygen tensions and hence most susceptible to injury. The initiation phase is followed by an extension phase, independent of the initial ischemic insult, mediated by microvascular endothelial injury and activation of inflammatory pathways. This phase is followed by a maintenance phase, during which the epithelial and endothelial cells undergo repair and redifferentiation, followed by recovery of renal function (Norbert, 2005).

Several mechanisms are thought to underlie the reduction in GFR during ATN. There is profound vasoconstriction, mediated directly by endothelial injury and indirectly through tubuloglomerular feedback, resulting in a direct reduction in glomerular filtration. In addition, sloughing of cells from the tubular epithelium denudes the tubular basement membrane and leads to formation of intratubular casts. These casts cause tubular obstruction, and the denuded basement membrane permits back leak of glomerular filtrate (Khalil et al., 2008).

The clinical course of ATN can be highly variable. There is typically an initial oliguric phase, beginning within 24 h of the inciting event and lasting 1–3 weeks, followed by a diuretic phase characterized by a progressive increase in urine volume that is usually indicative of renal recovery. Many patients, however, may be nonoliguric throughout their course.

4.3.3.2 Acute Interstitial Nephritis

Acute interstitial nephritis (AIN) represents a frequent cause of AKI, accounting for 15%–27% of renal biopsies performed. This is likely an underestimate since biopsies are not performed in majority of patients. By and large, drug-induced AIN is currently the most common etiology of AIN, with antimicrobials and NSAIDs being the most frequent offending agents. Other causes include systemic diseases like lupus, sarcoidosis, and infection. AIN is a hypersensitivity reaction with resultant immune-mediated injury to the tubules. Specifically, cell-mediated immunity plays a major role in the pathogenesis of AIN. AIN is characterized histologically by the presence of inflammatory infiltrates and edema within the interstitium. The interstitial infiltrates are mostly composed of lymphocytes, macrophages, eosinophils, and plasma cells. AIN usually spares the glomeruli (Praga and Gonzalez, 2010).

Removal of the offending drug is the mainstay of the treatment. However, a significant proportion of patients, ranging from 30% to 70%, do not fully recover their baseline renal function, likely because of the rapid transformation of interstitial cellular infiltrates into large areas of fibrosis. Although prospective randomized trials in AIN are lacking, recent retrospective studies suggest that early steroid treatment (within 7 days after diagnosis) improves the recovery of renal function.

4.3.3.3 Glomerulonephritis

The two types of glomerulonephritis that cause AKI are rapidly progressive glomerulonephritis and acute proliferative glomerulonephritis. In primary glomerulonephritis, disease is almost entirely restricted to the kidneys (as in IgA nephropathy or poststreptococcal glomerulonephritis), whereas in secondary glomerulonephritis it occurs in association with more diffuse inflammation (as in systemic lupus erythematosus or systemic vasculitis). The hallmark findings of GN-associated AKI are related to damage to the glomerular basement membrane (GBM) and glomerular bleeding. Besides hematuria, patients usually have hypertension, edema, and proteinuria. Serologic studies and a renal biopsy assist in making the diagnosis. The specific findings on kidney biopsy depend on the underlying glomerular process; proliferative lesions in the glomerulus are characteristic. Prompt recognition of these entities is critical because prompt initiation of therapy is essential to preserve kidney function and prevent irreversible renal damage.

4.3.3.4 Vascular Diseases

Renal artery occlusion by thrombosis, emboli, or dissection may cause AKI. Patients will typically have sharp abdominal pain and hematuria. Diagnosis is established by contrast computed tomography (CT) scans, angiograms, or renal scintiscans.

Small-vessel disease is a more common cause of AKI. Cholesterol embolization syndrome refers to embolization of the contents of an atherosclerotic plaque (primarily cholesterol crystals) from a proximal large-caliber artery to distal small to medium arteries, causing end-organ damage by mechanical plugging and an inflammatory response. This condition develops subsequent to large-vessel manipulation either by endovascular procedures or during surgery, or secondary to trauma. On occasion, cholesterol embolism may occur spontaneously or following thrombolytic therapy. These crystals lodge in small arteries and arterioles where they usually are nonobstructing but incite an inflammatory reaction that ultimately leads to narrowing or obliteration of the vascular lumen. Patients may develop constitutional manifestations, livedo reticularis (a mottled bluish discoloration of the skin with a lacelike pattern), blue toe syndrome, gut ischemia, pancreatitis, retinal emboli, and central nervous system manifestations (Kronzon and Saric, 2010).

Thrombotic angiopathies such as thrombotic thrombocytopenic purpura, hemolytic uremic syndrome, malignant hypertension, and scleroderma renal crises are characterized by the presence of microangiopathic hemolytic anemia and thrombocytopenia in addition to renal involvement.

4.3.3.5 Crystal Nephropathies

Intratubular precipitation of either exogenously administered medications or endogenous crystals (induced by certain drugs) can promote chronic and AKI, termed crystal nephropathy. Among endogenous substances, uric acid can precipitate in the setting of tumor lysis syndrome. In multiple myeloma, light chains that are filtered can precipitate in the tubules with Tamm Horsfall proteins and form dense, obstructing casts in the distal and collecting tubules. These casts induce a characteristic inflammatory reaction around the casts, which is referred to as *myeloma cast nephropathy*. Several medications that are insoluble in human urine are known to precipitate within the renal tubules. Examples of these drugs include sulfadiazine, acyclovir, indinavir, triamterene, methotrexate, ciprofloxacin, and oral phosphate solutions (Yarlagadda and Perazella, 2008). Clinical settings that enhance the risk of drug or endogenous crystal precipitation within the kidney tubules include true or effective intravascular volume depletion, underlying kidney disease, and metabolic disturbances that promote changes in urinary pH favoring crystal precipitation.

Ethylene glycol poisoning causes oxalate to precipitate in the tubules resulting in AKI.

4.4 EVALUATION OF A PATIENT WITH AKI

The first step is to differentiate AKI from chronic kidney disease (CKD). Prior laboratory assessments of kidney function, if available, are the most useful for this. Presence of anemia and an elevated parathyroid hormone support the diagnosis of CKD. Most patients with CKD have small kidneys on ultrasound. The normal size of an adult human kidney is about 10–13 cm (4–5 in.) long and about 5–7.5 cm (2–3 in.) wide. Patients with CKD due to amyloid, diabetes, obstructive uropathy, HIV nephropathy, and polycystic kidney disease have preserved kidney size.

The clinical evaluation of the patient who has AKI begins with assessing whether the patient has prerenal, postrenal, or intrinsic disease. An excellent history and examination combined with laboratories, urine studies, and radiological examination can establish the diagnosis in most patients. A history of exposure to drugs that effect renal hemodynamics including radiocontrast media, nonsteroidals, ACE inhibitors, angiotensin receptor blockers, and calcineurin inhibitors must be elicited. Skin rash may suggest an interstitial nephritis, vasculitis, or systemic lupus erythematosus. Hemoptysis or epistaxis suggests a pulmonary-renal syndrome such as Wegner's granulomatosis. Bone pain and anemia may indicate a myeloma.

Although postrenal AKI can present with anuria, some patients with partial obstruction may have polyuria (urine output > 3 L/day). Symptoms of prostatic hypertrophy include frequency, nocturia, hesitancy, and urgency. The patient may complain of pain due to ureteric colic (sharp, stabbing, flank pain) or suprapubic pain due to a bladder obstruction. Bladder outlet obstruction is assessed by measuring a postvoid residual bladder volume using an ultrasonic bladder scanner or by placement of a bladder catheter after the patient attempts to void. A postvoid bladder volume >100 mL is highly suggestive of bladder outlet obstruction. Upper tract obstruction should be assessed using renal ultrasound or CT (Khalil et al., 2008).

Prerenal azotemia is suggested by a history of volume depletion, including diarrhea, vomiting or poor intake. Examination will find tachycardia, orthostatic hypotension, hypotension, poor skin turgor, dry mucous membranes, and absent axillary sweat. Patients with decreased effective circulating volume from congestive heart failure and cirrhosis may appear volume overloaded.

Urinary indices are often used to differentiate between prerenal azotemia and ATN (Klahr and Miller, 1998). In prerenal azotemia, the kidney tries to conserve sodium to preserve intravascular volume and excrete wastes in a limited quantity of urine. This makes the urine very concentrated (high osmolality) but very low in urinary sodium. In ATN, the cells lose their functional capability; hence

TABLE 4.5
Urinary Indices in Prerenal Azotemia and Acute Tubular Necrosis

Index	Prerenal	Acute Tubular Necrosis
Urinary sodium (mEq/L)	<20	>40
Fractional excretion of sodium (%)[a]	<1	>2
Urine osmolality (mOsm/L)	>500	<350
BUN/Serum creatinine ratio	>20:1	10:1
Fractional excretion of urea (%)[b]	<35	>50

[a] Fractional excretion of sodium = [(urinary Na/plasma Na)/(urine creatinine/plasma creatinine)] × 100.

[b] Fractional excretion of urea = [(urinary urea/plasma urea)/(urine creatinine/plasma creatinine)] × 100.

the urine is similar in osmolality to plasma, and urinary sodium is high. The fractional excretion of sodium (FENa) is a commonly used index in differentiating prerenal azotemia and ATN. FENa is the percentage of the sodium filtered by the kidney that is excreted in the urine. The use of diuretics can decrease the sensitivity of FENa by inhibiting tubular sodium reabsorbtion. In contrast, the fractional excretion of urea nitrogen (FEUN) is primarily dependent on passive forces and is therefore less influenced by diuretic therapy. Thus, in some studies, a low FEUN ($\leq$35%) has been found to be consistent with a diagnosis of prerenal azotemia (Carvounis et al., 2002). The ultimate determination of whether a patient has prerenal or intrinsic AKI may require a diagnostic trial of intravenous fluids. The differences between prerenal azotemia and ATN are highlighted in Table 4.5.

The urinalysis is an extremely useful tool in the diagnosis. The urine is typically bland in prerenal azotemia and postrenal etiologies. The presence of dysmorphic red blood cells and red-blood-cell casts is strongly indicative of an acute glomerular process. The presence of heme-positive urine with no red blood cells on microscopy suggests rhabdomyolysis or hemolysis. The presence of white blood cells, white-blood-cell casts, and eosinophiluria supports the diagnosis of AIN. Tubular epithelial cells and muddy brown granular casts are present in ATN. Heavy oxalate or uric acid crystalluria or the presence of drug crystals suggests intratubular crystal deposition, and the presence of nonalbumin proteinuria suggests a diagnosis of myeloma kidney.

Eosinophilia may be seen in atheroembolic disease, acute interstitial nephritis, or Churg–Strauss disease. Thrombocytopenia and fragmented red cells suggest the diagnosis of a microangiopathy, such as thrombotic thrombocytopenic purpura, hemolytic uremic syndrome, disseminated intravascular coagulation, malignant hypertension, or scleroderma renal crisis. Serological studies including antistreptolysin-O titers, antinuclear antibodies, antineutrophil cytoplasmic antibody, anti-GBM antibodies, and complement levels are indicated to diagnose certain vasculitis and glomerulonephritis.

A kidney biopsy may be indicated when the diagnosis remains uncertain, especially if there is suspicion of acute glomerulonephritis or acute interstitial nephritis or if there is failure of kidney function to improve.

4.5 MANAGEMENT OF AKI

The therapy for AKI needs to be tailored to the clinical circumstances.

4.5.1 Prerenal AKI and ATN

4.5.1.1 Restoration of Effective Circulatory Volume

The initial fluid of choice is normal saline in most situations. If severe hemorrhage is responsible for volume depletion, the transfusion of packed red blood cells may be indicated. Therapy should also be directed to prevent further volume/blood loss. Patients, especially those with cardiac compromise, oliguria, or elderly patients, need to be closely monitored during aggressive fluid resuscitation. Some patients may need invasive hemodynamic monitoring with either a central venous catheter or a Swan-Ganz catheter to guide therapy.

Prerenal azotemia is often seen in congestive heart failure. Optimizing the treatment of heart failure can improve kidney perfusion. Sometimes, especially with advanced heart failure, one has to accept some amount of prerenal azotemia. In hospitalized patients who have decompensated heart failure, inotropic agents such as dobutamine or milrinone, or vasodilators such as nitroglycerine, nitroprusside, or nesiritide may be used to optimize renal perfusion, although usually such treatment are only a temporizing measure (House et al., 2010).

Hepatorenal syndrome needs to be differentiated from volume depletion and a host of other conditions. Rehydration and intravenous albumin are often used in such patients. The definitive cure lies in either liver transplantation or spontaneous recovery of the diseased liver. The use of drugs that induce splanchnic vasoconstriction (octreotide) and renal vasodilatation (midodrine) have been beneficial in treating hepatorenal syndrome. Some patients benefit from transjugular intrahepatic portosystemic shunts, which cause a decrease in the portal pressures.

4.5.1.2 Identifying and Discontinuing Nephrotoxins

NSAIDs, ACE inhibitors, angiotensin receptor blockers, and calcineurin inhibitors such as cyclosporine and tacrolimus should be discontinued, if possible. Iodinated radiocontrast media should be avoided.

4.6 POSTRENAL AKI

Relief of urinary obstruction is the key to treating postrenal AKI. Placement of a foley catheter or a suprapubic catheter will relieve obstruction at the level of the bladder outlet or urethra. Upper tract obstruction requires either ureteral stenting or placement of a percutaneous nephrostomy. Prompt relief of obstruction is necessary to prevent irreversible renal injury. Some patients develop a postobstructive diuresis and may need intravenous saline to maintain hydration.

4.6.1 Intrinsic AKI

Acute interstitial nephritis often resolves with removal of the antigen. Recent studies strongly suggest that early steroid administration (within 7 days after diagnosis) improves the recovery of renal function, decreasing the risk of chronic renal impairment. Delayed steroid treatment, when interstitial fibrosis has taken place, has a less pronounced or no therapeutic benefit (Praga and Gonzalez, 2010).

Glomerulonephritides and vasculitides need a kidney biopsy for diagnosis and are treated by immunosuppressive drugs. Plasmapheresis is indicated in thrombotic thrombocytopenic purpura and hemolytic uremic syndrome.

4.7 GENERAL SUPPORTIVE THERAPY

Drug doses should be adjusted to level of kidney function. One should remember that the serum creatinine lags the loss of kidney function. Anuric and oliguric patients should receive drug dosing based on a GFR < 10 mL/min. Drug dosing also needs to be adjusted if the patient is receiving renal replacement therapy and the modality of therapy. Drug level monitoring may be required for certain drugs like vancomycin and aminoglycosides.

Electrolyte disorders need to be addressed. Mild hyperkalemia may be treated medically. Metabolic acidosis can be temporized using a sodium bicarbonate infusion if the $pH < 7.2$ and/or $HCO_3^- < 15$ mEq/L. Diuretics may be utilized to control hypervolemia.

4.8 RENAL REPLACEMENT THERAPIES

Indications for RRT include refractory hyperkalemia, metabolic acidosis, and volume overload as well as overt uremia with pericarditis, encephalopathy, or bleeding diatheses.

There are inadequate data to provide definitive recommendations regarding the optimal timing of initiation of RRT in AKI. The predominantly retrospective data from the first three decades of clinical dialysis strongly support the prophylactic initiation of dialysis prior to the onset of advanced uremia. While these studies support initiation of treatment by the time the BUN reaches 80–100 mg/dL, there are limited data addressing the question of earlier initiation of therapy (Palevsky, 2006).

In the early 1980s, the options for RRT were limited to intermittent hemodialysis (IHD) and acute peritoneal dialysis (PD). Patients with AKI in the intensive care unit often receive high volumes of fluid in the form of parenteral nutrition, sedation, and antibiotics necessitating the removal of large volumes of fluid during IHD in a relatively short period of time, which can cause hypotension. PD has the advantage of not requiring anticoagulation and better hemodynamic stability. It requires placement of a peritoneal access. PD is not an option in patients with recent abdominal surgery, fecal or fungal peritonitis, abdominal wall cellulitis, peritoneo-pleural communications, and severe respiratory failure. Because of its lower clearances, it is not indicated in severe hyperkalemia or catabolic states. Also, lactate is the buffer in most PD solutions and needs to be processed to bicarbonate in the liver. In some patients with advanced liver disease and in patients with lactic acidosis, these solutions can worsen metabolic acidosis (Passadakis and Oreopoulos, 2007).

Continuous forms of RRT (CRRT) were developed to address the problems with IHD and PD. These modalities are typically used in intensively ill patients with hemodynamic instability. The types of CRRT are named after the vascular access (arteriovenous or venovenous) and the modality of waste removal (diffusion or dialysis, convection or hemofiltration, or a combination of diffusion and convection or hemodiafiltration). Initially, continuous arteriovenous hemofiltration (CAVH) was described using arterial access and blood pressure to maintain blood flow through the system. However, the clearances derived from such circuits were often insufficient and dialysate was added (CAVHD) to increase efficiency. Now, pump-driven venovenous circuits (continuous venovenous hemofiltration and continuous venovenous hemodiafiltration) are used for CRRT. Recently, "hybrid" therapies—modalities of "slow" hemodialysis that combine conventional IHD machine technology with the extended duration and more gradual volume removal of CRRT—have been developed. Sustained low-efficiency dialysis can provide high clearances with improved hemodynamic stability without the need for special CRRT machines and customized solutions.

The continuous and hybrid therapies offer several advantages over intermittent hemodialysis, including increased time-averaged dose, more stable volume management, enhanced drug clearance, and, possibly, removal of higher-molecular-weight solutes, including inflammatory cytokines (Davenport et al., 2008). However, data do not support a survival advantage to using CRRT over IHD. Further, a systematic review of the literature found that increased dosing of CRRT is not associated with a decrease in the mortality of patients with AKI in an intensive care unit setting (Casey et al., 2010). There may, however, be better recovery of renal function with CRRT (Bell, 2008).

4.9 METABOLIC CHANGES IN AKI

AKI rarely occurs in isolation. It is frequently accompanied with hypotension, sepsis, and multiorgan failure. Besides the effect on the water and electrolytes, it exerts impact on various aspects of fat, carbohydrate, and protein metabolism. AKI is also a pro-inflammatory state impacting the antioxidative system (Druml, 2005). The initiation of extracorporeal therapy adds to the metabolic changes already occurring in the setting of AKI. Thus, the goals of nutritional therapy in patients with AKI vary depending on the nature and the severity of the initiating disease, the kidney failure, and the chosen modality of RRT.

Severe malnutrition can be seen in as many as 42% patients with AKI. Protein energy wasting is associated with an increased risk of complications like sepsis, bleeding and arrhythmias, and heightened mortality (Fiaccadori et al., 1999). Nutritional therapy should not only cover the energy, protein, and micronutrient requirements but also preserve lean body mass and support immune function and wound healing.

4.10 ENERGY METABOLISM AND ENERGY REQUIREMENTS

The energy requirements in patients with AKI are usually more a reflection of the underlying disease process causing the kidney injury rather than of the kidney failure itself. In most uncomplicated cases of AKI, the energy requirements tend to be no different than in healthy individuals. In sepsis or multiorgan failure, the basal energy requirements tend to be up to 30% higher determined by the underlying sepsis rather than the AKI (Druml, 2005; Faisy et al., 2003). There is no major benefit of increasing the energy intake over 30 kcal/kg body weight/day. Any extra caloric intake over this level is not utilized and results in hyperglycemia and hypertriglyceridemia (Druml, 2005). Hyperglycemia has an important role in increasing the risk of complications; maintenance of normoglycemia is a priority in these patients. All efforts should be undertaken to avoid any overfeeding to patients with AKI and multiorgan failure.

There are not enough data available to address the optimal energy to nitrogen ratio in patients with AKI. The only available data were from an observational study in patients with RRT in which it was felt that patients with ARF may require a high-protein (approximately 1.5–1.8 g/kg/day) and relatively low-energy content (approximately 25–35 kcal/kg/day; Macias et al., 1996). While reduced protein intake caused a negative nitrogen balance, increasing the energy intake in comparison to protein intake increased the risk of hyperglycemia and hypertriglyceridemia.

4.10.1 Carbohydrate Metabolism

Carbohydrate metabolism is frequently altered in patients with AKI, and hyperglycemia is frequently seen (Druml, 2005; Fiaccadori et al., 1999). In patients with sepsis and AKI, there is increased release of inflammatory mediators and counter regulatory hormones like epinephrine and cortisol. This along with use of exogenous steroids and adrenergic agents augments the insulin resistance. Despite increased circulating levels, there is decreased suppression of hepatic gluconeogenesis. Reduced skeletal muscle uptake of glucose also contributes to the hyperglycemia in these patients.

Hyperglycemia in diabetics and even nondiabetics has shown to have deleterious consequences. It causes direct toxic effects to the endothelial and epithelial cells (Fiaccadori et al., 1999). Hyperglycemia results in generation of reactive oxygen species, impairs immunity, and causes hypercoagulability (Rao et al., 1999). Maintenance of normoglycemia has been shown to reduce the incidence of AKI in intensive care units (Schetz et al., 2008). Hyperglycemia is one of the predictors of mortality in patients with AKI (Basi et al., 2005). Even though avoidance of hyperglycemia is a priority during nutritional support of patients, avoidance of hypoglycemia is also important. Recent studies have indicated that maintaining strict glycemic control in critically ill patients may be associated with increased risk of hypoglycemia and increased morbidity and mortality (D'Ancona et al., 2011). The absolute targets of glycemic control may need to be individualized. Further studies are needed in this regard.

4.10.2 Lipid Metabolism

As with carbohydrate metabolism, lipid metabolism undergoes various changes in patients with AKI. The triglyceride content of all plasma lipoproteins, especially very-low-density lipoproteins

(VLDL) and low-density lipoproteins increases. The total cholesterol and HDL levels decrease (Druml, 2005; Fiaccadori et al., 2008). The activity of both peripheral lipoprotein lipase and hepatic triglyceride lipase is reduced by about 50% and this causes impairment of lipolysis. Metabolic acidosis that frequently accompanies AKI in the hospital setting also causes inhibition of lipoprotein lipase and impairment of lipolysis. In addition, the clearance of the infused lipids is reduced in patients receiving parenteral nutrition.

4.10.3 Protein and Amino Acid Metabolism

Protein synthesis as well as degradation is altered in patients with AKI. The excessive catabolism results from increased breakdown of the skeletal muscle and stimulation of amino acid oxidation. Insulin resistance and metabolic acidosis are major factors in stimulating muscle breakdown with catabolic hormones and hyperparathyroidism also contributing to the process (Druml, 2005). Insulin resistance causes decreased anabolism of proteins and increased breakdown in the skeletal muscle. Independent of azotemia and hyperglycemia, acidosis causes increased oxidation of amino acids (Btaiche et al., 2008). The amino acid concentrations of phenylalanine, methionine, taurine, and cysteine are increased, and valine and leucine concentrations are decreased (Btaiche et al., 2008). The net result is increased circulating amino acids which are extracted by the liver and increased gluconeogenesis and ureagenesis occurs. Most nonessential amino acids like arginine and tyrosine become conditionally indispensible and need to be replaced along with the essential amino acids. Overall protein synthesis decreases except for acute-phase reactants. If there is inadequate replacement of calories, protein catabolism increases.

RRT can stimulate protein catabolism. Water-soluble amino acids are lost through hemodialysis, and bio-incompatibility of dialyzer membranes lead to increased reactive oxygen species that enhance protein catabolism.

In terms of amino acids, both essential and nonessential amino acids are required in patients with AKI. The previously developed specialized parenteral and enteral amino acid formulations primarily provided essential amino acids. The aim was to force the recycling of urea nitrogen for the synthesis of nonessential amino acids. However, the recycling of urea is ineffective under stress, and some of these nonessential amino acids can become conditionally essential during periods of stress.

4.10.4 Metabolism and Requirements of Micronutrients

Micronutrients are present in the blood in very low concentrations, and some of these are essential. Serious illnesses and death are the consequence of severe deficiencies. Not many studies have analyzed the magnitude of alterations of micronutrients and their impact in patients with AKI. The presence of concurrent illnesses and the shorter duration of AKI in comparison to chronic maintenance hemodialysis make this even harder to study. Most of the alterations in trace elements are related to the RRT because of their small molecular weight and easy passage though dialysis membranes.

RRT affects the levels of the micronutrients based on their protein binding and on the duration and frequency of dialysis therapy. Convective losses of these micronutrients may be significant with CRRT and high-flux therapies. Hemodialysis patients usually have lower levels of most micronutrients, such as zinc, manganese, cooper and selenium, because of increased clearance. Manganese removal by CRRT appears to be least affected, whereas significant selenium clearance occurs. Selenium concentrations in plasma and erythrocytes are profoundly decreased. As selenium is a cofactor for glutathione peroxidase, this can result in decreased antioxidant activity (Wooley et al., 2005). Although zinc is lost during the dialytic therapy, there is usually not a serious deficiency probably as a result of addition of zinc to the parenteral nutrition therapies (Wooley et al., 2005).

4.10.5 Electrolytes

4.10.5.1 Potassium

Potassium levels are frequently abnormal in patients with AKI. The impairment of potassium excretion frequently occurs with oliguric kidney failure. The contribution of increased cell death and turnover and increased extracellular shifts as a result of acidosis are also contributing factors. Hypokalemia may also occur in patients with ARF because of the use of diuretics and during the recovery phase of ATN, especially if potassium intake is restricted. Dialytic therapies are very effective in controlling hyperkalemia in most patients with AKI.

4.10.5.2 Phosphorus

Phosphorus levels are usually high in patients with kidney failure. The impaired renal excretion along with increased release from the cells and increased bone turnover all contribute to the process. Usually patients with AKI will need binders to reduce serum phosphorus levels.

The duration of dialysis is a significant factor in determining the clearance of phosphorus. Increasing the duration of dialysis treatment typically increases clearance of phosphorus. Continuous RRTs commonly cause hypophosphatemia requiring replacement.

4.10.5.3 Calcium

Calcium has a variety of roles that go beyond bone metabolism. It helps to maintain the electrophysiological characteristics of both the smooth muscles and the cardiac muscles and plays an important role in blood coagulation and platelet adhesion. Most patients with AKI develop hypocalcemia. Patients with AKI usually have hyperphosphatemia along with hypocalcemia because of impaired production of 1, 25 dihydroxy vitamin D. The decreased intestinal calcium absorption and skeletal resistance to parathyroid hormone are also thought to play a part. On the other hand, immobilization leads to hypercalcemia. Other contributing factors include calcium concentrations in the dialysate and hyperparathyroidism. Severe hypocalcemia may be seen in acute pancreatitis and rhabdomyolysis due to precipitation of calcium. Conditions like multiple myeloma and milk alkali syndrome can cause AKI as well as hypercalcemia.

Calcium levels should always be interpreted in the light of albumin levels and the acid-base status. It may be beneficial to obtain an ionized calcium level.

4.10.5.4 Magnesium

Reduced magnesium excretion is typically seen with oliguric AKI. Hypermagnesemia in patients with AKI usually tends to be mild unless there is evidence of rapid cell breakdown. The symptoms of hypermagnesemia are usually related to neuromuscular irritability or cardiac arrhythmias. Treatment usually involves intravenous calcium, which can rapidly resolve these symptoms. RRT can be used to control hypermagnesemia. Low serum magnesium levels are seen as side effects of some medications. Loop diuretics and certain nephrotoxic drug, such as amphotericin and cisplatin, are associated with urinary magnesium wasting. Hypomagnesemia may develop in patients on CRRT owing to dialytic losses with prolonged duration of therapy. These can be easily treated with oral or parenteral replacement.

4.10.6 Vitamins

The levels of water-soluble vitamins are generally low in patients with AKI who require dialysis support. These vitamins are mainly lost in the dialysate and need to be replaced. The magnitude of loss varies and can be significant, with up to 100 mg of vitamin C being lost per day in the dialysate. The losses can be even higher when continuous RRT are used and higher intakes of vitamin C up to 150–200 mg/day are needed. However, the metabolism of vitamin C is different from most other water-soluble vitamins, as its metabolic products can accumulate and cause secondary oxalosis. The total intake of vitamin C should not exceed 250 mg/day. Significant losses of B vitamins including thiamine tend to occur during renal replacement therapies (Wooley et al., 2005). In general, patients on dialysis and severely malnourished patients should receive double the normal dose of water-soluble vitamins.

Some of the fat-soluble vitamins can also be deficient, especially vitamin D, which depends on the kidneys to be hydoxylated to the active form. The levels of vitamin A and E can also be low in AKI patients. However, hypervitaminosis A has been recently documented in pediatric patients with AKI on RRT (Lipkin and Lenssen, 2008). Vitamin K does not need any special replacement in patients with AKI as its levels are generally increased in patients with AKI.

4.11 ASSESSMENT OF NUTRITIONAL STATUS

Various methods can be used to assess the nutritional status of patients with AKI. Each of these has limited specificity in patients who are critically ill. The anthropometric measurements like body mass index are of little use in critically ill patients. Mid-arm circumference measurement can change because of fluid overload and patient positioning. Subjective global assessment, although not widely used as an assessment tool in the intensive care setting, has been utilized in some studies, and it has been noted that preexisting malnutrition was an independent predictor of negative hospital outcomes.

The levels of serum proteins (albumin, pre-albumin, retinol-binding protein, transferrin) are clinically useful, but their levels are affected by the nonnutritional factors such as stress levels, inflammation, and the hydration status of critically ill patients.

Nitrogen balance is used to assess the extent of protein balance that the person is able to achieve. This is based on the assumption that when the supply is adequate to replace the losses that occur in urine and stools, the excess is excreted as urea. The desired positive nitrogen balance is usually in the range of 4–6 g/day (Btaiche et al., 2008). Positive nitrogen balance is typically difficult to achieve until metabolic stress resolves. However, even with the improvement of nitrogen balance, some patients may not achieve increased protein synthesis.

Measurement of the nitrogen balance is usually done with the help of urine urea nitrogen with some degree of adjustment for nonurea nitrogen components. This is not possible in patients with AKI and oliguria. In patients undergoing dialysis, urea nitrogen appearance (UNA) is used and calculated as follows:

UNA (g/day) = UUN (g/day) + dialysate urea nitrogen (g/day) + change in body urea nitrogen (g/day)

Change in body urea nitrogen (g/day) = $[(BUN_f - BUN_i) \times BW_i \times 0.6 \text{ L/kg}] + [(BW_f - BW_i) \times BUN_f \times 1 \text{ L/kg}]$,

where i and f represent the initial (immediately after dialysis) and final (immediately before the second dialysis session) values for the period of measurement. The factor of 0.6 is an estimate of the fraction of adult body weight as water, and 1.0 is the fractional distribution of urea in the gained or lost weight (Btaiche et al., 2008).

Protein catabolic rate (PCR) is a measure of net protein degradation. PCR is based on edema-free body cell mass. It can be normalized to protein degraded divided by the dry body weight and is labeled as normalized PCR (nPCR). PCR is calculated as

PCR (g/day) = 6.25 × UNA (g/day).

The limitations of wide applicability of nPCR are due to its variable values in metabolically unstable patients and its rapid fluctuations with changes in protein intake. It also tends to underestimate protein intake when the intake is high and overestimates it when protein intake is less than 1 g/kg/day. It tends to be most accurate in state of equilibrium, and in critically ill patients daily measurements of PCR are sometimes needed to make an accurate assessment (Btaiche et al., 2008). Higher PCR is expected in highly catabolic patients such as those with severe burn injuries.

4.11.1 Patient Classification

There are three major categories that have been identified in planning for nutritional support for patients with AKI. They are largely based on the severity of the underlying illness and the extent of catabolism that is seen.

Group 1 consists of patients with UNA < 6 g/day. They have low mortality, rarely need dialysis support, can be given oral feedings, and do not have any excess energy or protein requirements over the baseline.

Group 2 consists of patients with UNA between 6 and 12 g/day who have a higher risk of mortality and the need for dialysis. These patients require tube feedings and parenteral nutritional support and often need dialysis to support volume and electrolyte status.

Group 3 consists of the severely sick patients with overwhelming multiorgan failure or sepsis and where the mortality rate is very high and the need for dialysis support is frequent. UNA is markedly increased over 12 g/day. Patients in Group 3 frequently need multiple modes of nutritional therapy and have increased protein requirements in the range of 1.5 g/kg/day.

4.12 NUTRITIONAL SUPPORT

The aim of nutritional support is to reduce the hypercatabolic state and eliminate malnutrition-related problems like nonhealing wounds. Goals of nutritional therapy in the acute situation are somewhat different from that of patients with CKD, and phosphorus restriction may not be as critical in this situation given its shorter duration. Two different forms of nutritional support exist based on the route of delivery.

4.12.1 Enteral Feeding

Oral feedings should be used in all patients whenever possible to maintain mucosal gut integrity and to decrease the risk of bacteremia and infection. Enteral nutrition increases renal plasma flow and has been shown to improve prognosis of experimental rats with AKI (Mouser et al., 1997). Whether this effect can be extrapolated to human subjects is not known given the paucity of studies that have looked at this issue. The enteral feeding is safe and does not carry many side effects. Because a significant proportion of patients with AKI are likely to have gastroparesis, small-bowel access may be preferable in these patients.

The formula used for enteral nutrition may be tailored to the specific needs of the patients.

There are many standard formulas available, and these may not be appropriate for patients with AKI because of the lower protein content and higher than required levels of certain electrolytes including potassium and phosphorus. Once CRRT or other forms of dialysis are utilized, there is no special need for renal-specific formulas as the metabolic parameters can be easily controlled.

The protein intake in patients with AKI should be usually in the range of 0.6–0.8 g/kg/day. It can be increased to 0.8 g/kg/day as long as BUN stays below 100 mg/dL. Patients requiring dialysis should have even higher protein intake, to 1–1.4 g/kg/day. With increased losses through the dialysate, supplementation of water-soluble vitamins is required. Increased losses of trace elements including zinc- and water-soluble vitamins would need to be provided in patients with CRRT. Using special formulas that are high in vitamins A and C should be avoided in patients with AKI because of the risk of hypervitaminosis A and oxalosis, respectively.

Even in patients who are unable to tolerate enteral feeding effectively to maintain their nutritional needs, trophic feedings to maintain gut mucosa are used effectively to decrease the risk of bacterial translocation and risk of infections. The combination of parenteral nutrition to provide the nutritional requirements and the enteral feedings for trophic purposes should be considered as they complement each other.

4.12.2 Parenteral Nutrition

Parenteral nutrition is indicated in AKI if enteral feeding is either not possible or inadequate to meet the energy requirements. Issues with delayed gastric emptying are often encountered in patients with AKI, and short-term parenteral nutrition may be required. The nutrition can be provided through enteral as well as parenteral route, but given the high osmolality of the formulas (given fluid restriction that is required in patients with AKI), central access is usually preferred.

The balanced parenteral nutrition consists of 20%–30% calories from lipids, 50%–60% from carbohydrates, and 10%–20% from protein sources/amino acids. The carbohydrates should be the main energy source and efforts must be made to avoid excessive intake, which can cause hyperglycemia and lipogenesis. The carbohydrate intake is usually restricted to 4–5 g/kg/day to avoid complications like hyperglycemia, increased lipogenesis, and increased CO_2 production. Insulin therapy is frequently required as there is insulin resistance in patients with AKI.

Lipid emulsions have high energy content and low osmolality and can be a useful energy source in patients with AKI. They decrease the risk of hyperglycemia, which is beneficial in all patients, and reduce CO_2 production, which is helpful in patients with a low respiratory reserve. Metabolism of the commercially available fat emulsions is similar to endogenous VLDL, and their clearance is decreased in patients with AKI, especially with high infusion rates. These lipid emulsions are usually given over a period of 18–24 h to avoid severe hypertriglyceridemia. The triglyceride levels should be monitored on a regular basis, and the lipid emulsion should be stopped if the level exceeds 400 mg/dL. Medium-chain triglycerides are metabolized at a faster rate, so giving a combination of medium- and long-chain triglycerides is usually considered to be better, even though there are no definitive pharmacokinetic studies to support this.

A standard mix of essential and nonessential amino acids is required for optimal nutrition of patients with AKI. Some of the nonessential amino acids become conditionally essential in patients with AKI, and therefore a balance of both is typically required. The formulation needs to provide an adequate amount of essential as well as nonessential amino acids.

Special amino acid solutions are available for patients with AKI. These solutions provide adequate dose of the required amino acids without the concomitant increase in urea concentration but have not been shown to improve survival endpoints. Maintaining lower levels of urea is less of a concern in AKI patients on dialysis because of the removal of urea during the process. The use of branched-chain amino acids in patients with AKI has not been shown to be of any particular benefit.

There have been studies in patients using additional glutamine supplementation for its antioxidant and immunomodulatory properties. Glutamine has been considered to be a conditionally essential amino acid in stressful illnesses. There is no current reason for special supplementation of glutamine except to compensate for increased losses in the dialysate during renal replacement therapy. The losses in the dialysate occurring during hemodialysis are based on the dialytic therapy; 10 g/day in intermittent dialysis and 3–5 g/day during the CRRT therapies (Wernerman, 2008). Even though the amino acid levels increase with supplementation, there are no data to determine any potential benefits from the increased levels of glutamine in patients with AKI.

The increase in amino acid intake in patients on dialysis support increases the net protein synthesis but does not prevent catabolism. Increased amino acid losses with dialysis may not result in significant change in concentrations in the blood (Btaiche et al., 2008). Intake of amino acids in amounts that exceed muscle protein synthetic capacity are utilized toward ureagenesis and gluconeogenesis and should be avoided.

The electrolyte balance is usually controlled efficiently in patients on dialysis. In patients undergoing CRRT, replacement of electrolytes like phosphorus and magnesium may be required.

4.12.3 Renal Replacement Therapy

RRT makes the nutritional support easier to maintain with regard to volume control and maintenance of urea clearance. RRT can, however, have other effects on the metabolism of these patients because of the increased losses of small- and medium-sized molecules. RRT has been shown to cause increased generation of reactive oxygen species and increased protein breakdown along with increased losses of amino acids in the dialysate. High-flux dialysis leads to loss of about 0.2 g/kg/day of amino acids in the dialysate, and this should be accounted for in calculating the nitrogen deficit in these patients. It also causes increased losses of water-soluble vitamins and micronutrients, which need to be replaced. Dialysate contains glucose and thus can be a source of carbohydrate load to patients. Electrolytes can be easily controlled in patients on RRT and need to be replaced or removed based on the individual's labs.

Patients on RRT typically require protein intakes in the range of 0.6–0.8 g/kg/day with addition for stress as needed. With severely catabolic patients with AKI, the protein intake should be increased in the range of 1–1.4 g/kg/day. As with other patients with AKI, an intake of both essential and nonessential amino acids is used to maintain nitrogen balance in these patients.

REFERENCES

Abernethy, V. and Lieberthal, W. 2002. Acute renal failure in the critically ill patient. *Crit Care Clin*, 18, 203–222.

Basi, S., Pupim, L., Simmons, E., et al. 2005. Insulin resistance in critically ill patients with acute renal failure. *Am J Physiol Renal Physiol*, 289, F259–F264.

Bell, M. 2008. Acute kidney injury: New concepts, renal recovery. *Nephron Clin Pract*, 109, c224–c228.

Bellomo, R., Ronco, C., Kellum, J., et al. 2004. Acute renal failure—Definition, outcome measures, animal models, fluid therapy and information technology needs: The Second International Consensus Conference of the Acute Dialysis Quality Initiative (ADQI) Group. *Crit Care*, 8, R204–R212.

Btaiche, I., Mohammad, R., Alaniz, C., et al. 2008. Amino acid requirements in critically ill patients with acute kidney injury treated with continuous renal replacement therapy. *Pharmacotherapy*, 28, 600–613.

Carvounis, C., Nisar, S. and Guro-Razuman, S. 2002. Significance of the fractional excretion of urea in the differential diagnosis of acute renal failure. *Kidney Int*, 62, 2223–2229.

Casey, E., Gupta, B., Erwin, P., et al. 2010. The dose of continuous renal replacement therapy for acute renal failure: A systematic review and meta-analysis. *Renal Fail*, 32, 555–561.

Cerda, J., Bagga, A., Kher, V., et al. 2008. The contrasting characteristics of acute kidney injury in developed and developing countries. *Nat Clin Pract Neph*, 4, 138–153.

D'ancona, G., Bertuzzi, F., Sacchi, L., et al. 2011. Iatrogenic hypoglycemia secondary to tight glucose control is an independent determinant for mortality and cardiac morbidity. *Eur J Cardiothorac Surg*, 40, 360–366.

Davenport, A., Bouman, C., Kirpalani, A., et al. 2008. Delivery of renal replacement therapy in acute kidney injury: What are the key issues? *Clin J Am Soc Nephrol*, 3, 869–875.

Druml, W. 2005. Nutritional management of acute renal failure. *J Ren Nutr*, 15, 63–70.

Faisy, C., Guerot, E., Diehl, J., et al. 2003. Assessment of resting energy expenditure in mechanically ventilated patients. *Am J Clin Nutr*, 78, 241–249.

Fiaccadori, E., Lombardi, M., Leonardi, S., et al. 1999. Prevalence and clinical outcome associated with preexisting malnutrition in acute renal failure: A prospective cohort study. *J Am Soc Nephrol*, 10, 581–593.

Fiaccadori, E., Parenti, E. and Maggiore, U. 2008. Nutritional support in acute kidney injury. *J Nephrol*, 21, 645–656.

Hoste, E. and Schurgers, M. 2008. Epidemiology of acute kidney injury: How big is the problem? *Crit Care Med*, 36, S146–S151. DOI: 10.1097/CCM.0b013e318168c590.

House, A., Haapio, M., Lassus, J., et al. 2010. Therapeutic strategies for heart failure in cardiorenal syndromes. *Am J Kid Dis Off J Natl Kid Found*, 56, 759–773.

Khalil, P., Murty, P. and Palevsky, P. 2008. The patient with acute kidney injury. *Prim Care*, 35, 239–264, vi.

Klahr, S. and Miller, S. 1998. Acute oliguria. *N Engl J Med*, 338, 671–675.

Kronzon, I. and Saric, M. 2010. Cholesterol embolization syndrome. *Circulation*, 122, 631–641.
Lipkin, A. and Lenssen, P. 2008. Hypervitaminosis A in pediatric hematopoietic stem cell patients requiring renal replacement therapy. *Nutr Clin Pract*, 23, 621–629.
Loo, M., Felsen, D., Weisman, S., et al. 1988. Pathophysiology of obstructive nephropathy. *World J Urol*, 6, 53–60.
Macias, W., Alaka, K., Murphy, M., et al. 1996. Impact of the nutritional regimen on protein catabolism and nitrogen balance in patients with acute renal failure. *J Parenter Enteral Nutr*, 20, 56–62.
Mouser, J., Hak, E., Kuhl, D., et al. 1997. Recovery from ischemic acute renal failure is improved with enteral compared with parenteral nutrition. *Crit Care Med*, 25, 1748–1754.
Norbert, L. 2005. The pathophysiology of acute renal failure. *Crit Care Clin*, 21, 197–210.
Palevsky, P. 2006. Unresolved issues in dialysis: Dialysis modality and dosing strategy in acute renal failure. *Semin Dialysis*, 19, 165–170.
Passadakis, P. and Oreopoulos, D. 2007. Peritoneal dialysis in patients with acute renal failure. *Adv Perit Dial*, 23, 7–16.
Praga, M. and Gonzalez, E. 2010. Acute interstitial nephritis. *Kidney Int*, 77, 956–961.
Rao, A., Chouhan, V., Chen, X., et al. 1999. Activation of the tissue factor pathway of blood coagulation during prolonged hyperglycemia in young healthy men. *Diabetes*, 48, 1156–1161.
Schetz, M., Vanhorebeek, I., Wouters, P., et al. 2008. Tight blood glucose control is renoprotective in critically ill patients. *J Am Soc Nephrol*, 19, 571–578.
Srisawat, N., Hoste, E., Kellum, J. 2010. Modern classification of acute kidney injury. *Blood Purif*, 29, 300–307.
Thadhani, R., Pascual, M., Bonventre, J. 1996. Acute renal failure. *N Engl J Med*, 334, 1448–1460.
Wernerman, J. 2008. Clinical use of glutamine supplementation. *J Nutr*, 138, 2040S–2044S.
Wooley, J., Btaiche, I. and Good, K.005. Metabolic and nutritional aspects of acute renal failure in critically ill patients requiring continuous renal replacement therapy. *Nutr Clin Pract*, 20, 176–191.
Yarlagadda, S. and Perazella, M. 2008. Drug-induced crystal nephropathy: An update. *Expert Opin Drug Saf*, 7, 147–158.

5 Nephrotic Syndrome

Tai-Gen Cui
Capital Medical University

Joseph Janicki and Taixing Cui
University of South Carolina School of Medicine

CONTENTS

5.1 INTRODUCTION

Nephrotic syndrome (NS) refers to a group of diseases characterized by heavy proteinuria, hypoalbuminemia, hyperlipidemia, and edema. It is usually classified as primary or secondary. Primary nephrotic syndrome is also known as idiopathic nephrotic syndrome, which is caused by a variety of primary glomerular diseases. In secondary nephrotic syndrome, kidney disease is part of an identifiable systemic disease (Orth and Ritz, 1998). Although nephrotic syndromes can be caused by various diseases, they have one common feature—injury to the glomerular filtration barrier resulting in the loss of a large amount of plasma protein in the urine and subsequent metabolic disorders (Falk, 2004).

5.2 ETIOLOGY

Theoretically, any injury to the glomerular capillary wall, regardless of etiology, may result in nephrotic syndrome. Patients with this syndrome typically have proteinuria with an otherwise bland urine sediment. Several systemic diseases such as diabetes mellitus and systemic lupus erythematosus or amyloidosis are associated with nephrotic syndrome. This syndrome can also be associated with primary renal disorders such as minimal change disease (MCD) (seen mostly in children), focal segmental glomerulosclerosis (FSGS), or membranous nephropathy. However, FSGS and membranous nephropathy can also be secondary to systemic diseases. Other nephritides such as membranoproliferative glomerulonephritis or IgA nephropathy can cause nephrotic syndrome, but patients with this type of nephrotic syndrome have an active urine sediment with red blood cells (RBCs) or RBC casts frequently found on microscopic analysis of urine (Myers et al., 1982).

The most common etiology of nephrotic syndrome varies according to age. In children with nephrotic syndrome, 90% of those below 10 years and 50% of those above 10 years will have MCD (A Report of the International Study of Kidney Disease in Children, 1978). Patients with MCD have findings of diffuse foot process effacement on electron microscopy and otherwise unremarkable changes on light microscopy. Adults with idiopathic nephrotic syndrome are most likely to have FSGS, which is found in about 35% of cases in the United States and 50% of cases among black adults (Haas et al., 1997). FSGS can be either primary or secondary, and it is very important to differentiate the types, as they require very different treatments. Membranous nephropathy is another common etiology of nephrotic syndrome in adults and can be either primary or secondary. Specific treatment and outcome of nephrotic syndrome depend on its etiology.

5.3 CLINICAL FEATURES AND PATHOGENESIS

Nephrotic syndrome typically presents with heavy proteinuria, hypoalbuminemia, edema, and hyperlipidemia. Among these, heavy proteinuria and hypoalbuminemia are of diagnostic importance. Although the exact mechanism behind nephrotic syndrome is not clear, glomerular injury leading to structural and/or functional damage of the glomerular filtration barrier is likely to be the key factor.

5.3.1 Glomerular Injury and Proteinuria

Proteinuria is an essential defining criteria of nephrotic syndrome. A urinary protein excretion rate of more than 3.5 g/day is usually referred to as "heavy proteinuria" or "nephrotic-range proteinuria," which is required for diagnosing nephrotic syndrome. Analysis of urinary proteins in nephrotic syndrome shows that urinary proteins are glomerular in origin, caused by injury to the glomerular filtration barrier in the development of the syndrome. The glomerular capillary wall is the anatomical basis of the glomerular filtration barrier, which consists of three components: fenestrated endothelial cells, the glomerular basement membrane (GBM), and epithelial cell (also known as podocyte) foot processes. Water and small solutes (glucose and urea) transverse the capillary wall freely, whereas filtration of large solutes such as albumin and IgG is restricted by two mechanisms: charge-selectivity and size-selectivity. The endothelial cells and GBM have a net negative charge owing to the presence of polyanions such as heparin sulfate proteoglycans, which create a charge barrier to the filtration of large anions such as albumin. The glomerular capillary wall is porous. Whereas the endothelial cell fenestrate is wide (radius approximately 375–400 Å), the pores in the GBM and at the slit diaphragms between the podocyte foot processes are much smaller (approximately 40–45 Å), which limit the filtration of large macromolecules such as IgG (radius approximately 50–55 Å). In glomerular diseases, injury to glomeruli may cause structural or functional changes of the glomerular filtration barrier, resulting in leakage of plasma proteins into urine.

5.3.2 Hypoalbuminemia

Serum albumin falls as a consequence of proteinuria. In nephrotic syndrome, the serum albumin level usually drops below 30 g/L. Generally, hepatic albumin synthesis increases in response to albumin loss in an attempt to normalize plasma albumin concentration (Ballmer et al., 1992). Usually, however, the increased synthesis is unable to compensate for the loss of albumin due to nephrotic syndrome. More importantly, since there is a substantial increase in renal tubular cell catabolism of filtered proteins in nephrotic syndrome, the urinary protein excretion rate will not be an accurate measure of the protein loss.

5.3.3 Urinary Loss of Other Plasma Proteins and Their Functional Consequences

In nephrotic syndrome, in addition to the loss of urinary albumin, other plasma proteins of similar molecular weight are filtered across the glomerular capillary wall. In contrast, some large proteins, such as IgM, fibrinogen, and large lipoproteins, do not transverse the glomerular capillary wall, and thus their plasma levels are either normal or high. In nephrotic syndrome, prominent changes take place in the level of coagulation-system proteins, including increased plasma fibrinogen and factors II, V, VII, VIII, X, and XIII and decreased antithrombin III, protein S, and factors IX, XI, and XII. These abnormalities may result in thrombosis, especially deep vein thrombosis (DVT) (Kendall et al., 1971). Moreover, patients with nephrotic syndrome, especially children and elderly, are susceptible to infection. This may be partly due to a decreased level of IgG and certain complement components such as factor B, C3, and C1q. Moreover, hormone-binding proteins, such as thyroid-binding globulin and vitamin D-binding protein, are typically lost in the urine, often resulting in a decreased level of these proteins (Koening et al., 1992). However, hypothyroidism and abnormal bone mineralization usually do not occur in nephrotic syndrome (Feinstein et al., 1982).

5.3.4 Hyperlipidemia

Hyperlipidemia is another typical feature of nephrotic syndrome. The abnormalities of lipid profile in nephrotic syndrome include hypercholesterolemia and hypertriglyceridemia with increases in both low-density lipoproteins (LDL) swelling and very low-density lipoproteins (VLDL). Decreased plasma osmotic pressure appears to stimulate hepatic lipoprotein synthesis, resulting in hypercholesterolemia. In addition, a defect in the LDL receptor results in a diminished clearance of LDL. Impaired metabolism rather than increased synthesis is responsible for hypertriglyceridemia (de Sain-vander Velden et al., 1998). Hyperlipidemia in nephrotic syndrome is an independent risk factor for atherosclerotic cardiovascular disease; it also aggravates renal disease and is associated with thrombosis.

5.3.5 Edema

Edema is the most common symptom of nephrotic syndrome. Fluid retention is limited mainly to the interstitial compartment. The severity of edema usually parallels the degree of hypoalbuminemia. Edema may manifest as periorbital swelling and/or bilateral pitting edema of legs. Also, pleural effusion and ascites are not uncommon in nephrotic patients and, in severe cases, anasarca and even pulmonary edema may occur. Two mechanisms have been proposed to explain the occurrence of edema in nephrotic syndrome. In some patients, a decrease in plasma osmotic pressure resulting from a low serum albumin level is thought to be the primary cause of fluid accumulation in the interstitial space; subsequent water and sodium retention is caused by activation of the nervous and endocrine systems secondary to a reduction in the effective circulatory volume. In other patients, there is a corresponding fall in the interstitial protein concentration and little change in the transcapillary osmotic pressure gradient, and circulatory volume is normal or even high. In these patients, edema appears to be the consequence of primary renal sodium retention in the collecting tubules (Ichikawa et al., 1983).

5.4 COMPLICATIONS

5.4.1 Acute Renal Failure

Acute renal failure can occur in some patients with nephrotic syndrome, particularly in those with a pathological type of MCD (Jennette and Falk, 1990). Its mechanism is not fully understood. Certain drugs, including antibiotics, diuretics, angiotensin-converting enzyme inhibitors (ACEIs), and nonsteroidal anti-inflammatory drugs (NSAIDs), may cause acute kidney injury by inducing acute tubulointerstitial nephritis. Bilateral renal vein thrombosis (RVT) may cause acute renal failure. Two other conditions are (1) collapsing FSGS, in which tubular injury is thought to play an important role, and (2) crescentic glomerulonephritis superimposed on membranous nephropathy, in which active urine sediment can be found. Acute renal failure may occur without any identifiable cause; several factors, including hypovolemia, interstitial edema, and ischemic tubular injury, have been suggested for this (Smith and Hayslett, 1992).

5.4.2 Thromboembolism

Patients with nephrotic syndrome have a greater risk of thromboembolism, particularly DVT and RVT. Cerebral vein thrombosis has been rarely reported. Although the mechanism of hypercoagulability has not been completely understood, it may be related to changes in plasma coagulation factors. Several other factors may also be involved, including hypovolemia, hyperlipidemia, and the use of diuretics, all of which lead to increased blood viscosity (Llach, 1985).

RVT occurs disproportionately in patients with membranous nephropathy. Acute RVT often presents with flank pain, gross hematuria, and a decline in renal function. However, most patients with RVT are asymptomatic, and RVT is suspected only when pulmonary thromboembolism develops. Although pulmonary thromboembolism is not common, it can be fatal.

5.4.2.1 Infection

Patients with nephrotic syndrome are susceptible to infection. Before the advent of antibiotics, infection was the leading cause of death in children with nephrotic syndrome (Taube et al., 1984). Pneumococcal infections, especially peritonitis, were particularly common (Krensky et al., 1982). Urinary tract and lung infections may also occur in nephrotic patients. Here too, the process of impairment of the normal defense mechanism of the body is not well understood. However, low levels of IgG due to urinary losses and decreased synthesis of IgG may be the reason (Heslan et al., 1982). Also, glucocorticoid and immunosuppressive drugs used for treating nephrotic syndrome predispose patients to infection.

5.4.3 Protein Malnutrition

A loss in lean body mass with negative nitrogen balance often occurs in patients with marked and persistent proteinuria, although it may be masked by concurrently increasing edema (Castellino and Cataliotti, 2002). This may be compounded by gastrointestinal symptoms of anorexia and vomiting, which are secondary to edema of the gastrointestinal tract.

5.5 DIAGNOSIS

Diagnosis of nephrotic syndrome is not difficult. Criteria include the presence of nephrotic-range proteinuria, in which urinary protein excretion rate exceeds 3.5 g/day as determined by 24-h urinary protein excretion, hypoalbuminemia (serum albumin level below 30 g/L), hyperlipidemia, and edema. Among these criteria, the first two are required for a confirmed diagnosis. However, one should not be content with the presence of such criteria, which can by caused by various other primary glomerular diseases or systemic diseases. A thorough knowledge of the patient's history, physical examination, and further serologic studies are needed, and in most cases, a kidney biopsy is usually required to establish the final diagnosis.

5.6 TREATMENT

Nephrotic syndrome calls for nonspecific and specific treatments. Nonspecific treatment aims at alleviating nutritional deficiencies, treating proteinuria, edema, hyperlipidemia, and hypercoagulability. Antiproteinuric medications such as angiotensin receptor blockers (ARBs) and ACEIs are often the mainstay of nonspecific treatment. Specific treatment aims at the underlying causes, which are determined by kidney biopsy, and can include steroids and immunosuppressant medications.

5.6.1 Nutritional Therapy

Patients with nephrotic syndrome have massive urinary protein loss and a negative nitrogen balance. However, a high-protein diet is usually not recommended. Dietary protein restriction may slow disease progression; however, this modality should not be used in patients with very low serum albumin levels (Nath et al., 1986). Apart from the amount of protein, its composition in the diet may be equally important. Studies have shown that a diet based on soy protein or flaxseed can reduce proteinuria and attenuate tubular interstitial injury (D'Amico et al., 1992). Polyunsaturated fats in the diet are beneficial as they improve the lipid profile and reduce proteinuria (Wheeler et al., 1991).

5.6.2 Proteinuria Treatment

In the absence of a specific therapy for the underlying disease, efforts should be made to reduce urinary protein excretion. This is usually done by administering ACEI or ARB. Both ACEI and ARB can reduce proteinuria by lowering systemic blood pressure and intraglomerular pressure (Heeg et al., 1987). Reducing urinary protein excretion may slow the rate of progression of kidney disease, resulting in renal protection (Praga et al., 1992). Potentially adverse effects of the aforementioned agents include acute renal failure and hyperkalemia; serum creatinine and potassium levels should be measured following the initiation and titration of drugs.

5.6.3 Edema Treatment

Edema in nephrotic syndrome is due to primary renal sodium retention in most patients, and therefore, it should be managed with both dietary-sodium restriction and diuretics. Dietary sodium should be limited to about 2 g of sodium per day. However, this is difficult for most patients, and therefore, diuretics are often the mainstay of treatment. Thiazides may be used successfully for mild edema in some patients; however, loop diuretics are usually required by most patients with nephrotic syndrome. Generally, there is less natriuresis in patients with nephrotic syndrome than in patients without the syndrome. The efficacy of diuretics is usually reduced by hypoalbuminemia (causing decreased delivery of protein-bound drugs to the kidney) and albuminuria (binding the drug within the tubular lumen). For these reasons, the diuretic dose often has to be increased, and infusion of albumin is occasionally needed if the serum albumin level is too low. However, albumin is a very expensive and short-acting solution. An important guide for evaluating diuretic therapy is serial measurement of body weight to avoid incidence of hypovolemia when treating edema with diuretics.

5.6.4 Hyperlipidemia Treatment

Treatment of hyperlipidemia is strongly recommended for patients with persistent nephrosis, as hyperlipidemia may not only increase the risk of cardiovascular diseases but also induce glomerulosclerosis. Dietary modification is generally of little use. Most patients are initially treated with an 3-hydroxy-3-methylglutaryl-coenzyme A (HMG CoA) reductase inhibitor, otherwise known as statin (Vega and Grundy, 1988).

5.6.5 Hypercoagulability Treatment

There is a relatively high incidence of venous thromboemboli among patients with nephrotic syndrome, particularly membranous nephropathy. At present, there is no consensus on whether routine prophylactic anticoagulation therapy should be used for treating hypercoagulability. If thrombosis occurs, it is typically treated with heparin followed by warfarin.

5.6.6 Specific Therapy

Patients with secondary nephrotic syndrome who have clearly identifiable etiology found by biopsy should receive specific treatment aimed at the underlying causes. For primary nephrotic syndrome, pathological findings are of prime importance in determining the proper therapeutic regimen. Although glucocorticoids are often used to treat nephrotic syndrome, cytotoxic drugs or immunosuppressive agents are also used either alone or in combination with glucocorticoids based on the pathological results. Specific treatments for individual etiologies of nephrotic syndrome are beyond the scope of this book. However, special attention should be paid to monitoring closely the adverse effects such as infection, elevation in blood sugar, or other comorbidities that occur with steroid treatment or other immunosuppressant medications.

REFERENCES

A Report of the International Study of Kidney Disease in Children. 1978. Nephrotic syndrome in children: Prediction of histopathology from clinical and laboratory characteristics at time of diagnosis. *Kidney Int.* 13:159.

Ballmer, P., Weber, B., Roy-Chaudhury, P., et al. 1992. Elevation of albumin synthesis rates in nephrotic patients measured with [1–13C] leucine. *Kidney Int.* 41:132–138.

Castellino, P. and Cataliotti, A. 2002. Changes of protein kinetics in nephrotic patients. *Curr Opin Clin Metab Care.* 5:51–54.

D'Amico, G., Gentile, M., Manna, G., et al. 1992. Effect of vegetarian soy diet on hyperlipidemia in nephrotic syndrome. *Lancet.* 339:1131–1134.

de Sain-vander Velden, M., Kaysen, G., Barrett, H., et al. 1998. Increased VLDL in nephrotic patients results from a decreased catabolism while increased LDL results from increased synthesis. *Kidney Int.* 53:994–1001.

Falk, R. 2004. *Primary Glomerular Disease. Brenner BM, Rector FC. The Kidney*, 7th edition. Philadelphia, PA: WB Saunders.

Feinstein, E., Kaptein, E., Nicoloff, J., et al. 1982. Thyroid function in patients with nephrotic syndrome and normal renal function. *Am J Nephrol.* 2:70–76.

Haas, M., Meehan, S., Karrison, T., et al. 1997. Changing etiologies of unexplained adult nephrotic syndrome: A comparison of renal biopsy findings from 1976–1979 and 1995–1997. *Am J Kidney Dis.* 30:621.

Heeg, J., de Jong, P., van der Hem, G., et al. 1987. Reduction of proteinuria by angiotensin converting enzyme inhibition. *Kidney Int.* 32:78–83.

Heslan, J., Lautie, J., Intrator, L., et al. 1982. Impaired IgG synthesis in patients with nephrotic syndrome. *Clinical Nephrol.* 18:144–147.

Ichikawa, I., Rennke, H., Hover, J., et al. 1983. Role for intrarenal mechanisms in the impaired salt excretion of experimental nephrotic syndrome. *J Clin Invest.* 71:91–103.

Jennette, J. and Falk, R. 1990. Adult minimal change glomerulopathy with acute renal failure. *Am J Kidney Dis.* 16:432–437.

Kendall, A., Lohmann, R., Dossetor, J. 1971. Nephrotic syndrome. A hypercoagulable state. *Arch Intern Med.* 127:1021–1027.

Koening, K., Lindeberg, J., Zerwekh, J., et al. 1992. Free and total 1,25-dihydroxyvitamin D levels in subjects with renal disease. *Kidney Int.* 41:161–165.

Krensky, A., Ingelfinger, J., Grupe, W. 1982. Peritonitis in childhood nephrotic syndrome. *Am J Dis Child.* 136:732–736.

Llach, F. 1985. Hypercoagulability, renal vein thrombosis, and other thrombotic complications of nephrotic syndrome. *Kidney Int.* 28:429.

Myers, B., Okarma, T., Friedman, S., et al. 1982. Mechanisms of proteinuria in human glomerulonephritis. *J Clin Invest.* 70:732–746.

Nath, K., Kre, S., Hostetter, T. 1986. Dietary protein restriction in established renal injury in the rat: Selective role of glomerular capillary pressure in progressive glomerular dysfunction. *J Clin Invest.* 78:1199–1205.

Orth, S. and Ritz, E. 1998. The nephrotic syndrome. *N Engl J Med.* 338:1202.

Praga, M. ,Hernandez, E., Montoyo, C., et al. 1992. Long-term beneficial effects of angiotensin-converting enzyme inhibition in patients with nephrotic proteinuria. *Am J Kidney Dis.* 20:240–248.

Smith, J. and Hayslett, J. H. 1992. Reversible renal failure in the nephrotic syndrome. *Am J Kidney Dis.* 19:201–213.

Taube, D., Brown, Z., Williams, D. 1984. Impaired lymphocyte and suppressor cell function in minimal change nephropathy, membranous nephropathy and focal segmental glomerulonephritis. *Clin Nephrol.* 22:176–782.

Vega, G. and Grundy, S. 1988. Lovastatin therapy in nephrotic hyperlipidemia: Effects on lipoprotein metabolism. *Kidney Int.* 33:1160–1168.

Wheeler, D., Nair, D., Persaud, J., et al. 1991. Effects of dietary fatty acids in an animal model of focal glomerulosclerosis. *Kidney Int.* 39:930–937.

6 Current Techniques for Dialysis

Jennifer Othersen
WJB Dorn VA Medical Center
and University of South Carolina School of Medicine

CONTENTS

6.1 INTRODUCTION

The decision to initiate hemodialysis is a complex one. Many factors must be considered, and the patient must be fully involved. According to the National Kidney Foundation Kidney Disease Outcomes Quality Initiative (KDOQI)™ guidelines, patients should be referred to a nephrologist when their glomerular filtration rate (GFR) is less than 30 (National Kidney Foundation, 2000). However, some patients have been shown to benefit from earlier referral, whereas late referral to a nephrologist has been shown to be strongly associated with early death in patients with end-stage renal disease (Kessler et al., 2003). Patients with rapidly changing renal function, proteinuria, or evidence of glomerular disease should be immediately referred to a nephrologist. Nephrologists are able to evaluate the etiology of renal disease as well as treat the multiple comorbidities, thereby improving outcomes. Early referral to a nephrologist also allows the patient and nephrologist time to develop a relationship. It is essential that patients be fully educated about chronic kidney disease (CKD) and the expected progression of their disease. This allows for patient-centered care and patient participation in the decision-making process.

6.2 VASCULAR ACCESS PLANNING

KDOQI recommends vascular access planning for hemodialysis at around a GFR or creatinine clearance < 25 mL/min, when the serum creatinine level is > 4 mg/dL, or within 1 year of the

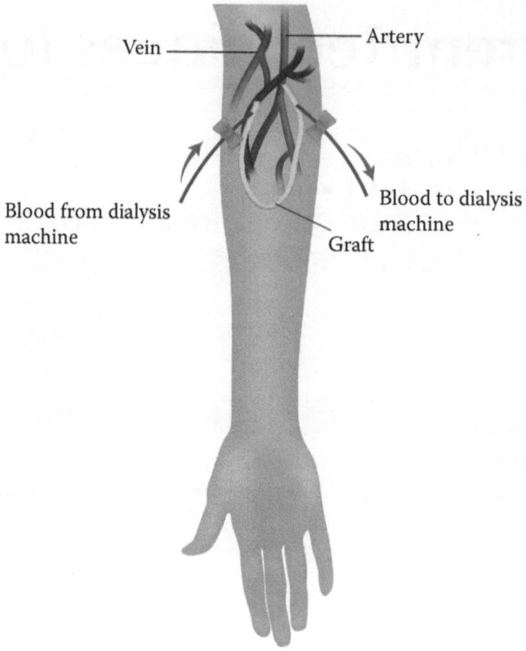

FIGURE 6.1 Access for dialysis. (From Guniita/Dreamstime.com, Dreamstime USA Headquarters, Brentwood, TN. With permission.)

anticipated need for dialysis (Figure 6.1; National Kidney Foundation, 2002). By the time patients meet these criteria, discussions should have occurred about the patient's wishes regarding dialysis and preference for dialysis modality. Ideally, patients should participate in formal dialysis education that provides information about the different modalities of dialysis, access to the various types of dialysis, and transplantation options. There are excellent online resources for patients if formal dialysis education is not an option. It is not uncommon for patients to initially refuse dialysis or dialysis access placement. However, after appropriate patient education or development of symptoms due to progression of disease, patients who initially refuse dialysis often decide to proceed with renal replacement therapy (RRT). Providers should be prepared to have continuing discussions with their patients regarding dialysis and dialysis planning. Outcomes are improved for patients who participate in early hemodialysis planning. It is important that all members of the health care team be involved in patient education, including nephrologists, nursing staff, social workers, vascular surgeons, and dieticians.

6.3 THE DIALYSIS DECISION

The decision to initiate hemodialysis can be emergent or elective. The mnemonic AEIOU is often used to denote the indications for hemodialysis, as follows:

A refers to acidemia which cannot be medically managed.
E refers to electrolyte abnormalities such as hyperkalemia.
I refers to ingestion of toxins (or intoxications) requiring dialysis for clearance.
O refers to volume overload that cannot be medically managed.
U refers to uremia.

The uremic symptoms often begin as mild fatigue, occasional nausea or vomiting, and dysgeusia. These may progress to persistent nausea or vomiting, bleeding diathesis, pericarditis, pleuritis,

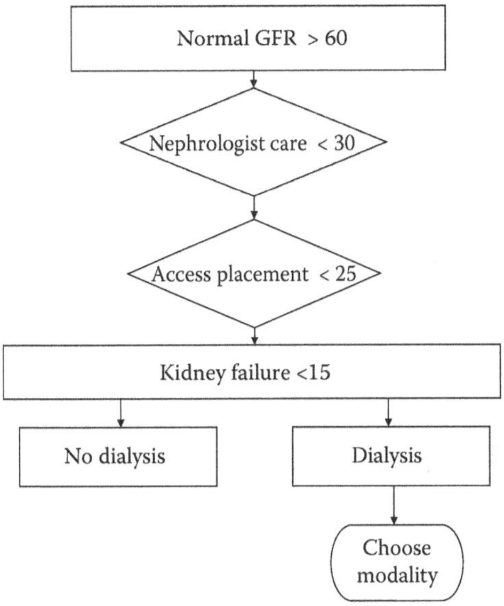

FIGURE 6.2 Decision stages leading to dialysis. (From Guniita/Dreamstime.com, Dreamstime USA Headquarters, Brentwood, TN. With permission.)

encephalopathy, or neuropathy. Progressive uremic symptoms or otherwise unmanageable AEIOU indications are urgent indications for hemodialysis. The decision to initiate dialysis may be made on a more selective basis in the presence of mild uremic symptoms or when there is increasing difficulty controlling complications using medical management alone (Figure 6.2).

There is an ongoing debate over the impact on survival of early versus late hemodialysis initiation. A recent randomized, controlled study did not find improved survival with initiation of early as opposed to late dialysis (Cooper et al., 2010). However, patients who delay the start of dialysis until an acute indication develops, such as severe hyperkalemia, metabolic acidosis, or volume overload, often require hospitalization for emergent initiation of dialysis. Elective initiation can prevent the need for hospitalization for acute hemodialysis.

6.3.1 Benefits

Dialysis may be used for correction of electrolyte abnormalities or acidosis, for clearance of "uremic" or other toxins from the body, and ultrafiltration or removal of excess fluids. Resolution of uremic symptoms with adequate dialysis often results in an increase of patients' oral intake and thus improvement of their nutritional status. Associated comorbidities such as anemia, iron deficiency, and renal osteodystrophy are often treated with medications during dialysis. In addition, nutritional status, lipid profiles, hypertension, and diabetes are monitored regularly as part of dialysis care. Many dialysis centers offer nutritional supplementations in conjunction with careful monitoring by the center's dietician.

6.4 MODALITY SELECTION

Once the decision has been made to initiate dialysis, it is necessary to choose the best modality for the patient. The two modalities for chronic RRT are hemodialysis and peritoneal dialysis. Based on 2009 data from the U.S. Renal Data System (USRDS), 94% of patients in the United States were started on hemodialysis and only 6% of patients were initiated on peritoneal dialysis (USRDS, 2010). The use of peritoneal dialysis is declining in the United States and in other countries (Blake, 2009). Both modalities are not offered in all locations.

In making a choice between hemodialysis and peritoneal dialysis, several factors must be considered, of which the first is availability. Peritoneal dialysis is only an option if there is a peritoneal dialysis program available with a staff that is capable of training patients and having someone available to troubleshoot problems that may arise at home. Patients who live in rural areas may not have easy access to in-center dialysis and may have difficulty traveling to the center three times a week for hemodialysis. Individual patient characteristics, such as the patient's medical comorbidities, compliance, ability to obtain vascular access, and social support, must also be considered.

6.4.1 Peritoneal Dialysis

Peritoneal dialysis as an option for the treatment of renal failure was first described in 1961 and has evolved over the years to the therapy available today (Boen, 1961). Peritoneal dialysis typically occurs in the home, 7 days a week, and involves fewer visits to the clinic, typically one to two visits per month. To be considered for peritoneal dialysis, patients must either be able to perform the procedure themselves or have a support person to assist them. The home environment must be sanitary, and patients must be compliant as they have the primary responsibility for their own RRT. One advantage of peritoneal dialysis is that patients are more independent; they may continue to work and travel, unencumbered by the restraints of hemodialysis. Typically, patients on peritoneal dialysis feel more involved in their care. Residual renal function has a more important role in peritoneal dialysis. Patients on peritoneal dialysis do not experience the frequent hemodynamic changes that patients on hemodialysis are subjected to during the course of treatment and thus often retain more residual renal function than patients on hemodialysis.

In peritoneal dialysis, the peritoneal membrane is used for the exchange of solutes and fluids (Figure 6.3). The peritoneal membrane lines the peritoneal cavity, and it consists of the visceral peritoneum, which lines the organs in the abdominal cavity, and the parietal peritoneum, which lines the peritoneal cavity. The peritoneum serves as the surface across which dialysis occurs; the exchange of solutes and fluids takes place between peritoneal capillaries and the dialysate, which is infused into the peritoneal cavity through a surgically inserted catheter in the patient's abdomen. Each dialysis exchange typically requires 2–3 L of dialysate. Electrolytes and uremic solutes cross the peritoneal membrane in accordance with the principle of diffusion of solutes from areas of high concentration to areas of low concentration. The rate of diffusion is dependent on the characteristics of the patient's peritoneal membrane, which may change over time. During the dwell—the time that the fluid remains in the abdomen—there is equilibration until the concentration of solutes in the dialysate reaches levels

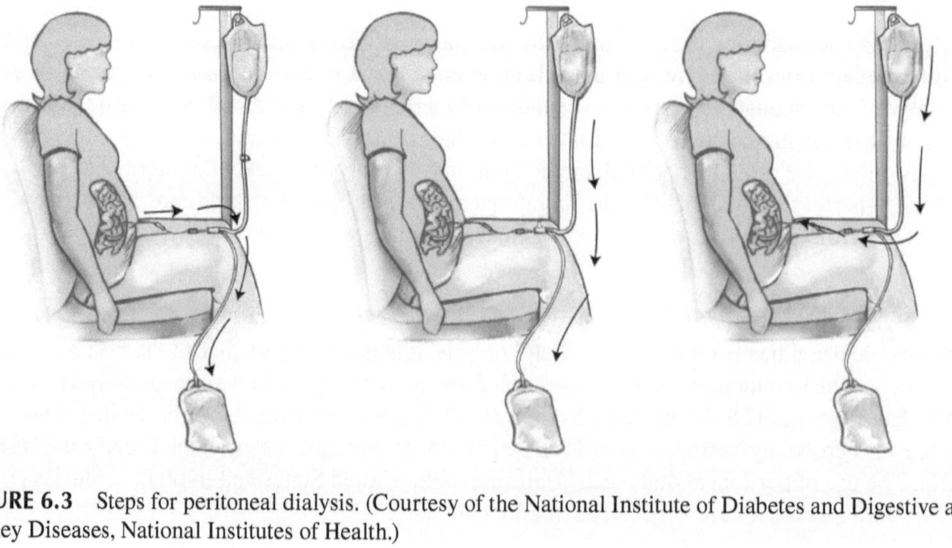

FIGURE 6.3 Steps for peritoneal dialysis. (Courtesy of the National Institute of Diabetes and Digestive and Kidney Diseases, National Institutes of Health.)

near those in the blood. At this point, the fluid should be exchanged, as the clearance or diffusion of solutes is much less effective. This loss of concentration gradient is what necessitates repeated exchanges of dialysate fluid. The transport characteristics of the peritoneal membrane can be determined using the peritoneal equilibration test. The results are then used to individualize a patient's prescription for peritoneal dialysis. High or rapid transporters require short dwells with frequent exchanges. Low or slow transporters have a less efficient membrane for exchange, and this results in the slower transport of solutes. Therefore, low transporters may require longer dwells.

In peritoneal dialysis, ultrafiltration of fluid (volume removal) is achieved using the osmotic force created by high osmolality dialysate solutions. Low (slow) transporters are more successful in obtaining adequate ultrafiltration because they maintain the osmotic gradient for a longer period, allowing better removal of fluid. High (rapid) transporters have a more rapid absorption of the solutes that create the osmotic gradient and therefore have more difficulty achieving adequate ultrafiltration.

6.4.2 Types of Peritoneal Dialysis

There are two main types of peritoneal dialysis: continuous ambulatory peritoneal dialysis (CAPD) and automated peritoneal dialysis (APD), also known as automated continuous cycling peritoneal dialysis. In CAPD, patients perform 4–6 manual fluid exchanges throughout the day. Patients who are on APD use a cycler machine that automatically performs the exchanges, typically at night, often with additional exchanges during the day. Patients who use a cycler machine should also be trained to do manual exchanges so that they will be able to dialyze in the event of a power outage, natural disaster, or cycler malfunction. The peritoneal catheter, used for this procedure, should be placed by an experienced surgeon or nephrologist (Figure 6.4). Patients typically perform exchanges at night and some may leave fluid in the abdomen during the day to allow for additional clearance of solutes. In rapid transporters, longer dwells carry the risk of fluid absorption; thus patients' therapy must be carefully monitored and adjusted as needed.

6.4.3 Complications

The main complication of peritoneal dialysis is peritonitis, signs of which include cloudy fluid in the drainage bag, abdominal pain, and fever. Cell counts and cultures of the peritoneal fluid are used

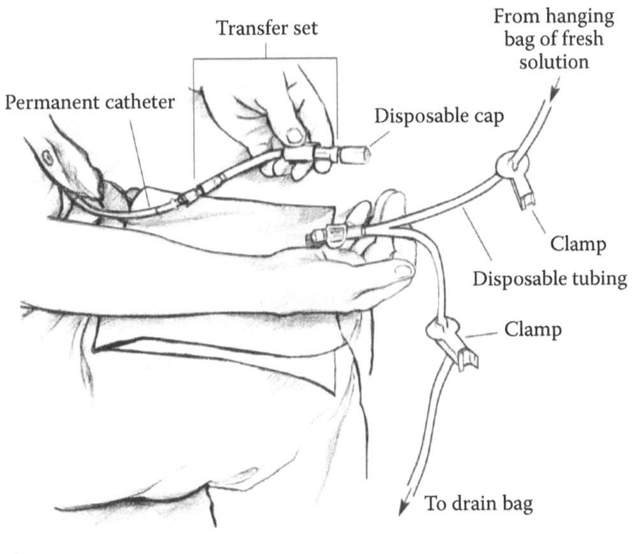

FIGURE 6.4 Peritoneal catheter. (Courtesy of the National Institute of Diabetes and Digestive and Kidney Diseases, National Institutes of Health.)

to confirm peritonitis while empiric antibiotics are started. The preferred method for administering antibiotics is intraperitoneal. Episodes of peritonitis may have detrimental effects on the functionality of the peritoneal membrane (Jovanović et al., 1999). After multiple episodes of peritonitis, the peritoneum may lose the ability to serve as an effective membrane for dialysis. Patients must also be monitored for signs of exit-site infection of the peritoneal catheter.

6.4.4 Adequacy of Dialysis

As with any form of dialysis, it is important to assess the clearance (*Kt*) achieved. In peritoneal dialysis, the total *Kt* = peritoneal *Kt* + renal *Kt* (residual renal function). Thus, the loss of residual renal function may have a significant negative impact on achieving adequate clearance in peritoneal dialysis patients. Clearance also depends on a patient's size (body surface area) as well as the peritoneal membrane transport characteristics (high, high average, low average, or low). Adjustments can be made to the frequency, number, or volume of exchanges as well as in the type of dialysis solution used. Patient comfort can limit the amount of volume used in exchanges, and compliance may be compromised if a high number of manual exchanges or increased time on the cycler machine is required.

6.4.5 Nutrition

Nutrition is very important for peritoneal dialysis patients. Poor nutrition has been shown to increase the relative risk of death, hospitalization, and technique failure in peritoneal dialysis patients (Canada-USA, 1996). There is significant protein loss associated with peritoneal dialysis. The loss of protein is thought to occur through large pores in the peritoneal membrane from the capillaries that supply the membranes. Peritoneal dialysis patients with high peritoneal membrane transport characteristics have more protein losses than patients with low peritoneal membrane transport characteristics (Daugirdas et al., 2006). Protein losses increase during episodes of peritonitis. During dwells, peritoneal dialysis patients have large volumes of dialysate in their peritoneal cavity. This may result in a feeling of fullness that may suppress the desire to eat, negatively impacting the patient's nutritional status. The dialysate fluids are typically dextrose-containing fluids. The glucose in the fluid is systemically absorbed and can impact blood glucose levels and affect appetite (Hylander et al., 1992). Dextrose-containing fluids can negatively impact diabetic control in diabetic patients. Icodextrin is a newer dialysate solution that has less systemic absorption of glucose and allows sustained ultrafiltration as it maintains the osmotic gradient for a longer time (Rodriguez-Carmona et al., 2007).

6.5 HEMODIALYSIS

In hemodialysis, blood passes through a dialyzer to achieve clearance of toxins and removal of fluid. In-center hemodialysis occurs three times per week, and each treatment typically lasts 3–4 h (Figures 6.5 and 6.6). A vascular access or "shunt" is required, as is discussed later. Blood drawn out of the patient through an arterial needle using a blood pump runs on a continuous circuit through the dialyzer and is then returned to the patient via a venous needle. The dialyzer is a tube with two compartments separated by a semipermeable membrane. The blood travels through hollow fibers on one side of the dialyzer's semipermeable membrane; the dialysate runs through the other compartment in the opposite direction on the other side of the dialyzer's semipermeable membrane (Figure 6.7). Dialysate consists of purified water mixed with electrolyte solutions of various concentrations. Solutes are cleared as the blood and dialysate pass in a countercurrent flow. The solutes are cleared from the patient by the process of diffusion from areas of high concentration to areas of low concentration. The properties of the dialysis membrane, the blood flow rate (typically 300–500 mL/min), and dialyzer flow rate (typically 500–800 mL/min), all help to determine the

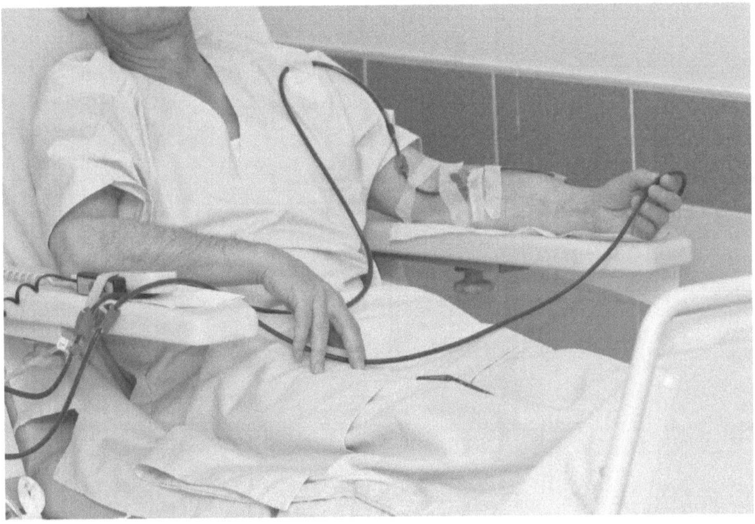

FIGURE 6.5 Patient on hemodialysis. (From Picsfive/Dreamstime.com, Dreamstime USA Headquarters, Brentwood, TN. With permission.)

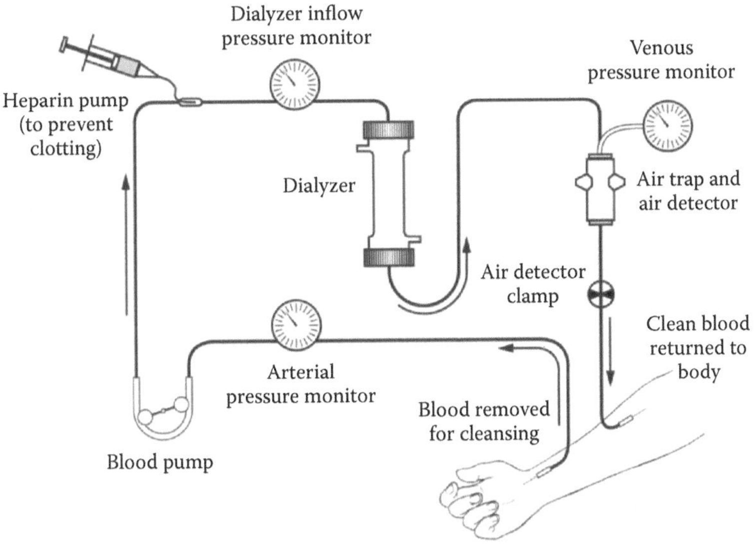

FIGURE 6.6 Mechanics of hemodialysis. (Courtesy of the National Institute of Diabetes and Digestive and Kidney Diseases, National Institutes of Health.)

efficiency of clearance of various solutes. The length of dialysis is adjusted as needed to ensure adequate clearance. Ultrafiltration refers to the removal of fluid using pressure applied across the membrane. Convective transport occurs as solutes move with the ultrafiltrate. Anticoagulation is often used during hemodialysis to prevent clotting of blood in the tubing or as the blood passes through the dialyzer (Figure 6.8).

In some instances, patients may receive hemodialysis at home. The patient's home environment, social support, compliance, and ability to be properly trained to perform dialysis and handle problems are all assessed before this modality is offered. Home hemodialysis may be done three times a week, on a daily basis, or on any schedule in between (Figure 6.9). Intensive dialysis involves increasing the frequency of dialysis or the duration of dialysis to improve clearance or volume removal. Dialysis

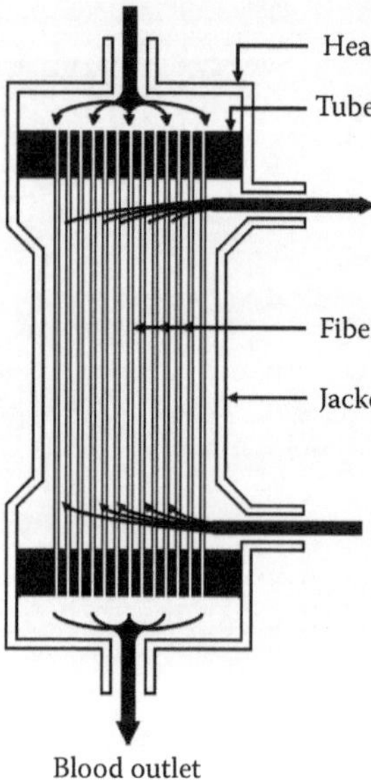

FIGURE 6.7 The dialysis membrane. (Courtesy of the National Institute of Diabetes and Digestive and Kidney Diseases, National Institutes of Health.)

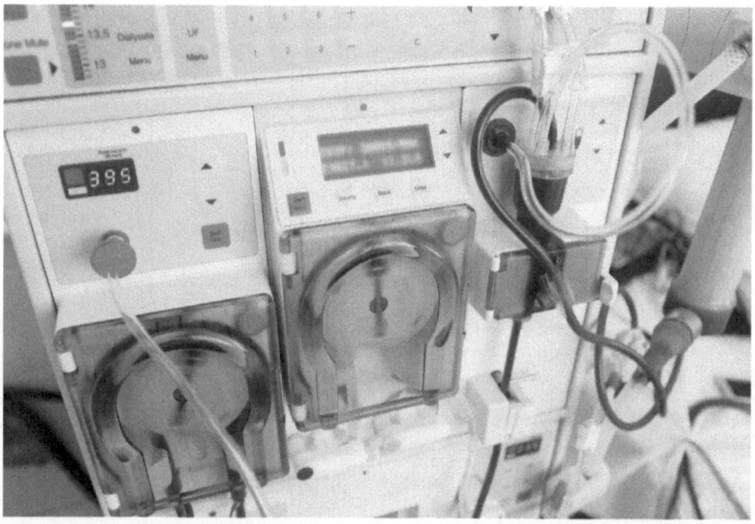

FIGURE 6.8 Typical hemodialysis machine. (From Andre Malov/Dreamstime.com, Dreamstime USA Headquarters, Brentwood, TN. With permission.)

may also be done while the patient sleeps; this is called *nocturnal hemodialysis*. Some centers offer in-center nocturnal hemodialysis, or it may be done in the home. Nocturnal hemodialysis typically has a longer duration and lower blood flow than standard hemodialysis. It is a good option for patients who wish to continue to work. Longer and more frequent dialysis sessions are more physiologic than the typical thrice-weekly short sessions of hemodialysis. Studies have shown improvements in hypertension, hyperphosphatemia, and left ventricular function with more intensive hemodialysis (Chan et al., 2002, 2005; Seabra et al., 2008; Toussaint and Boddington, 2006). Patients receiving nocturnal

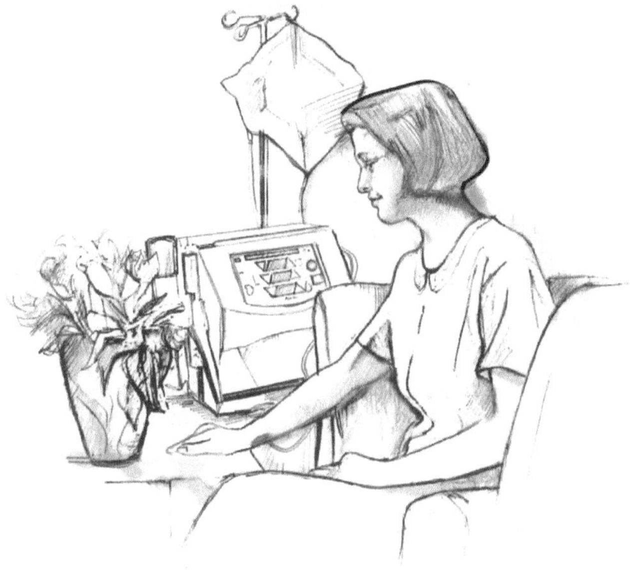

FIGURE 6.9 Patient on home hemodialysis. (Courtesy of the National Institute of Diabetes and Digestive and Kidney Diseases, National Institutes of Health.)

hemodialysis may have improved clearance of fluid, phosphorous, and electrolytes such as potassium allowing for liberalization of the patient's diet. The dietary restrictions imposed during hemodialysis are a frequent source of complaints from dialysis patients. However, a recent study did not demonstrate any significant improvement in measures of quality of life with nocturnal hemodialysis as compared to patients on conventional hemodialysis (Manns and Walsh, 2009).

Serious complications of hemodialysis include hypotension, bleeding, infection, and vascular access issues. Hypotension may occur due to rapid fluid or electrolyte shifts during hemodialysis. Hypotension on hemodialysis is typically treated by decreasing the ultrafiltration rate or giving a fluid bolus. Blood pressure (BP) medications often need to be adjusted after initiation of hemodialysis to avoid intradialytic hypotension. There is a risk of bleeding and blood loss due to the cannulation of large blood vessels, the use of a blood pump to achieve high blood flow rates, and the use of anticoagulation to prevent clotting. Careful monitoring of access sites and monitoring for venous needle dislodgement can help prevent bleeding complications. Sterile technique should always be used to access vascular access sites, and all reusable equipment must be carefully sterilized. To reduce complications, patients must also be educated about how to care for their vascular access or catheters. Serious complications including death may occur if proper care is not taken to avoid contamination and to ensure proper balance and purification by the water delivery systems used in hemodialysis. Less serious, but perhaps the most common complication, is cramping during hemodialysis. Cramping is typically related to fluid and electrolyte shifts and can be improved by limiting weight gains and avoiding high sodium foods. The temperature of dialysate must also be closely monitored. Dialysate above physiologic temperatures may result in hemolysis and patient death. Cooler dialysate temperatures have been shown to improve hemodynamic measures in otherwise unstable patients, but use of this can be limited by patient intolerance.

Labs are monitored and patients are assessed, typically on a monthly basis for hemodialysis patients. The nephrologist provides oversight for the management of lipids, hypertension, electrolytes, anemia, iron deficiency, renal osteodystrophy, and clearance. Adequacy of dialysis is measured and reported as Kt/V, where K is the coefficient of the dialyzer being used, t is the time on hemodialysis, and V is the volume of distribution of urea of the dialyzed patient. Typically, larger patients require more time on hemodialysis to achieve adequate clearance. There is debate about whether there is a better way to scale dialysis dose, such as correcting for metabolic rate, and whether the current *Kt*/*V* gives accurate information for women (Baslie and Vernaglione, 2010; Morton and Singer, 2007; Spalding, 2008). However, for now, *Kt*/*V* remains the accepted standardized measure of adequacy of dialysis.

6.6 VASCULAR ACCESS

A hemodialysis patient's vascular access is considered their lifeline. If one considers that a patient has forearm and upper-arm sites for vascular access in each arm, then there are limited sites for vascular access. Although there are other possible sites for vascular access such as femoral vessels, these are used only as salvage sites once a patient's main access sites have been exhausted. These lifelines must be treated as such. To prevent complications, clotting, and contamination, only trained medical personnel should access a patient's dialysis access. Once patients develop advanced CKD, they should be instructed to protect the future planned vascular access sites. In most cases, this means instructing patients to avoid blood draws or BP checks in their nondominant arm in preparation for vascular access placement. This special consideration is even more critical after the access has been placed. The preferred access for hemodialysis is a fistula, which is a surgically created connection between a vein and artery. It utilizes native vessels that have been surgically reconfigured. Fistulas are the preferred option for dialysis access because they have a lower risk of complications and long duration of use. An alternative vascular access is a graft that uses synthetic material to connect a native artery and vein. A graft is used, if patients are not candidates for fistula placement due to vessel inadequacy or other reasons. However, grafts typically do not have the longevity of a good fistula, and because they involve the implantation of synthetic material, they are more likely to become infected. Temporary or tunneled dual lumen catheters may be used if a fistula or graft is not present at the time hemodialysis is initiated. Catheters have the highest risk of infection and other complications, and should be avoided if possible. There is increasing awareness of the importance of avoiding catheters and obtaining fistulas in all patients who are candidates. The Fistula First initiative has been instrumental in increasing the awareness of this important issue. Obtaining functional vascular access for CKD patients prior to the initiation of hemodialysis is essential. The vascular surgeons who place fistulas or grafts should have experience placing dialysis access and be invested in obtaining good outcomes with close monitoring and follow-up.

6.7 CONTINUOUS RENAL REPLACEMENT THERAPY

Continuous renal replacement therapy (CRRT) is a broad term for various slow, continuous dialysis modalities available at some hospitals for critically ill patients who are not able to tolerate conventional hemodialysis. Various types of CRRT include continuous venovenous hemofiltration (CVVH), continuous venovenous hemodialysis (CVVHD), and continuous venovenous hemodiafiltration (CVVHDF). Please see "Acute Kidney Injury" (Chapter 4) for further information about these modalities. Once initiated, CRRT is typically for 24 h per day, requiring high-intensity intensive care unit (ICU) care. During CRRT, the blood flow and dialysate flow are slower, and the volume and electrolyte removal are at a lower, continuous rate. This modality may be better tolerated by acutely ill, hemodynamically unstable patients, and it may be more successful for patients who require significant volume removal especially those who are hemodynamically unstable. However, CRRT is not available in all hospitals and requires significant resources including ICU staff who are trained to monitor patients on this modality. Given the slow blood flow rates, anticoagulation using heparin- or citrate-based protocols is typically used in CRRT to prevent clotting.

6.8 OUTCOMES IN DIALYSIS

Patients with end-stage renal disease have significantly reduced life expectancy. According to 2009 USRDS data, ESRD patients have a 5-year survival between 30% and 50% (for nondiabetics) and

25% in diabetics (National Kidney Foundation, 2000). Therefore, there has been significant interest in exploring different aspects that may improve patient outcomes. The vast majority of data has involved comparisons between peritoneal and in-center hemodialysis as these are the two primary dialysis modalities. The results have been controversial. Studies that attempted to correct for age and comorbidities have shown conflicting results. One prospective study found that mortality risk was the same during the first year for both hemodialysis and peritoneal dialysis patients, but during the second year, mortality was higher for peritoneal dialysis patients (Jarr et al., 2005). One study found that the survival was less dependent on modality and more influenced by the *Kt*/*V* or the adequacy of dialysis (Keshaviah and Collins, 2002). This finding supported earlier studies that indicated that of all the factors impacting mortality, the most important was dose of dialysis (Collins and Ma, 1994). An Italian study showed similar findings indicating that the most important factors were age and predialysis comorbidity as well as predialysis nutritional status and adequacy of dialysis (Maiorca et al., 1996). A large Canadian study found that the survival advantage of peritoneal dialysis was related to differences in comorbidities at the time of initiation of dialysis. Overall, this study did not determine that there was a difference in survival rates between hemodialysis and peritoneal dialysis patients (Murphy and Foley, 2000).

One study compared the hospitalization rates between patients on the home modalities of daily hemodialysis as compared to peritoneal dialysis. Patients treated with daily hemodialysis had lower rate of hospitalization and shorter length of stay than patients on peritoneal dialysis (Kumar et al., 2008).

Multiple studies have compared intermittent hemodialysis (IHD) to CRRT for acute kidney-injury patients who require RRT. One study found that the modality of RRT did not affect the outcomes of ICU patients with acute kidney injury (Lins et al., 2009). Another study found similar outcomes, but significantly increased ICU-related costs for patients treated with CRRT rather than IHD (Rauf et al., 2008). The lack of significant improvement in outcomes with CRRT has been supported by meta-analyses (Ghahrmani and Shadrou, 2008). However, according to recently published data, the proportion of patients who receive CRRT has increased over time (Afshinnia and Straight, 2009). One systematic review in 2008 found that early initiation of RRT in acute renal failure may be associated with improved survival (Seabra et al., 2008).

6.9 SUMMARY

Deciding to initiate dialysis is a complex process to which patients are often initially resistant. Proper patient education may improve patient outcomes and will improve a patient's ability to participate in the decision making regarding this difficult process. Early nephrology referral and proper dialysis planning will improve outcomes for patients. The main chronic dialysis modalities are hemodialysis and peritoneal dialysis. Individual patient characteristics and social issues must be considered when determining the best modality for a given patient. Alternative dialysis therapies are available, both in the chronic and acute setting, each of which has advantages and disadvantages.

REFERENCES

Afshinnia, F., Straight, A. 2009. Trends in dialysis modality for individuals with acute kidney injury. *Renal Failure* 31(8):647–654.

Baslie, C., Vernaglione, L. 2010. Comparison of alternative methods for scaling dialysis dose. *Nephrol Dial Transplant*. 25(4):1232–1239.

Blake, P. 2009. Proliferation of hemodialysis units and declining peritoneal dialysis use: An international trend. *Am J Kidney Dis*. 54(2):194–196.

Boen, S.T. 1961. Kinetics of peritoneal dialysis. *Medicine* 40:243.

Canada-USA Peritoneal Dialysis Study Group. 1996. Adequacy of dialysis and nutrition in continuous peritoneal dialysis: Associate with clinical outcomes. *J Am Soc Nephrol*. 7:198.

Chan, C., Flores, J., Miller, J., et al. 2002. Improvement in ejection fraction by nocturnal hemodialysis in end stage renal failure patients with coexisting heart failure. *Nephrol Dial Transplant.* 17:1518–1521.

Chan, C., Jain, V., Picton, P. 2005. Nocturnal hemodialysis increases arterial baroreflex sensitivity and compliance and normalizes blood pressure of hypertensive patients with end-stage renal disease. *Kidney Int.* 68:338–344.

Collins, A., Ma, J. 1994. Urea index and other predictors of hemodialysis patient survival. *Am J Kidney Dis.* 23 (2):272–282.

Cooper, B., Branley, P., Bulfone, L., et al. 2010. A randomized, controlled trial of early versus late initiation of dialysis for the IDEAL study. *N Engl J Med.* 363:609–619.

Daugirdas, J., Blake, P., Ing, T. 2006. *Handbook of Dialysis*, 4th edn. Lippincott Williams & Williams.

Ghahrmani, N., Shadrou, S. 2008. A systematic review of continuous renal replacement therapy and intermittent hemodialysis in management of patients with acute renal failure. *Nephrology* 13(7):570–578.

Hylander, B., Barkeling, B., Rossner, S. 1992. Eating behavior in continuous ambulatory peritoneal dialysis and hemodialysis. *Am J Kidney Dis.* 20:592.

Jarr, B., Coresh, J., Plantinga, L. 2005. Comparing the risk for death with peritoneal dialysis and hemodialysis in a national cohort of patients with chronic kidney disease. *Ann Intern Med.* 143:174.

Jovanović, D., Nesić, V., Dimitrijevic, Z. 1999. The effect of the number of peritonitis episodes on peritoneal membrane function. *Srp Arh Celok Lek.* 127(1–2):28–31.

Keshaviah, P., Collins, A. 2002. Survival comparison between hemodialysis and peritoneal dialysis based on matched doses of delivered therapy. *Am Soc Nephrol.* 13(Suppl):S48–S52.

Kessler, M., Frimat, L., Panescu, V., et al. 2003. Impact of nephrology referral on early and midterm outcomes in ESRD: EPidémiologie de l'Insuffisance REnale chronique terminale en Lorraine (EPIREL): Results of a 2-year, prospective, community-based study. *Am J Kidney Dis.* 42(3):474–485.

Kumar, V., Ledezma, M., Idroos, M. 2008. Hospitalization rates in daily home hemodialysis versus peritoneal dialysis patients in the United States. *Am J Kidney Dis.* 52(4):737–744.

Lins, R., Eiseviers, M., Van der Niepen, P. 2009. Intermittent versus continuous renal replacement therapy of acute kidney injury patients admitted to the intensive care unit: Results of a randomized clinical trial. *Nephrol Dial Transplant.* 24(2):512–518.

Maiorca, R., Cancarini, G., Brunori, G. 1996. Comparison of long-term survival between hemodialysis and peritoneal dialysis. *Adv Perit Dial.* 12:79–88.

Manns, B., Walsh, M. 2009. Nocturnal hemodialysis does not improve overall measures of quality of life compared to conventional hemodialysis. *Kidney Int.* 75(5):542–549.

Morton, A., Singer, M. 2007. The problem with Kt/V: Dialysis dose should be normalized to metabolic rate not volume. *Semin Dial.* 20(1):12–15.

Murphy, S., Foley, R. 2000. Comparative mortality of hemodialysis and peritoneal dialysis in Canada. *Kidney Int.* 57:1720–1726.

National Kidney Foundation. 2006. K/DOQI Clinical Practice Guidelines for Vascular Access. Guideline 8, Timing of Access Placement. *Am J Kidney Dis.* 48:S176–S247, Suppl 1.

National Kidney Foundation. 2007. K/DOQI Clinical Practice Guidelines for Chronic Kidney Disease Evaluation, Classification, and Stratification. Part 5. Definition and Classification of Stages of Chronic Kidney Disease. *Am J Kidney Dis.* 49(2):S12–S154, Suppl 2.

Rauf, A., Long, K., Gajic, O., et al. 2008. Intermittent hemodialysis versus continuous renal replacement therapy for acute renal failure in the intensive care unit: An observational outcomes analysis. *J Intensive Care Med.* 23(3):195–203.

Rodriguez-Carmona, A., Perez Fontan, M., Garcia Lopez, E., et al. 2007. Use of icodextrin during nocturnal automated peritoneal dialysis allows sustained ultrafiltration while reducing the peritoneal glucose load: A randomized crossover study. *Periton Dialysis Int.* 27(3):260–266.

Seabra, V., Balk, E., Liangos, O., et al. 2008. Timing of renal replacement therapy initiation in acute renal failure: A meta-analysis. *Am J Kidney Dis.* 52(2):272–284.

Spalding, E. 2008. Kt/V underestimates the hemodialysis dose in women and small men. *Kidney Int.* 74(3):348–355.

Toussaint, N., Boddington, J. 2006. Calcium phosphate metabolism and bone mineral density with nocturnal hemodialysis. *Hemodial Int.* 10:280–286.

United States Renal Data System. 2010. Excerpts from the USRDS 2009 annual data report: Atlas of end-stage renal disease in the United States. *Am J Kidney Dis.* 1(Suppl 1):S1.

7 Nutrition Care Process
Screening and Assessment

Claire Moise
WJB Dorn VA Medical Center

Lynn K. Thomas
University of South Carolina School of Medicine

CONTENTS

7.1 KIDNEY DISEASE: PAST AND PRESENT—INTRODUCTION

Nutrition problems of patients with chronic kidney disease (CKD) should be addressed in all medical care settings. Nutrition screening and assessment are the building blocks of planning nutrition intervention for patients with CKD. Nutrition care process (NCP) starts with screening by a qualified health-care provider who will identify individuals at nutrition risk who have the need for a more detailed assessment. If the screening instrument's criteria indicate the need for a detailed assessment, then a comprehensive nutrition evaluation will follow.

In CKD, nutrition assessment encompasses the same elements across all stages. It provides dietary information that is more than pertinent. A complete assessment encompasses the patient's current medical history, past medical history, environmental concerns, medications, physical examination, diet history, and current food intake.

Ideally, a renal dietitian will complete the nutrition assessment, especially in the later stages of CKD. When a renal dietitian is not available, an experienced clinical dietitian is also capable of completing an inclusive review of a patient's nutrition status. The use of an electronic medical record allows for ready access to all the information provided by many team members in a physician practice setting, a hospital setting, or a dialysis clinic. A thorough search of the entries will ensure a complete nutrition assessment.

The American Dietetic Association (2008) supports the use of standardized terminology for the NCP. The NCP includes four steps: assessment, diagnosis, intervention, and monitoring/evaluation. In this chapter, the discussion on NCP is limited to assessment.

7.2 NUTRITION SCREENING

In the early stages of CKD, nutrition screening may be used to identify individuals who are at the risk for malnutrition. The American Dietetic Association Evidence Based Library (ADA, 2011) defines screening as the process of identifying patients, clients, or groups who may have a nutrition diagnosis and benefit from nutrition assessment and intervention by a registered dietitian (RD). Key considerations for screening are as follows (ADA, 2011):

- Nutrition screening may be conducted in any practice setting as appropriate.
- Nutrition screening tools should be quick; easy to use; and valid and reliable for the patient, population, or setting. Usually screenings are completed in less than 10 min.
- Nutrition screening tools and parameters are established by RDs, but the screening process may be carried out by others who have been trained in nutrition screening.
- Nutrition screening and rescreening should occur within an appropriate time frame for the setting.

Typical criteria used for screening include history of weight loss (% of usual body weight, body mass index [BMI], etc.), loss of appetite, malnourished appearance, laboratory indices, and effect of current medical problems. Several inclusive screening instruments such as the Malnutrition Universal Screening Tool (Weekes et al., 2004), the Mini Nutritional Assessment—Short Form (Kaiser et al., 2009), and the Short Nutritional Assessment Questionnaire (Kruizenga et al., 2005) are available. They are useful for screening patients in the early stages of CKD in which the focus is on control of comorbidities (Figure 7.1). An appropriate follow-up time frame should be in place for rescreening.

7.3 NUTRITION ASSESSMENT

The comprehensive nutrition assessment is composed of many individual components, which when put together build a picture of a patient's nutrition risk, allow for an accurate nutrition diagnosis to be made, and help formulate a plan of care. Food-intake interview should be conducted with as much privacy as possible. In a clinic or in an outpatient setting, a separate office can be used, if available, for the interview. A pull curtain can help increase privacy in shared spaces. Start the interview with introductions; explain to the patient the purpose of the assessment and also why certain questions will be asked. Acknowledge the answers and thank the patient and/or the patient's family for cooperating.

7.3.1 Subjective Global Assessment

The subjective global assessment (SGA) is a very popular assessment tool for the general adult population. It has been validated and found to be reliable many times. The SGA is often used to assess patients in the early stages of CKD. It is comprehensive and requires no laboratory testing. Steiber et al. (2007) found the SGA tool to be valid and reliable for use among patients with stage 5 CKD hemodialysis. The KDOQI™ Clinical Practice Guidelines (2000) also recommends the use of this

Nestlé Nutrition Institute

Mini Nutritional Assessment
MNA®

Last name:		First name:		
Sex:	Age:	Weight, kg:	Height, cm:	Date:

Complete the screen by filling in the boxes with the appropriate numbers. Total the numbers for the final screening score.

Screening

A Has food intake declined over the past 3 months due to loss of appetite, digestive problems, chewing or swallowing difficulties?
0 = severe decrease in food intake
1 = moderate decrease in food intake
2 = no decrease in food intake

B Weight loss during the last 3 months
0 = weight loss greater than 3 kg (6.6 lbs)
1 = does not know
2 = weight loss between 1 and 3 kg (2.2 and 6.6 lbs)
3 = no weight loss

C Mobility
0 = bed or chair bound
1 = able to get out of bed / chair but does not go out
2 = goes out

D Has suffered psychological stress or acute disease in the past 3 months?
0 = yes 2 = no

E Neuropsychological problems
0 = severe dementia or depression
1 = mild dementia
2 = no psychological problems

F1 Body Mass Index (BMI) (weight in kg) / (height in m^2)
0 = BMI less than 19
1 = BMI 19 to less than 21
2 = BMI 21 to less than 23
3 = BMI 23 or greater

IF BMI IS NOT AVAILABLE, REPLACE QUESTION F1 WITH QUESTION F2.
DO NOT ANSWER QUESTION F2 IF QUESTION F1 IS ALREADY COMPLETED.

F2 Calf circumference (CC) in cm
0 = CC less than 31
3 = CC 31 or greater

Screening score
(max. 14 points)

12-14 points: Normal nutritional status
8-11 points: At risk of malnutrition
0-7 points: Malnourished

Ref. Vellas B, Villars H, Abellan G, et al. *Overview of the MNA® - Its History and Challenges.* J Nutr Health Aging 2006;10:456-465.
Rubenstein LZ, Harker JO, Salva A, Guigoz Y, Vellas B. *Screening for Undernutrition in Geriatric Practice: Developing the Short-Form Mini Nutritional Assessment (MNA-SF).* J. Geront 2001;56A: M366–377.
Guigoz Y. *The Mini-Nutritional Assessment (MNA®) Review of the Literature - What does it tell us?* J Nutr Health Aging 2006; 10:466–487.
Kaiser MJ, Bauer JM, Ramsch C, et al. *Validation of the Mini Nutritional Assessment Short-Form (MNA®-SF): A practical tool for identification of nutritional status.* J Nutr Health Aging 2009; 13:782–788.

FIGURE 7.1 Mini Nutrition Assessment—Short Form. (From Nestlé S.A., Mini nutrition assessment, N67200 12/99 10M, 1994, Revision 2009. With permission.)

tool. The SGA uses these core categories: weight status, dietary intake, gastrointestinal symptoms, functional status, metabolic stress, and physical examination (Detsky et al., 1987; Figure 7.2).

7.3.2 Medical History

Medical history usually includes the chief complaint or the most current diagnosis. Comorbidities, past illnesses, and surgeries that might affect present nutrition status are recorded in the history. Previous gastrointestinal diseases and gastric surgeries should also be identified. Questions regarding the past weight and the rate of any recent weight loss and whether the patient is experiencing nausea, vomiting, constipation, or diarrhea should be posed to the patient. Any reported food allergies or intolerances should be documented. Questions regarding physical activity and sleep patterns should be asked. Limb amputations, organ transplants, ostomies, slow wound healing, and complications during past medical procedures should be recorded if there is any likelihood that these would affect the nutrition status of the patient.

SUBJECTIVE GLOBAL ASSESSMENT OF Nutrition STATUS

TABLE I

Features of subjective global assessment (SGA)

(Select appropriate category with a checkmark, or enter numerical value where indicated by "#."

A. History

1. Weight change

Overall loss in past 6 months: amount = # ________ kg; % loss = #

Change in past 2 weeks: ________ increase,

________ no change,

________ decrease.

2. Dietary intake change (relative to normal)

________ No change,

________ Change ________ duration = # ________ weeks

________ type: ________ suboptimal liquid diet,

________ full liquid diet

________ hypocaloric liquids,

________ starvation.

3. Gastrointestinal symptoms (that persisted for >2 weeks)

________ none, ________ nausea, ________ vomiting, ________ diarrhea, ________ anorexia

4. Functional capacity

________ No dysfunction (e.g., full capacity),

________ Dysfunction ________ duration = # ________ weeks.

________ type: ________ working suboptimally,

________ ambulatory,

________ bedridden.

5. Disease and its relation to nutrition requirements

Primary diagnosis (specify) ________

Metabolic demand (stress): ________ no stress, ________ low stress,

________ moderate stress, ________ high stress.

B. Physical (for each trait specify: 0 = normal, 1+ = mild, 2+ = moderate, 3+ = severe).

________ loss of subcutaneous fat (triceps, chest)

________ muscle wasting (quadriceps;, deltoids)

________ ankle edema

________ sacral edema

________ ascites.

C. SGA rating (select one]

________ A = Well nourished

________ B = Moderately (or suspected of being) malnourished

________ C = Severely malnourished

FIGURE 7.2 Subjective Global Assessment. (Reproduced from Detsky, A. et al., *J. Parenteral Enteral Nutr.*, 11, 9, 1987. With permission of American Society for Parenteral and Enteral Nutrition.)

7.3.3 The Effect of Comorbidities

Comorbidities have a profound effect on nutrition risk. Cardiovascular disease and diabetes mellitus complicate the nutrition care plan by compounding dietary restrictions over and above the various therapeutic renal diets. Disease or surgery of the gastrointestinal tract alters absorption of nutrients. Cancer can increase metabolic needs, and cancer treatments can cause malabsorption. Autoimmune diseases increase the risk of malnutrition. Diminished sight or hearing loss can alter the ability to shop and prepare food. In the early stages of CKD, the control of comorbidities can delay the rate of kidney failure.

7.3.4 Medications and Drug–Nutrient Interactions

The dietitian should document all medications and over-the-counter supplements used by the patient. The dietitian should pose questions such as "How are medications taken?" "How many medications are being taken?" "Are they taken as prescribed?" and "Was there recent use of antibiotics?" to the patient, ask specifically about laxative use, and note specifically the vitamin and mineral supplements taken by the patient. The dietitian should also ask about the timing of intake of phosphate binders and about any "home-grown" or herbal supplements. The nutrition assessment can be a time of education on the safe and appropriate selection and use of nutrition supplements (ADA, 2009). Medications can affect nutrition status by altering the taste of foods, changing appetite, and causing dry mouth, nausea, diarrhea, constipation, or altered absorption.

The dietitian should be alert to possible loss of vitamins, minerals, and electrolytes. Low albumin should also be noted. Low serum values will provide fewer binding sites for protein-bound drugs, resulting in more unbound drug and a larger pharmacologic effect. Any drug–nutrient/food interactions should always be documented. For example, eating high-vitamin-K foods such as spinach and kale will lower effectiveness of anticoagulant medications. Another example, iron supplements should be taken on an empty stomach since some foods will bind the iron and lower absorption (Pronsky and Crowe 2008).

7.3.5 Psychosocial History

Psychosocial history can provide insights to the way mental status or the environment affects dietary intake. Alcohol and recreational drug use are often identified in this portion of the assessment. The dietitian should record whether a recent crisis or a change in stress level has affected food intake. Physical or psychiatric impairments that affect the activities of daily living should also be recorded. In an older patient, mental status exam can be helpful to determine the patient's ability to comply with recommendations. The dietitian should also record whether the patient is undergoing any medical therapies, such as dialysis, chemotherapy, physical therapy, or radiation therapy, and whether it has been difficult for the patient to access health-care services.

An effort should be made to establish literacy level, uncover any language barriers, and look for cultural and religious factors that might affect food intake. Answers to questions such as "Is family support adequate?" "Does the patient live alone?" "Who does the shopping and cooking?" "Are there transportation problems?" "Is housing adequate?" "Inside plumbing available?" "Are there financial difficulties?" and "Does the patient know where to find help?" should be sought (Cresci, 2004).

7.3.6 Diet History

The start of a diet history can overlap with certain questions from the medical history. Details about food intolerances and allergies are often entered in the medical history by other members of the medical team. Frequently, inquiries about recent weight loss and whether or not the change was intentional are also found in the medical history. Questions about over-the-counter supplements might be documented in the medication review. Questions for the diet history include the following: "When was the last complete meal?" "Are there any chewing and swallowing difficulties?" "Is there a problem with dryness, pain, or sores in the mouth?" "Are teeth/dentures in good condition?" Questions about appetite are important. Information about any special diets needs to be documented. Details regarding meal patterns and whether the patient has anything else to tell about diets or foods should be documented.

Although many patients will readily give an accurate account of a day's food intake, it would be helpful to quantify intake over time. Recording the intake of certain items over time is also important. A food frequency questionnaire or 3–7-day food diaries can be beneficial when looking for deficiencies or overages. Food models and food pictures are ways patients can show meal patterns and portion amounts. Once the data are obtained, the dietitian can then do the analysis either manually or using a computerized analysis program. The U.S. Department of Agriculture offers a free analysis program on http://www.choosemyplate.gov and an accessible nutrient database on http://www.nal.usda.gov/fnic/foodcomp/search (USDA, 2011; Williams, 2003).

7.3.7 Physical Examination

A focused physical examination will help alert the dietitian or other health practitioner to signs of nutrition deficiencies. Muscle and fat wasting are usually readily identified. Other macrosigns include overall appearance, ascites, decreased skin turgor, liver enlargement, and parotid gland hypertrophy. Table 7.1 lists many of the more common signs of malnutrition. Blood pressure and radial pulse readings should be obtained or documented if those readings have been previously obtained by other team members. Physical examination is also an integral part of the SGA.

7.3.8 Height, Weight, and Other Anthropometric Measures

A patient's height should be measured from a standing position if at all possible. If one is unable to obtain an accurate height, then other approaches should be considered (Table 7.2). Knee height and arm span are often used to predict stature (Chumlea et al., 1998; Hwang et al., 2009; Figure 7.3). These measures are close estimates, not exact.

Frame size can be determined by elbow breadth (Frisancho, 1984). Wrist circumference is also widely used, but it is not as statistically accurate as elbow breadth (Mitchell, 1993). Elbow breadth is determined by measuring the breadth of the epicondyle (two prominent bones) on either side of the elbow while the elbow is flexed in an upward position (Table 7.3).

Weight should also be documented from measurement, not from report. Once actual body weight or dry weight is obtained, it should be evaluated in relationship to height, usual body weight, BMI, and body composition. Adjustments for amputation should be made (Figure 7.4) as needed (Osterkamp, 1995). BMI is calculated by using Quetelet's formula (weight in kilograms/height in square meters). Results are assessed using a nomogram or a table (Table 7.4). A waist circumference of over 40 in. for men and over 35 in. for women is an indicator of increased risk in persons with BMI >24.9 or persons who are overweight. The measurement should be done 1 in. below the umbilicus (NIDDK, 2011). The Hamwi Method for Desirable Body Weight (DBW) or Ideal Body Weight (IBW) can help evaluate current weight status also (Hamwi, 1964; Table 7.5).

The KDODI™ guidelines (KDOQI, 2000) recommend the use of standard body weight for nutrient calculations, but the BMI tables are preferred now. Usual body weight is a useful consideration in the estimation of fluid status and the percentage of any recent weight change. The Blackburn (1977) formula is widely used: significant weight loss = 5% in 1 month, >7.5% in 3 months, and >10% in 6 months. Another weight-change formula by Dr. Blackburn is also used as a predictor of malnutrition risk: percent usual body weight: 85%–95% = mild malnutrition, 75%–84% = moderate malnutrition, and <74% = severe malnutrition.

TABLE 7.1
Physical Examination Findings and Possible Deficiencies

	Findings	Deficiency	Excess
Eyes	Xerophthalmia	Vitamin A	
	Blurred vision		Vitamin A
	Pale conjunctiva	Iron	
Mouth	Cracking teeth	Vitamin A	
	Decreased saliva	Riboflavin, folate	
	Glossitis	Cobalamin	
	Cheilosis	Ascorbic acid	
	Bleeding gums	Niacin	
	Atrophic papillae		
Hair	Alopecia	Protein-calorie, biotin	
	Brittle, pluckable	Zinc	
	Color change	Vitamin A	
	Dryness		
Nails	Transverse ridging	Protein	
	Koilonychia	Iron	
Extremities	Osteomalacia	Vitamin D	
	Muscle twitching	Thiamine	
	Muscle weakness	Riboflavin	
Skin	Dry, scaly, keratinization	Vitamin A	
	Dermatitis	Riboflavin	
	Cheilosis	Ascorbic acid	
	Ecchymosis		
	Petchiae		
	Flushing and yellow pigmentation of palms with normal white sclera		Niacin Excess beta carotene
Systems	Kidney stones		Vitamin D
	Increased prothrombin time	Vitamin K	
	Enlarged heart	Thiamine	
	Beriberi	Niacin	
	Pellagra	Cobalamin, Thiamine	
	Neurological	Vitamin A	
	Decrease immune function		

Source: Food and Nutrition Board, Institute of Medicine, *Dietary Reference Intakes*, National Academies Press, Washington, DC, 2006. With permission; Food and Nutrition Board, Institute of Medicine, . *Dietary Reference Intake: Water,* 2011. Online: http://iom.edu/Activities/Nutrition/SummaryDRIs/~/media/Files/Activity%20Files/Nutrition/DRIs/DRI_Electrolytes_Water.ashx (accessed 30 May 2011). With permission.

Triceps skin fold (TSF) thickness and arm muscle area (AMA) measurements are useful in predicting body composition. TSF is an index of body fat stores, and AMA represents muscle protein. Both measurements are taken using the midpoint of the patient's arm (Figure 7.5). A caliper is used for measuring the TSF, and a measuring tape is used for determining the AMA. Further calculations are required for deriving the AMA: mid-arm circumference − (TSF × 0.314) = mid-arm muscle circumference (MAMC). AMA = (MAMC) 2/12.56. Tables of reference data are used to determine percentile ranks (Table 7.6). In the elderly, change in body composition over time can decrease the reliability of these assessments (Frisancho, 1989).

TABLE 7.2
Determination of Height

	Method	Comments
Arm span	Fully extend the upper extremities including hands; hold parallel to the ground; measure the distance between the tip of one middle finger to the tip of the opposite middle finger	Measurement will be within 10% of adult height
Knee height	Equation: Men = (2.02 × knee height in cm) – (0.04 × age) + 64.19 Women = (1.83 × knee height in cm) – (0.24 × age) + 84.88 Convert to inches by dividing the result by 2.54	Used for those with curvature of the spine, who are bedridden or who are using wheel chair
Stature prediction in the elderly using knee height (cm) (Chumlea et al., 1998)	Non-Hispanic white men: Stature = 78.31 + (1.94 knee height) – (0.14 age) Non-Hispanic black men: Stature = 79.69 + (1.85 knee height) – (0.14 age) Mexican American men: Stature = 82.77 + (1.83 knee height) – (0.16 age) Non-Hispanic white women: Stature = 82.21 + (1.85 knee height) – (0.21 age) Non-Hispanic black women: Stature = 89.58 + (1.61 knee height) – (0.17 age) Mexican American women Stature = 84.25 + (1.82 knee height) – (0.26 age)	

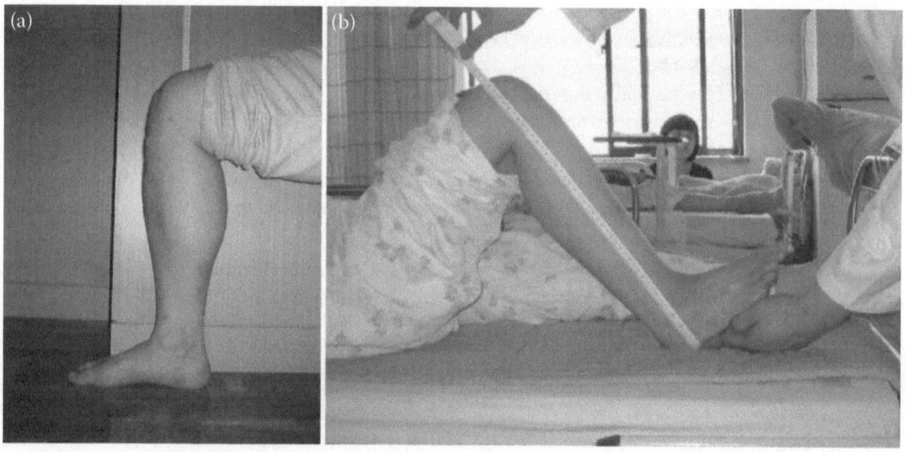

FIGURE 7.3 Knee height calculations. (Adapted from Hwang, C., et al., *Epidemiol. Health,* 31, 1–6, 2009.) Body position for the measurement of knee height in clinical validation group: (a) healthy elderly group and (b) mobility-impaired group. In both groups, knee height was measured using a flexible tape, whereas the knee and ankle joints were flexed at 90°. (a) It was measured in the sitting position with a tape attached to the wall and was defined as the distance between the floor and suprapatellar point. This method is identical to the one used in "Size Korea 2004." (b) In recumbent position, the measured distance is between landing point and suprapatellar point from lateral side.

7.3.9 Nutrient Calculations

Total daily energy needs are based on best estimates using one of the many formulas available. An experienced renal dietitian will choose the appropriate formula once the stage of CKD and other factors are identified in the complete nutrition assessment. One of the more challenging variables is the adjustment for physical activity for patients on hemodialysis. One recent study suggested that

TABLE 7.3
Frame Size from Elbow Breadth in Centimeters

Age (years)	Small Frame	Medium Frame	Large Frame
Males			
25–34	≤6.7	>6.7 – <7.9	≥7.9
35–44	≤6.7	>6.7 – <8.0	≥8.0
45–74	≤6.7	>6.7 – <8.1	≥8.1
Females			
25–34	≤5.7	>5.7 – <6.8	≥6.8
35–44	≤5.7	>5.7 – <7.1	≥7.1
45–54	≤5.7	>5.7 – <7.2	≥7.2
55–64	≤5.8	>5.8 – <7.2	≥7.2

Source: Frisancho, A. *Am. J. Clin. Nutr.*, 40, 808–819, 1984.

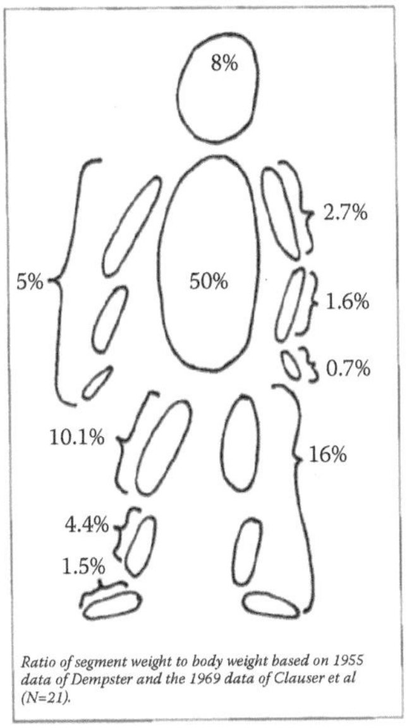

FIGURE 7.4 Adjustments for amputees. (Reprinted from *Journal of the American Dietetic Association,* 95, Osterkamp, L., Current perspective on assessment of human body proportions of relevance to amputees, 217, 1995, with permission from Elsevier.)

activity-related energy expenditure is as much as 53% lower on days on which the patient is on dialysis and 28% lower on days on which the patient is not on dialysis (Baria et al., 2011).

Most calculations for daily energy expenditure will equate to 30–35 cal/kg for patients with CKD. Besides the formulas for energy estimation, formulas for estimation of adjusted weight and dry weight are available.

The National Kidney Foundation (NFK) KDOQI™ Clinical practice guidelines recommends a range of 30–50 cal/kg actual or dry weight categorized based on the stage of CKD and on variations for age, weight, stress, etc. (Masud and Mitch, 2010; NKF, 2000). Other equations such as the Harris–Benedict formula with adjustments for stress can be used for calculating the total energy expenditure (Harris and Benedict, 1919).

Men: Basal energy expenditure (BEE) = 66.42 + 13.75 (weight) + 5.0 (height) – 6.8 (age).

Women: BEE = 655.1 + 9.65 (weight) + 1.85 (height) – 4.68 (age)

TABLE 7.4
BMI Table

	Normal						Overweight					Obese		
	19	**20**	**21**	**22**	**23**	**24**	**25**	**26**	**27**	**28**	**29**	**30**	**35**	**40**
Height (in.)							**Weight (lb)**							
58	91	96	100	105	110	115	119	124	129	134	138	143	167	191
59	94	99	104	109	114	119	124	128	133	138	143	148	173	198
60	97	102	107	112	118	123	128	133	138	143	148	153	179	204
61	100	106	111	116	122	127	132	137	143	148	153	158	185	211
62	104	109	115	120	126	131	136	142	147	153	158	164	191	218
63	107	113	118	124	130	135	141	146	152	158	163	169	197	225
64	110	116	122	128	134	140	145	151	157	163	169	174	204	232
65	114	120	126	132	138	144	150	156	162	168	174	180	210	240
66	118	124	130	136	142	148	155	161	167	173	179	186	216	247
67	121	127	134	140	146	153	159	166	172	178	185	191	223	255
68	125	131	138	144	151	158	164	171	177	184	190	197	230	262
69	128	135	142	149	155	162	169	176	182	189	196	203	236	270
70	132	139	146	153	160	167	174	181	188	195	202	207	243	278
71	136	143	150	157	165	172	179	186	193	200	208	215	250	286
72	140	147	154	162	169	177	184	191	199	206	213	221	258	294
73	144	151	159	166	174	182	189	197	204	212	219	227	265	302
74	148	155	163	171	179	186	194	202	210	218	225	233	272	311
75	152	160	168	176	184	192	200	208	216	224	232	240	279	319
76	156	164	172	180	189	197	205	213	221	230	238	246	287	328

Source: Parameters for normal based on *Federal Obesity Clinical Guidelines, National Heart Lung and Blood Institute*, 2000.

TABLE 7.5
Hamwi Method for DBW or IBW

Men: 106 pounds for first 5 feet and 6 pounds for every additional inch
Women: 100 pounds for first 5 feet and 5 pounds for every additional inch
Add or subtract 10% to accommodate large or small frame size
Subtract 5%–10% from DBW for paraplegia
Subtract 10%–15% from DBW for quadriplegia

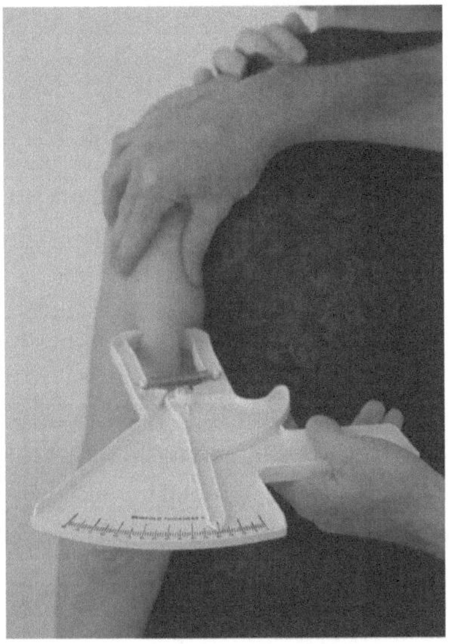

FIGURE 7.5 TSF measurement illustration. (From Shaun Riffle, USC School of Medicine, Columbia, SC. With permission.)

In the aforementioned formulas, weight, height, and age are expressed in kilograms, centimeters, and years, respectively.

Total energy expenditure (TEE) = BEE × stress factor. The stress factor varies from 0.85 in simple starvation to 1.4 in sepsis. Most patients with CKD fall in the 1.0–1.2 range (Barak et al., 2002).

The Ireton–Jones energy equation for spontaneously breathing patients is also widely used:

Estimated energy expenditure (EEE) calories per day = 629 − 11 (age/years) + 25 (weight/kg) − 609 (presence of obesity factor)

Presence of obesity factor = 30% > IBW (absent = 0, present = 1) (Ireton–Jones and Jones, 1998).

Adjusted-weight formulas are recommended when a patient is above 125% of DBW. This recommendation is based on the premise that in an obese patient not all fat is metabolically active. The usual adjustment is as follows: DBW + [(actual BW − IBW × 0.25)] (Frankenfield et al., 2003). If nutrient recommendations are based on actual body weight, then an overestimation might occur (Frisancho, 1984). Upon review, the Mifflin–St. Jeor formula has been found to have one of the smallest overestimation errors (Frankenfield et al., 2005). The formula is as follows (Mifflin et al., 1990):

Men: RMR = 9.99 × weight + 6.25 × height − 4.92 × age + 5.

Women: RMR = 9.99 × weight + 6.25 × height − 4.92 × age − 161.

Here, RMR is the resting metabolic rate in calories per day. Weight is expressed in kilograms and height in centimeters.

TABLE 7.6
TSF and AMA: Abbreviated Reference Table

TSF Adult Male (18–65 Years; Measured in mm)	Percentile (%)	AMAC Adult Male (18–65 Years; Measured in cm)
4.0–5.0	10	37.3–38.7
10.0–11.5	50	49.4–52.1
17.5–20.0	85	61.8–64.8
TSF Adult Female (18–65 Years; Measured in mm)		**AMAC Adult Female (18–65 Years; Measured in cm)**
11.0–16.0	10	21.5–24.5
12.0–17.5	50	28.3–34.5
18.5–26.0	85	36.4–45.6

Source: Frisancho, A. *Anthropometric Standards for the Assessment of Growth and Nutrition Status*, University of Michigan Press, Ann Arbor, MI, 1989.

Fluid management is dependent on the severity of acute kidney failure or on the stage of CKD. Goals include balanced hydration and normalized electrolytes. Insensible losses, input/output measures, and any fevers, sweating, or gastric/kidney fluid losses secondary to the current medical problem should all be considered when establishing a daily fluid limit for the patient (Whitmire, 1998). The Holliday–Segar equation (1957) is used to estimate general fluid needs:

For weight >20 kg, use 1500 mL + 20 mL/kg for each kg >20.

The Food and Nutrition Board, Institute of Medicine (2011) sets the dietary reference intake of all fluids as 3.7 L/day for men and 2.7 L/day for women.

Daily protein, vitamin, and mineral requirements vary based on the stage of CKD. Each of these elements is discussed in later chapters for both pediatric and adult indications.

7.3.10 Laboratory Data

Laboratory assessment is essential for complete nutrition assessment. Values will vary from laboratory to laboratory depending on analytical methods and procedures. Target ranges will change based on the stage of CKD and the goals of the physician or the clinic. Table 7.7 presents a list of laboratory tests often used in nutrition assessment. Values are given in SI units (NFK 2000; Khan et al., 2002). Accurate interpretation of data is important. Progress in one parameter may only indicate a trend or a partial benefit, whereas decline in a parameter could indicate reduced oral intake. The overarching goals of the assessment are to achieve improvement in nutrition status and clinical outcome.

There is no single test for malnutrition. Serum protein concentrations are often used in combination with other findings to indicate nutrition status. The acute-phase response to inflammation and the complicated interactions with body processes will alter the analysis of hepatic transport protein test results (Table 7.8). Malnutrition may not always be the cause of reduced values (Russell and McAdams, 1998; Litchford, 2008).

7.4 MONITORING

Once the assessment is complete, it is important to monitor the tolerance and the benefits of the recommendations. A timely follow-up should always be scheduled to make certain that any changes in the nutrition status are documented and that adjustments to the intervention are made quickly.

TABLE 7.7
Common Laboratory Data

Blood Test	Target Value (Varies with Lab)	Kidney Disease Target	Comments
Albumin (g/L)	35–55 (depends on assay bromcresol green [BCG] vs. bromcresol purple [BCP])	35–50	High in dehydration. Low in fluid overload and infection.
Alkaline phosphatase (U/L)	42–128	42–128	Monitored for suspected bone disease.
Blood urea nitrogen (mmol/L)	3.6–7.1	14.4–21.4	Varies with various stages of chronic kidney disease (CKD) and dialysis adequacy
Calcium (Ca++) (mmol/L)	2.3–2.8	2.3–2.8	Low with insufficient vitamin D; high with excess. With low albumin, use corrected Ca++ formula or obtain ionized Ca++ value.
C-reactive protein (mg/dL)	<0.8	<0.8	A sign of inflammation. If high, look for the cause: infection, malignant disease, autoimmune
Creatinine (μmol/L)	Male: 53–106 Female: 44–97	176.8–1326	High in catabolism Low in wasting
Ferritin (pmol/L)	Male: 12–300 Female: 10–150	CKD or PD: >224.7 HD: >449.4	High in inflammation Low in iron deficiency
Glucose (mmol/L)	3.9–5.8	3.9–5.8	High: diabetes mellitus Low: Malnutrition Note: Clinic labs values are usually nonfasting values
Hemoglobin (Hgb) (mmol/L)	Male: 8.7–1.2 Female: 7.4–9.9	CMS targets: 6.2–7.44	Low: Fluid overload, anemia, CKD, blood loss
Carbon dioxide (mmol/L)	23–31	23–31	High: Metabolic acidosis Low: Metabolic alkalosis
Cholesterol (mmol/L)	<5.2	<5.2	Low: Acute infection, malnutrition
High-density lipoprotein cholesterol (HDL-C)	>1.5	>1.5	
Low-density lipoprotein cholesterol (LDL-C)	<2.6	<2.6	
Triglycerides (mmol/L)	<1.7	<1.7	
Iron (μmol/L)	13–31	13–31	
Magnesium (mmol/L)	0.6–1.0	0.6–1.0	Low: Malnutrition, diarrhea, alcohol abuse
Phosphorus (mmol/L)	0.97–1.45	0.97–1.45	High: CKD, vitamin D intoxication, inadequate binder Low: Vitamin D deficiency, malabsorption, refeeding syndrome, osteomalacia
Plasma intact parathyroid hormone (PTH; pg/mL)	10–65	150–300	High: Hyperparathyroidism, vitamin D deficiency Low: Hypoparathyroidism, vitamin D intoxication
Potassium (mmol/L)	3.5–5.0	3.5–6.0	High: CKD, tissue trauma, hyperglycemia Low: Diuretic therapy, ETOH abuse, vomiting, and diarrhea
Pre-albumin/transthyretin (mg/L)	150–360	≥30	Low: Inflammation, malnutrition
Sodium (mmol/L)	136–145	136–145	High: Dehydration Low: Overhydration, starvation, hyperglycemia
Transferrin saturation (%)	16–48	20–50	High: Iron overload Low: Malnutrition

TABLE 7.8
Serum Hepatic Transport Proteins

Protein	Change	
Albumin (Half life = 14–20 days) Prealbumin (Half life = 2 days)	*Increases* with intravascular volume depletion and use of steroids	*Decreases* with inflammation, liver failure, pregnancy, volume overload, protein wasting diseases, exudates, and severe zinc deficiency
Prealbumin (Half life = 2 days)	*Increases* with intravascular volume depletion, use of steroids, and some cases of nephritic syndrome	*Decreases* with inflammation, malignancies, protein wasting diseases, and severe zinc deficiency
Retinol-binding protein (Half life = 12 h)	*Increases* in renal failure	*Decreases* in uncomplicated protein calorie malnutrition and low vitamin A
Transferrin (Half life = 8 days)	*Increases* with iron deficiency, pregnancy, and alcoholism	*Decreases* with liver disease, chronic disease, inflammation, malignancies, and collagen vascular diseases
C-reactive protein (CRP) and highly sensitive CRP are best used to measure the presence of inflammation		

7.5 SUMMARY

The NCP starts with screening and expands into a thorough nutrition assessment when necessary. The paramount goals of both screening and assessment are to ensure that the resulting nutrition treatment is optimal for the patient. There are many parts to the nutrition assessment process, and no part is the best. Experience, clinical recommendations from the American Dietetic Association, the Council on Renal Nutrition, and the KDOQI guidelines, and the literature on evidence-based medicine will help the practitioner to decide on the NCP for a patient.

REFERENCES

American Dietetic Association Evidence Library. 2011. Nutrition care process: Nutrition screening. Online: www.adaevidencelibrary.com (accessed May 2011).

American Dietetic Association Position Paper. 2009. Nutrient supplementation. *J Am Dental Assoc.* 109:2073–2085.

American Dietetic Association Writing Group for the Nutrition Care Process/ Standardized Language Committee. 2008. Nutrition care process and model part I: The 2008 update. *J Am Dental Assoc.* 108:1113–1117.

Barak, N., Wall-Alonso, E., Sitrin, M. 2002. Evaluations of stress factors and body weight adjustments currently used to estimate energy expenditure in hospitalized patients. *J Parenteral Enteral Nutr.* 26:231–238.

Baria, F., Kamimura, M., Avesani, C., Lindholm, B., Stenvinkel, P., Draibe, S., Cuppari, L. 2011. Activity-related energy expenditure of patients undergoing hemodialysis. *J Renal Nutr*. 21:226–234.

Blackburn, G. 1977. Nutrition and metabolic assessment of the hospitalized patient. *J Parenteral Enteral Nutr.* 1:11–22.

Chumlea, W., Guo, S., Wholihan, K., Cockram, D., Kuczmarski, R., Johnson, C. 1998. Stature prediction equations using knee height for elderly Americans from NHANES III. *J Am Diet Assoc*. 98:137–142.

Cresci, G. 2004. Patient history. In Charney, P., Malone, A., eds. *ADA Pocket Guide to Nutrition Assessment.* Chicago, IL: American Dietetic Association.

Detsky, A., McLaughlin, J., Baker, J., Johnston, N., Whittaker, S., Mendelson, R., Jeejeebhoy, K. 1987. What is subjective global assessment of nutrition status? *J Parenteral Enteral Nutr.* 11:8–13.

Federal Obesity Guidelines. 2000. National Heart Lung and Blood Institute. Online: http://www.nhlbi.nih.gov/guidelines/obesity/prctgd_c.pdf (accessed 05 January 2012).

Food and Nutrition Board, Institute of Medicine. 2011. Dietary reference intake: Water. Online: http://iom.edu/Activities/Nutrition/SummaryDRIs/~/media/Files/Activity%20Files/Nutrition/DRIs/DRI_Electrolytes_Water.ashx (accessed 30 May 2011).

Food and Nutrition Board, Institute of Medicine. 2006. *Dietary Reference Intakes*. Washington, DC: National Academies Press.

Frankenfield, D., Roth-Yousey, L., Compher, C. 2005. Comparison of predictive equations for resting metabolic rate in healthy non-obese and obese adults: A systematic review. *J Am Dental Assoc.* 105(5):775–789.

Frankenfield, D., Rowe, W., Smithe, J., Cooney, R. 2003. Validation of several established equations for resting metabolic rate in obese and non-obese people. *J Am Dental Assoc.* 103:1152–1159.

Frisancho, A. 1984. New standards of weight and body composition by frame size and height for assessment of nutrition status of adults and the elderly. *Am J Clin Nutr.* 40:808–819.

Frisancho, A. 1989. *Anthropometric Standards for the Assessment of Growth and Nutrition Status.* Ann Arbor, MI: University of Michigan Press.

Hamwi, G. 1964. Therapy: Changing dietary concepts. In: Danowski, T. ed., *Diabetes Mellitus: Diagnosis and Treatment,* Volume 1. New York: American Diabetes Association, 73–78.

Harris, J., Benedict, F. 1919. *Biometric Studies of Basal Metabolism in Man.* Washington, DC: Carnegie Institution of Washington. Publication number 279, 227–228.

Holliday, M., Segar, W. 1957. The maintenance need for water in parenteral fluid therapy. *Pediatrics.* 19:823–832.

Hwang, C., Kim, K., Kang, H., Kang, D. 2009. Validity of stature-predicted equations using knee height for elderly and mobility impaired persons in Koreans. *Epidemiol Health* 31:1–6.

Ireton-Jones, C., Jones, J. 1998. Should predictive equations or indirect calorimetry be used to design nutrition support regimens? *Nutr Clin Pract.* 13:141–143.

Kaiser, M., Bauer, J., Ramsch, C., Uter, W., Gudgoz, Y., Cederhome, T., Thomas, D., Anthony, P., Charlton, K., Maggio, M., Tsai, A., Grathwohl, D., Vellas, B., Sieber, C. 2009. Validation of the mini nutrition assessment short form (MNA®-SF): A practical tool for identification of nutrition status. *J Nutr Health Aging.* 13:782–788.

Khan, F., Sachs, H., Pechet, L., Snyder, L. 2002. *Guide to Diagnostic Testing.* Philadelphia, PA: Lippincott, Williams & Wilkins.

Kruizenga, H., Seidell, J., de Vet, H., Wierdsma, N., van Bokhorst-de van der Schueren, M. 2005. Development and validations of a hospital screening tool for malnutrition: the short nutrition assessment questionnaire (SNAQ©). *Clin Nutr.* 24:75–82.

Litchford, M. 2008. Assessment: Laboratory data. In Mahan, L., Escott-Stump, S. *Krause's Food & Nutrition Therapy.* Philadelphia, PA: Saunders Elsevier, 411–431.

Masud, T., Mitch, W. 2010. Requirements for protein, calories, and fat in the predialysis patient. In Mitch, W., Ikizler, T. *Handbook of Nutrition and the Kidney,* 6th edition. Philadelphia, PA: Lippincott Williams & Wilkins, 92–108.

Mifflin, M., St. Jeor, S., Hill, L., Scott, B., Daugherty, S., Koh, Y. 1990. A new predictive equation for resting energy expenditure in healthy individuals. *Am J Clin Nutr.* 51:241–247.

Mitchell, M. 1993. Comparison of determinants of frame size in older adults. *JADA.* 93(1):53–57.

National Institute of Diabetes and Digestive and Kidney Diseases (NIDDK). 2011. U.S. Department of Health and Human Services. Weight and waist measurement tools. Online: http://win.niddk.nih.gov/Publications/tools.htm#circumf (accessed 26 May 2011).

National Kidney Foundation (NKF). 2000. NKF KDOQI™ Clinical practice guidelines for nutrition in chronic renal failure. *Am J Kidney Disease.* 35(6 Suppl 2):S1–140.

Osterkamp, L. 1995. Current perspective on assessment of human body proportions of relevance to amputees. *J Am Diet Assoc.* 95:215–218.

Pronsky, Z., Crowe, J. 2008. Assessment: Food-drug interactions. In Mahan, L., Escott-Stump, S. *Krause's Food & Nutrition Therapy.* Philadelphia, PA: Saunders Elsevier, 432–453.

Russell, M., McAdams, M. 1998. Laboratory monitoring of nutrition status. In Matarese, L., Gottschlich, M. *Contemporary Nutrition Support Practice.* Philadelphia, PA: Saunders, 47–63.

Steiber, A., Leon, J., Secker, D., McCarthy, M., McCann, L., Serra, M., Sehgal, A., Kalantar-Zadeh, K. 2007. Multicenter study of the validity and reliability of subjective global assessment in the hemodialysis population. *J Renal Nutr.* 17(5): 336–342.

U.S. Department of Agriculture (USDA). 2011. Online: www.choosemyplate.gov (accessed 2 June 2011).

Weekes, C., Elia, M., Emery, P. 2004. The development, validation, and reliability of a nutrition screening tool based on the recommendations of the British Association for parenteral and enteral nutrition. *Clin Nutr.* 23:1104–1112.

Whitmire, S. 1998. Fluids and electrolytes. In Matarese, L., Gottschlich, M. *Contemporary Nutrition Support Practice.* Philadelphia, PA: Saunders, 121–144.

Williams, S. 2003. Nutrition assessment and medical nutrition therapy in patient care. In Williams, S., Schlenker, E., eds. *Essentials of Nutrition and Diet Therapy*, 8th edition. St Louis, MO: Mosby, 373–390.

8 Nutrition for Chronic Kidney Disease, Stages 1–3

Kim S. Stote
State University of New York

CONTENTS

8.1 GENERAL PRINCIPLES: CHRONIC KIDNEY DISEASE, STAGES 1–3

Chronic kidney disease (CKD) is recognized as a global public health problem (Saran et al., 2010). Prevalence for adults in the United States is approximately 15% of the general population (Whaley-Connell et al., 2008). In addition, data from Europe, Australia, and Asia verify the high prevalence of CKD (Zhang et al., 2008). In the United States, disease-stage prevalence of CKD Stages 1, 2, and 3 is estimated to be 1.8%, 3.2%, and 7.7%, respectively (Whaley-Connell et al., 2008). Stages 1–3 account for most individuals with CKD. Individuals in the early stages of CKD have a higher risk of cardiovascular disease (CVD) morbidity and mortality than their risk of progression to kidney failure (Saran et al., 2010). A systematic review of population-based studies reported that prevalence of CKD was 7.2% in persons aged 30 years or older and 23.4%–35.8% in persons older than 64 years (Zhang et al., 2008). The high prevalence of CKD, chiefly among older adults and those with diabetes and hypertension, implies that CKD is a definite threat to public health. New objectives from Healthy People 2010 show a greater emphasis on CKD versus the end-stage renal disease from Healthy People 2010. These new objectives recognize this by proposing a reduction in the percentage of the U.S. population with CKD; reducing death rates among individuals with CKD; and increasing the percentage of individuals with CKD who know they have impaired renal function (Healthy People, 2010). Moreover, the establishment of a World Kidney Day in 2006 by the International Society of Nephrology and International Federation of Kidney Foundations was the result of recognition that CKD is a threat to global public health (Collins et al., 2006).

8.2 NUTRITION CARE

8.2.1 NKF-KDOQI™ Clinical Practice Guidelines for Nutrition

A standard for classification of stages of CKD has been determined by the National Kidney Foundation Kidney Disease Outcomes Quality Initiative (NKF-KDOQI) guidelines to assist in the treatment of those with CKD (2002). The nonprofit foundation Kidney Disease: Improving Global Outcomes (KDIGO™) was established in 2003 by an international board of directors with the mission "to improve the care and outcomes of kidney disease patients worldwide through promoting coordination, collaboration, and integration of initiatives to develop and implement clinical practice guidelines" (Levey et al., 2005). KDIGO has previously recommended accepting the definition and classification of CKD proposed by NKF KDOQI (Eckardt et al., 2009).

In addition, the NKF-KDOQI suggests the use of standardized practices in renal nutrition and that dietitians with expertise in the care of individuals with CKD provide those services. A registered dietitian with renal experience should be an essential component of the dietary management of individuals with CKD (Kopple, 2001).

8.2.2 Medical Nutrition Therapy

Nutrition interventions may include basic nutrition education and medical nutrition therapy (MNT). Basic nutrition education can be provided by most health care professionals. MNT, however, is a more rigorous approach to the nutrition management of chronic disease. MNT requires greater training in food and nutrition sciences than is commonly provided by the curriculum of other health professionals to translate complex diet prescriptions into individualized dietary modifications (Fox, 2000). Registered dietitians are the distinctly specialized group of health care professionals with the most standardized education, clinical training, continuing education, and national credentialing requirements necessary to be reimbursed as a provider of MNT. MNT is an integral component of CKD management. Goals of MNT for CKD Stages 1–3 include maintaining a good nutritional status, delaying the rate of progression of renal failure, and reducing the risk factors for comorbidities. MNT provided by a registered dietitian is recommended for individuals with CKD Stages 1–3. MNT prevents and treats protein-energy malnutrition and mineral and electrolyte disorders, and minimizes the impact of other comorbidities, such as diabetes, hypertension, and lipid metabolism disorders, on the progression of kidney disease (Escott-Stump, 2008). NKF KDOQI guidelines recommend that the nutritional status of individuals with CKD be monitored at regular intervals (e.g., at 1- to 3-month intervals). Research on the effectiveness of MNT report significant improvements in anthropometric and biochemical measurements sustained at least for 1 year (Kopple, 2001).

8.2.2.1 Medicare Reimbursement

In 2002, a Medicare Part B benefit was established covering MNT services provided by a registered dietitian or nutrition professional for Medicare beneficiaries with diabetes or renal disease. The Centers for Medicare and Medicaid Services defines "renal disease" as "chronic renal insufficiency, end-stage renal disease when dialysis is not received, or the medical condition of a beneficiary for 36 months after kidney transplant." Chronic renal insufficiency is defined as "the stage of renal disease associated with a reduction in function not severe enough to require dialysis or transplantation (glomerular filtration rate [GFR] 13–50 mL/min/1.73 m^2)." Registered dietitians or nutrition professionals are allowed to bill Medicare Part B for MNT services for CKD Stages 3–5, that is, patients not receiving renal replacement therapy (Infante et al., 2002). MNT includes an initial assessment of nutrition and lifestyle; nutrition counseling; information on managing lifestyle factors that affect diet; and follow-up visits to monitor patient progress in managing diet. Medicare covers 3 h of one-on-one counseling services the first year and 2 h each year after that. More hours of treatment with a physician's referral may be required if the individual's condition, treatment, or diagnosis changes. A physician must prescribe these services and renew their referral yearly if the need for continuing treatment extends into another calendar year. Private third-party insurance carriers may or may not follow similar diagnostic guidelines for coverage. Interestingly, reimbursement through Medicare for CKD MNT may be underutilized. This may be due to underdiagnosed and undertreated CKD (Aase, 2010; Infante and Michael, 2002).

8.3 NUTRITION INTERVENTION: NUTRITION PRESCRIPTION

8.3.1 Protein

Low-protein diets have been shown to slow the rate of progression in CKD (Aparicio, 2009; Kasiske et al., 1998). The largest and most well-controlled clinical trial to date, however, showed inconclusive results. The Modification of Diet in Renal Disease (MDRD) Study was a randomized, controlled clinical trial conducted from 1989 to 1993 that determined the effects of dietary protein restriction and strict blood pressure control on the progression of kidney disease. The study included two randomized multicenter trials with 840 adults, aged 18–70 years, with differing chronic renal diseases, excluding diabetes requiring insulin therapy. Subjects were randomized into two groups according to GFR. Study 1 subjects included those with GFRs of 25–55 mL/min/1.73 m^2, who were randomly assigned to either a usual protein diet (1.3 g protein/kg/day) and usual phosphorus intake (16–20 mg/kg/day), or, to a low-protein diet (0.58 g/kg/day), with approximately 65% of dietary protein of high biological value (from animal sources), and a low-phosphorus diet (5–10 mg/kg/day). Study 2 subjects included those with GFRs of 13–24 mL/min/1.73 m^2 randomly assigned to either a low-protein diet (0.58 g/kg/day) or a very low-protein diet (0.28 g/kg/day) supplemented with a mixture of keto acids and amino acids (0.28 g/kg/day) and a low-phosphorus diet (4–9 mg/kg/day). Subjects were also randomly assigned to either a low or usual blood pressure goal. Protein intake was measured every 2 months from the urea nitrogen excretion rate in 24-h urine collections. Protein intake was also estimated monthly from 3-day diet records; dietary regimens were altered as required to attain dietary protein goals. Average follow-up for the study was 2.2 years. Results of the study showed no statistical significance suggesting that protein restriction specifically slows the progression of kidney failure (Klahr et al., 1994). A primary limitation of this study was the short follow-up period; a longer duration of follow-up may have detected a significant difference on disease progression. Secondary analysis of the data from the MDRD study showed that strict control of blood pressure and modification of protein 0.6 g/kg/day with a GFR < 25 helped delay disease progression by as much as 41% (Levey et al., 2006).

A previously conducted well-controlled clinical trial showed that intensive diabetes therapy decreased albuminuria. Decreased albuminuria is associated with slower progression of CKD, particularly in those with diabetes mellitus (Hemmelgarn et al., 2010). The Diabetes Control and Complications Trial was a multicenter, randomized clinical trial designed to compare intensive (three or more insulin injections and frequent blood glucose monitoring) with conventional (two insulin injections per day and occasional blood glucose monitoring) diabetes therapy with regard to their effects on the development and progression of the early vascular and neurologic complications of insulin-dependent diabetes mellitus. Study subjects were 1441 individuals with insulin-dependent diabetes mellitus followed for a mean of 6.5 years. Results of the study showed that intensive diabetes therapy reduced the risk of microalbuminuria (defined as urinary albumin excretion, measured annually, = 40 mg per 24 h) and albuminuria (urinary albumin excretion = 300 mg per 24 h) by 39% and 59%, respectively (DCCT, 1993). In addition, this trial showed that strict blood-glucose control may be more significant than protein restriction in delaying the onset of renal failure in individuals who have diabetes.

Consumption of high-protein diets in the short term leads to increased renal workload and an increase in GFR (Brenner et al., 1982; Friedman, 2004). However, there is a paucity of research on the long-term impact of protein intake on renal function in individuals with normal renal function or mild renal insufficiency. Knight et al. examined the influence of protein intake on rate of renal function change in 1624 females, aged 42–68 years, over an 11-year period in the Nurse's Health Study. Protein intake was assessed using food-frequency questionnaires. In women who began the study with normal kidney function, the results showed no association between amounts of type of protein and decrease in kidney function over time. Even so, women who began with mildly decreased kidney function showed a worsening in renal function with increasing amounts of nondairy animal protein intake. Interestingly, vegetable and dairy proteins were not associated with a decrease in kidney function (Knight et al., 2003). More research is required on the long-term impact of protein intake in CKD Stages 1–3.

The NKF KDOQI Clinical Practice Guidelines for Nutrition in Chronic Renal Failure suggest 0.6 g of protein/kg/day when the GFR is <25 mL/min/1.73 m^2, which corresponds approximately to CKD Stages 4–5. However, dietary protein intake may be increased up to 0.75 g protein/kg/day if dietary energy intake cannot be maintained (Kopple, 2001). Previous research found no favorable effect from dietary protein intake more than the Dietary Reference Intakes (DRI; 0.8 g/kg/day); therefore, it may be practical to recommend that dietary protein intake be increased to this level for individuals in CKD Stages 1–3 with at least 50%–60% of high-biologic-value protein to ensure an adequate amount of essential amino acids. Protein consumption in Western diets shows that adults typically consume 1.0–1.5 g of protein/kg/day (Fulgoni, 2008; Klahr et al., 1994; Mitch and Ikizler, 2010; Otten et al., 2006).

Current guidelines from The National Kidney Disease Education Program (NKDEP) recommend limiting excessive dietary protein to 0.8 g protein/kg/day in persons without diabetes and to 0.8–1.0 g/kg/day of protein in persons with diabetes to slow progression of kidney disease (NKDEP, 2010). NKDEP is an initiative of the National Institutes of Health (NIH), United States, founded in 2001. Its mission is to reduce the morbidity and mortality caused by kidney damage and its complications. Recently, NKDEP, with the assistance of registered dietitians specializing in renal disease, have developed strategies on how best to educate general practice dietitians, physicians, other health professionals, and individuals with CKD. NKDEP has provided an overview guide for dietitians for treating CKD patients who are not on dialysis. In addition, user-friendly education materials for general practice dietitians have been developed. NKDEP (2010) has also supplied a wide array of tools and resources for other health professionals, such as physicians, physician assistants, registered nurses, and laboratory professionals.

Updated standards of practice and standards of professional practice have been published for general practice dietitians who see individuals with CKD (Brommage et al., 2009; Byham-Gray et al., 2006). The American Dietetic Association also provides, through its Evidence Analysis Library, current evidence-based renal guidelines for nutrition therapy (Blumberg-Kason et al., 2006). In addition, practice recommendations for assisting patients with CKD have been published for primary-care providers (Linden et al., 2010). These recommendations include a patient referral to a dietitian for guidance on nutrition therapy for CKD.

One of the primary goals of nutrition therapy is to maintain the individual's nutritional status. It is essential to maintain body protein stores to prevent protein-energy malnutrition. Decline of nutritional status is present when GFR falls below 60 mL/min, which begins at CKD Stage 2. Protein-energy malnutrition is a risk factor for morbidity and mortality in individuals with CKD (American Dietetic Association, 2010; Byham-Gray et al., 2008; Mitch et al., 2010).

8.3.2 Energy

Total energy expenditure (TEE) includes resting energy expenditure (REE), physical activity, and thermogenesis (the thermic effect of food). Resting expenditure accounts for 60%–75%; physical activity accounts for 15%–30%; and thermogenesis accounts for 10% of TEE (Cuppari and Avesani, 2004).

Previous research with individuals with CKD not receiving renal replacement therapy shows that the energy requirements are comparable to the general population. Research indicates that a diet providing approximately 35 kcal/kg/day is needed to maintain a neutral nitrogen balance, to maintain a higher serum albumin concentration, to support a more normal body composition, and to improve protein utilization. In CKD individuals ≥ 60 years of age who are less physically active, an energy intake of 30–35 kcal/kg/day may be appropriate (Kopple, 2001; KDOQI, 2000).

The use of REE prediction equations such as the Harris and Benedict and the Schofield equations has been shown to overestimate REE in individuals with CKD. More research is required to develop population-specific equations that can adequately estimate the energy requirements of individuals with CKD, though the prediction equations may be useful as an initial guide for dietary planning (Kamimura et al., 2011). Ultimately, the energy requirements for CKD Stages 1–3 should be determined by age, gender, physical activity, nutritional status, and other comorbidities. It is also recommended that the individual's nutritional status be monitored on a regular basis and adjustments for energy requirements be made as needed.

Obesity is an escalating major health problem in the world. It contributes to increased hypertension and type 2 diabetes, which are the major causes of end-stage renal disease. The energy requirements of obese (body mass index ≥ 30 kg/m^2) or overweight (body mass index 25.0–29.9 kg/m^2) individuals should be decreased. Structured programs emphasizing lifestyle changes including moderate weight loss (7% of body weight) and regular physical activity should be encouraged (Kopple, 2010). In addition, dietary strategies, including decreasing calories and fat, may reduce the risk for developing diabetes (American Diabetes Association, 2011).

8.3.3 Lipids

During CKD Stages 1–3, there is a high prevalence of dyslipidemias and CVD. Controlling dyslipidemia may reduce the rate of decline in the GFR (Beto, 2004b; Fried et al., 2001; K/DOQI, 2002). While few studies have examined the effects of fat modification on CKD progression among individuals with CKD, it is practical to recommend the National Cholesterol Education Program (NCEP) Adult Treatment Panel (ATP III) to individuals with CKD Stages 1–3. The NKF KDOQI recommended that NCEP ATP III guidelines are generally applicable to CKD Stages 1–3 (KDOQI, 2000). The National Heart, Lung, and Blood Institute of the NIH began the NCEP in November 1985. The goal of NCEP was to decrease illness and death from CVD in the United States by ultimately decreasing the percentage of Americans who have elevated cholesterol levels. The NCEP strived to raise awareness about high blood cholesterol through education aimed at the American public and health professionals (NCEP, 2001).

In 1988, the ATP of the NCEP released clinical guidelines for the dietary and drug management of hypercholesterolemia. These guidelines were revised in 1993 and in 2000. The Third Report of the Expert Panel on Detection, Evaluation, and Treatment of High Blood Cholesterol in Adults (ATP III) presents the most recent updated clinical guidelines. The NCEP periodically produces ATP clinical updates as determined by advances in the science of cholesterol management. Each of the ATP reports, ATP I, ATP II, and now ATP III, have had a major theme. ATP I outlined a strategy for primary prevention of CVD in individuals with elevated levels of low-density lipoprotein (LDL) cholesterol (≥160 mg/dL) or those with borderline high LDL cholesterol (130–159 mg/dL) with more than two risk factors. ATP II acknowledged the importance of this approach and added a new feature, which was the intensive management of LDL cholesterol in individuals with established CVD. For individuals with CVD, ATP II set forth a new lower LDL cholesterol goal of

≤ 100 mg/dL. While the core recommendations in ATP III remain as previously defined, the main features are a greater focus on primary prevention in individuals with multiple risk factors, which calls for more-intensive LDL cholesterol–lowering therapy and identification of LDL cholesterol < 100 mg/dL as optimal. According to ATP III, candidates for cholesterol diet therapy are those with:

1. LDL cholesterol > 160 mg/dL with zero to one heart-disease risk factors and a 10-year risk for CVD of <10%;
2. LDL cholesterol > 130 mg/dL with two or more heart-disease risk factors and a 10-year risk of CVD of ≤ 20%;
3. LDL cholesterol level > 100 mg/dL and established CVD.

The 10-year risk is estimated from the Framingham risk scores. The risk factors included in the calculation are age, total cholesterol, high-density lipoprotein cholesterol, systolic blood pressure, treatment for hypertension, and smoking (NCEP, 2001).

As in the previous NCEP guidelines, lowering LDL cholesterol is the goal of dietary management, and the aim is to achieve an LDL cholesterol level that is 30 mg/dL below the initial value. ATP III recommends the lifestyle approach, termed Therapeutic Lifestyles Changes (TLC), which includes reducing the intake of saturated fatty acids to <7% of energy and reducing the intake of dietary cholesterol to <200 mg/day, for those individuals with elevated LDL cholesterol prior to the initiation of drug therapy. These dietary guidelines are generally consistent with other dietary recommendations in the United States. The TLC diet recommends total fat intake may range from 25% to 35% of energy with polyunsaturated fatty acids providing up to 10% of energy and monounsaturated fatty acids providing up to 20% of energy. *Trans* fatty acids should also be limited. Carbohydrate intake should be 50%–60% of total energy and derived mostly from foods high in complex carbohydrates. Fiber intake should be 20–30 g/day (NCEP, 2001).

Omega-3 fatty acids have been shown in epidemiological and clinical trials to reduce the incidence of CVD. Epidemiological studies suggest that individuals at risk for CVD benefit from the consumption of plant- and marine-derived omega-3 fatty acids. However, the recommended intake remains uncertain. The American Heart Association Dietary Guidelines recommends the general population to include at least two servings of fish per week (particularly fatty fish) along with vegetable oils (soybean, canola, walnut, flaxseed) and food sources (walnuts, flaxseeds) that are high in α-linolenic acid (Kris-Etherton et al., 2003). It may be practical to recommend these guidelines as there is limited research on the effects of consuming foods high in omega-3 fatty acids in individuals with CKD Stages 1–3. Long-term omega-3 fatty acid supplement use has not been rigorously studied in individuals with CKD Stages 1–3 (Friedman, 2010).

8.3.4 Minerals

8.3.4.1 Sodium

Sodium is freely filtered by the glomerulus. In healthy individuals, 99.5% of sodium is reabsorbed. The GFR and fractional tubular reabsorption decrease gradually as CKD progresses. Many individuals with CKD, therefore, are able to maintain sodium balance with normal sodium intake (Mitch et al., 2010). The INTERSALT Study was an international epidemiological study that included 10,079 men and women, aged 20–59 years, from 52 places around the world. Results showed a positive correlation between sodium excretion and both systolic and diastolic blood pressure; the average level of blood pressure of individuals in a country increases with salt intake (Stamler, 1997). For individuals with hypertension, reduction of dietary sodium has also been associated with improved blood pressure control (Appel et al., 2010).

The major source of sodium in the diet is added salt in the form of sodium chloride. Sodium comprises 40% by weight of sodium chloride. One teaspoon of salt has 2300 mg of sodium. Processed foods account for approximately 77% of total sodium consumed as salt is used extensively in food processing and manufacturing; 10% comes from table salt and cooking. Sodium intake varies throughout Western countries from 1500 mg/day to more than 5000 mg/day. The estimated amount of sodium consumed by adults in the United States ranges from 3000 to 5000 mg/day (Mitch et al., 2010; Shils et al., 2006). The Dietary Guidelines for Americans recommend a daily sodium intake of less than 2300 mg for the general adult population. Moreover, hypertensive individuals, blacks, and middle-aged and older adults would benefit from reducing their sodium intake even further. Because these groups collectively make up approximately 70% of adults in the United States, the recommended sodium intake for the general population is 1500 mg/day. (Dietary Guidelines, 2010; Savica et al., 2010). This recommendation is particularly challenging given food processing methods and patterns of sodium consumption. Strategies for reducing sodium intake should provide for a gradual reduction to allow taste perception to adjust.

Guidelines from NKDEP recommend limiting dietary sodium to 2300 mg/day or less to slow progression of kidney disease. It should be noted, however, that reduced sodium intake has been associated with further renal impairment in some renal diseases; thus, each individual with CKD Stages 1–3 will need to be managed individually. The NKDEP website provides user-friendly education materials for lowering dietary sodium (NKDEP, 2010).

The importance of dietary modification in the prevention and treatment of hypertension is well recognized. The Dietary Approaches to Stop Hypertension (DASH) eating plan incorporates reduction in sodium; inclusion of fruits, vegetables, and whole grains; and limitation of fats consistent with the TLC diet to lower blood cholesterol. The DASH diet provides an eating pattern that limits sodium levels between 1500 and 2400 mg/day. In addition, it is high in potassium, calcium, magnesium, and fiber (Appel et al., 2010). While the DASH diet is beneficial in lowering blood pressure, the increased potassium and phosphorus intakes that may result may lead to hyperkalemia and hyperphosphatemia in individuals with GFR < 60 mL/min/1.73 m^2, corresponding to the beginning of CKD Stage 2. Persons with CKD will require individualized nutrition therapy (Byham-Gray et al., 2008).

The 7th Report of the Joint National Treatment of High Blood Pressure also provides lifestyle modification guidelines to manage hypertension. These include weight loss, reducing sodium intake to 2400 mg/day, limiting alcohol consumption to no more than two drinks per day, and increasing physical activity (Chobanian et al., 2003; Cushman, 2007).

8.3.4.2 Potassium

Dietary potassium is typically not restricted in CKD Stages 1–3. The prevalence of hypertension and hyperlipidemia with risk for CVD, coronary artery disease (CAD), and left ventricular hypertrophy is higher in individuals with CKD compared to the general population; therefore, serum potassium should be monitored because of the effect of some antihypertensive agents, such as renin-angiotensin system antagonists, on potassium excretion. Serum potassium concentrations should be maintained between 3.5 and 5.0 mEq/L. Dietary potassium should be limited when serum potassium > 5.0 mEq/L (Beto et al., 2004a; Kent, 2005; NKDEP, 2010).

8.3.4.3 Phosphorus

The optimal intake of dietary phosphorus for individuals with CKD Stages 1–3 has not been well established. Hyperphosphatemia, elevated parathyroid hormone (PTH), secondary parathyroidism with depressed serum calcium and vitamin D deficiency are metabolic disturbances that require early detection and treatment to prevent CKD mineral and bone disorder (CKD-MBD). CKD-MBD is a systematic disorder of mineral and bone metabolism due to CKD manifested by either one or a combination of abnormalities of calcium, phosphorus, PTH, or vitamin D metabolism; abnormalities in bone turnover, mineralization, volume, linear growth, or strength; and vascular or other soft-tissue calcification. Current guidelines on management of CKD-MBD reflect consensus rather than high-grade evidence. According to NKF KDOQI U.S. Commentary on the 2009 KDIGO Clinical Practice Guideline for the Diagnosis, Evaluation, and Treatment of CKD-MBD, changes in levels of the biomarkers of CKD-MBD (phosphorus, calcium, PTH, and alkaline phosphatase) may begin in CKD Stage 3. Treatment of CKD-MBD needs to be individualized and may include nutrition counseling and education on dietary phosphate restriction, use of phosphate binders, and calcium and vitamin D supplementation. Serum phosphorus concentrations should be maintained between 2.7 and 4.6 mg/dL. If serum phosphorus is elevated, dietary phosphorus restriction may be indicated (Uhlig et al., 2010). Assessing dietary intake, especially protein intake, is recommended. Phosphorus is present in a several foods, mainly protein sources. Dietary protein restriction decreases phosphorus intake. If further restriction of dietary phosphorus is required, nutrition counseling and education may be provided to teach the individual to reduce consumption of foods with added phosphorus such as fast foods, convenience foods, and processed foods. Individuals with elevated phosphorus should be educated to read ingredient lists for "phos" to identify foods with phosphate additives, as these additives may be more readily absorbed versus food sources. Phosphorus additives are used by food manufacturers to enhance flavor and stability (NKDEP, 2010). Average phosphorus consumption of the general population in the United States ranges from approximately 1550 and 1100 mg, in men and women aged 20 years and older, respectively (USDA, 2010). NKDEP (2010) provides user-friendly education materials for lowering dietary phosphorus on its website.

8.3.4.4 Calcium

Dietary calcium recommendations for CKD Stages 1–3 have yet to be established (NKDEP, 2010). Serum calcium concentrations should be maintained within 8.5–10.2 mg/dL or reference range. NKF KDOQI U.S. Commentary on the 2009 KDIGO Clinical Practice Guideline for the Diagnosis, Evaluation, and Treatment of CKD-MBD suggests monitoring serum calcium concentrations in individuals with CKD Stage 3 every 6–12 months. In addition, the committee did not recommend discarding the corrected calcium measurement, although data have suggested that this measurement is not more accurate than total calcium alone. Ionized calcium is considered a more accurate measure, but it is currently not practical or cost-efficient. Hypoalbuminemia may contribute to falsely low calcium concentration because the calcium is bound to protein (Uhlig et al., 2010). A common formula to determine corrected calcium as is (Kent, 2005):

$$\text{Corrected serum calcium in mg/dL} =$$

$$[(4 - \text{serum albumin concentration in mg/dL}) \times 0.8] + \text{serum calcium concentration in mg/dL}$$

The DRI (the standards in use for the United States and Canada as determined by the committee of the Food and Nutrition Board of the National Academy of Sciences' Institute of Medicine working in association with Health Canada) for calcium indicate for the general population, women aged 19–50 years and men up to 71 years require on average 800 mg of calcium per day. Women over 50 and both men and women 71 years and older should take 1000 mg/day on average (IOM, 2010).

8.3.4.5 Trace Elements

Nutrient requirements for trace elements have not been well established in CKD Stages 1–3 (Shils et al., 2006). Previous research suggests that zinc requirements may be greater than the recommended DRI. Urinary and fecal excretion of zinc may be increased in uremic individuals; however, further research is needed (Mafra et al., 2004). In addition, iron supplementation should be individualized and iron stores monitored in CKD Stages 1–3 (Mitch et al., 2010).

8.3.5 Vitamins

8.3.5.1 Fat-Soluble Vitamins

Vitamin D supplementation should be individualized in CKD Stages 1–3. Vitamin D metabolism is disordered in CKD. Abnormalities may begin in CKD Stage 3. The renal tubular cell primarily activates 25-hydroxyvitamin D (calcidiol) to 1,25-dihydroxyvitamin D (calcitriol or active vitamin D). Reduction of kidney function results in decreased production and conversion of calcidiol to calcitriol. Furthermore, there may be related imbalances of calcium, phosphorus, and PTH. Adequacy of vitamin D is typically measured by the circulating concentrations of 25-hydroxyvitamin D, which is the combined product of synthesis from sun exposure and dietary sources. In adults, the majority of circulating 25-hydroxyvitamin D originates from ultraviolet B ray exposure. If the serum level of 25-hydroxyvitamin D is less than 30 ng/mL supplementation may be indicated (Mitch, 2010; NKDEP, 2010; Uhlig, 2010). The dietary supplement cholecalciferol (vitamin D_3) may be used in early stages of CKD to increase vitamin D concentrations. NKF KDOQI U.S. Commentary on the 2009 KDIGO Clinical Practice Guideline for the Diagnosis, Evaluation, and Treatment of CKD-MBD suggest that individuals with CKD vitamin D deficiency and insufficiency should use treatment strategies recommended for the general population. In addition, 25-hydroxyvitamin D (calcidiol) may be measured with repeated testing determined by baseline values and therapeutic interventions. There are limited data about whether vitamin D concentrations should differ between the general population and those with CKD. Vitamin D deficiency or insufficiency may cause individuals with CKD to have increased PTH concentrations (Uhlig et al., 2010). Epidemiological studies show an association between low vitamin D concentrations and adverse clinical outcomes such as cancer and increased mortality (Holick, 2007). There is, however, a lack of data from clinical trials with vitamin D to confirm these clinical outcomes. It is recommended that clinicians individualize the decision to measure vitamin D. A practical approach would be to occasionally measure 25-hydroxyvitamin D in individuals with CKD and start treatment if the concentration is low. Recommendations for the general population for vitamin D repletion specify cholecalciferol dose of 1000–2000 IU/day. Serum concentrations of calcium, phosphorus, and PTH concentrations should be monitored when vitamin D dietary supplements are utilized (Uhlig et al., 2010).

In 2010, the DRI for vitamin D for the general population in the United States and Canada were updated by an appointed committee from the Institute of Medicine, utilizing current research on clinical outcomes associated with vitamin D. Previous recommendations for the vitamin suggested an adequate intake for vitamin D of 200 IU for men and women aged 19–50 years. The 2010 recommendation for vitamin D has increased to 400 IU/day. Individuals aged 71 years and older may require as much as 800 IU/day. The committee reported that there is not yet sufficient research about the health benefits of vitamin D beyond bone health. They also reported that the measurements, or cut-points, of sufficiency and deficiency used by laboratories to report vitamin D concentrations have not been set based upon rigorous scientific research. No central authority has determined which cut-points to use. An individual may be determined to be vitamin D sufficient or deficient, depending upon the laboratory where the serum was tested. The committee concluded that the number of individuals with vitamin D deficiency in North America may be overestimated as a result of laboratories using cut-points that may be higher than recommended. Laboratories should assist clinicians in interpretation of vitamin D concentrations by reporting assay characteristics and methodology utilized (IOM, 2010).

Supplementation of other fat-soluble vitamins such as vitamins A, E, and K has not been well established in CKD Stages 1–3. Current recommendations suggest that supplementation of vitamins A, E, and K should be avoided, as these may accumulate more rapidly in CKD (Mitch et al., 2010; Shils et al., 2006).

8.3.5.2 Water-Soluble Vitamins

Water-soluble vitamin supplementation is not well defined in CKD Stages 1–3. It is practical to recommend that vitamin supplements should contain the DRI for the water-soluble vitamins. Vitamin C is typically not supplemented above the DRI as it may cause oxalosis. CKD Stage 3, however, may be more prone to vitamin deficiencies due to suboptimal dietary intake, changes in metabolism of certain water-soluble vitamins, and medication interaction with intestinal absorption and metabolism of vitamins (Table 8.1). In addition, the process of aging may reduce nutrient absorption,

TABLE 8.1
Nutrient Recommendations Composite for Chronic Kidney Disease Stages 1–3

Stage	Protein (g/kg/day)	Energy	Sodium (g/day)	Potassium (g/day)	Phosphorus (g/day)	Calcium (mg/day)	Vitamins
1. GFR 90–130 mL/min	Nondiabetic: 0.8 g/kg/day, Diabetic: 0.8–1.0 g/kg/day, ≥50% high biologic value	Determined by energy expenditure	2300 mg or less	Typically no restriction, restrict if serum level is ≥5.0 mEq/L	Monitor and restrict if serum level >4.6 mg/dL	DRI, individualize, maintain serum calcium within reference range	DRI, individualize for vitamin D
2. GFR 60–89 mL/min	Same as Stage 1	Same as Stage 1	Same as Stage 1	Same as Stage 1	Same as Stage 1	Same as Stage 1	DRI, individualize for vitamin D
3. GFR 30–59 mL/min	Same as Stage 1	Same as Stage 1	Same as Stage 1	Same as Stage 1	Same as Stage 1	Same as Stage 1	DRI, B-complex and vitamin C, individualize for vitamin D, zinc, iron

Abbreviations: GFR, glomerular filtration rate; DRI, dietary reference intake.
Sources: Kopple, 2001; Mitch, 2010; NKDEP, 2010; American Dietetic Association, 2010; Uhlig, 2010; Byham-Gray and Wiesen, 2004.

increase urinary nutrient loss, and alter normal pathways of nutrient metabolism (Mitch et al., 2010; Shils et al., 2006).

The use of nutrient and dietary supplements is prevalent and increasing. Clinicians should regularly assess the individual's intake of vitamin supplements, other dietary supplements, and fortified foods that may be a part of dietary intake (Marra and Boyar, 2009; Skeie et al., 2009).

8.3.6 Fluid

Fluid requirements in CKD Stages 1–3 are typically unrestricted with normal urine output (Byham-Gray and Wiesen, 2004; Byham-Gray et al., 2008).

8.3.7 Fiber

Fiber recommendations for the general population are that individuals should consume adequate amounts of dietary fiber from a variety of plant foods. Research in the general population suggests that a high dietary fiber intake may reduce the incidence of constipation, irritable bowel syndrome, diverticulitis, and colon cancer. In addition, fiber may improve glucose tolerance in those with diabetes. Fiber consumption in the United States is approximately 15 g/day. The recommended DRIs call for consumption of 14 g of dietary fiber per 1000 calories, or 25 g of fiber per day for women and 38 g of fiber per day for men (Slavin, 2008). The appropriate amount and kinds of fiber have not been clearly established in CKD Stages 1–3. Fiber intake should be individualized for those with CKD Stages 1–3 based upon assessment of current dietary intake, gender, age, nutritional status, and other comorbidities.

8.4 WEBSITES

American Dietetic Association
http://www.eatright.org/
American Dietetic Association—Nutrition Care Manual
http://nutritioncaremanual.org/
American Dietetic Association—Evidence Analysis Library
http://www.adaevidencelibrary.com/
American Dietetic Association—Renal Dietitians Practice Group
http://www.renalnutrition.org/
National Kidney Disease Education Program
http://nkdep.nih.gov/
National Kidney Disease Education Program—Education materials and resources for health professionals
http://nkdep.nih.gov/professionals/index.htm
National Kidney Foundation
http://www.kidney.org/
National Kidney Foundation Kidney—Kidney Disease Outcomes Quality Initiative (NKF-KDOQI)
http://www.kidney.org/Professionals/kdoqi/
National Kidney Foundation—Council on Renal Nutrition
http://www.kidney.org/professionals/CRN/
International Society of Renal Nutrition and Metabolism
http://www.kidney.org/ISRNM/
Canadian Association of Nephrology Dietitians
http://www.renalrd.ca/
Kidney Disease Improving Global Outcomes
http://www.kdigo.org/

International Federation of Kidney Foundations
http://www.ifkf.net/
Annual World Kidney Day
http://www.worldkidneyday.org/
The American Association of Kidney Patients
http://www.aakp.org/

REFERENCES

Aase, S. 2010. Kidney friendly: What the National Kidney Disease Education Program strategic plan means for dietetic practice. *J Am Diet Assoc*. 110: 346–351.

American Diabetes Association. 2011. Executive summary: Standards of medical care in diabetes—2011. *Diabetes Care*. 34(Suppl 1): S4–S17.

American Dietetic Association. 2010. *Nutrition Care Manual, Chronic Kidney Disease*. Chicago, IL: American Dietetic Association.

Aparicio, M. 2009. Protein intake and chronic kidney disease: Literature review, 2003 to 2008. *J Renal Nutr*. 19: S5–S8.

Appel, L., Wright, J., Jr., Greene, T., et al. 2010. Intensive blood-pressure control in hypertensive chronic kidney disease. *N Engl J Med*. 363: 918–929.

Brenner, B., Meyer, T., Hostetter, T. 1982. Dietary protein intake and the progressive nature of kidney disease: The role of hemodynamically mediated glomerular injury in the pathogenesis of progressive glomerular sclerosis in aging, renal ablation, and intrinsic renal disease. *N Engl J Med*. 307: 652–659.

Brommage, D., Karalis, M., Martin, C., et al. 2009. American Dietetic Association and the National Kidney Foundation Standards of Practice and Standards of Professional Performance for registered dietitians (generalist, specialty, and advanced) in nephrology care. *J Renal Nutr*. 19: 345–356.

Beto, J., Bansal, V. 2004a. Medical nutrition therapy in chronic kidney failure: Integrating clinical practice guidelines. *J Am Diet Assoc*. 104: 404–409.

Beto, J., Bansal, V. 2004b. Nutrition interventions to address cardiovascular outcomes in chronic kidney disease. *Adv Chronic Kidney Dis*. 11: 391–397.

Blumberg-Kason, S., Lipscomb, R. 2006. Evidence-based nutrition practice guidelines: A valuable resource in the evidence analysis library. *J Am Diet Assoc*. 106: 1935–1936.

Byham-Gray, L., Wiesen, K., eds. 2004.*A Clinical Guide to Nutrition Care in Kidney Disease*. Chicago, IL: American Dietetic Association.

Byham-Gray, L., Burrowes, J., Chertow, G., eds. 2008. *Nutrition in Kidney Disease*. Totowa, NJ: Humana Press.

Byham-Gray, L., Wiesen, K., Goode, J. 2006. Scope of practice in renal nutrition. *J Renal Nutr*. 16: 160–167.

Chobanian, A., Bakris, G., Black, H., et al. 2003. The Seventh Report of the Joint National Committee on Prevention, Detection, Evaluation, and Treatment of High Blood Pressure: The JNC 7 report. *JAMA*. 289: 2560–2572.

Collins, A., Couser, W., Dirks, J., et al. 2006. World Kidney Day: An idea whose time has come. *Kidney Int*. 69: 781–782.

Cuppari, L., Avesani, C. 2004. Energy requirements in patients with chronic kidney disease. *J Renal Nutr*.14: 121–126.

Cushman, W. 2007. JNC-7 guidelines: Are they still relevant? *Curr Hypertens Rep*. 9: 380–386.

Diabetes Control and Complications Trial Research Group. 1993. The effect of intensive treatment of diabetes on the development and progression of long-term complications in insulin-dependent diabetes mellitus. *N Engl J Med*. 329: 977–986.

Dietary Guidelines for Americans. 2010. http://www.cnpp.usda.gov/Publications/DietaryGuidelines/2010/PolicyDoc/Chapter3.pdf (accessed June 8, 2011).

Eckardt, K., Berns, J., Rocco, M., et al. 2009. Definition and classification of CKD: The debate should be about patient prognosis—a position statement from KDOQI and KDIGO. *Am J Kidney Dis*. 53: 915–920.

Escott-Stump, S. 2008. *Nutrition and Diagnosis-Related Care*, 6th edn. Philadelphia, PA: Lippincott, Williams & Wilkins.

Fox, T. 2000. Institute of Medicine urges Medicare coverage of medical nutrition therapy. *J Am Diet Assoc*. 100: 166.

Fried, L., Orchard, T., Kasiske, B. 2001. Effect of lipid reduction on the progression of renal disease: A meta-analysis. *Kidney Int*. 59: 260–269.

Friedman, A. 2004. High-protein diets: Potential effects on the kidney in renal health and disease. *Am J Kidney Dis.* 44: 950–962.

Friedman, A. 2010. Omega-3 fatty acid supplementation in advanced kidney disease. *Semin Dial.* 23: 396–400.

Fulgoni, V. 2008. 3rd. Current protein intake in America: Analysis of the National Health and Nutrition Examination Survey, 2003–2004. *Am J Clin Nutr.* 87: 1554S–1557S.

Healthy People. 2010. http://www.healthypeople.gov/hp2020/ (accessed December 1, 2010).

Hemmelgarn, B., Manns, B., Lloyd, A., et al. 2010. Relation between kidney function, proteinuria, and adverse outcomes. *JAMA.* 303: 423–429.

Holick, M. 2007. Vitamin D deficiency. *N Engl J Med.* 357: 266–281.

Infante, M., Michael, P. 2002. Medicare Part B coverage and billing for medical nutrition therapy. *J Am Diet Assoc.* 102: 32.

Institute of Medicine (IOM). 2010. Dietary reference intakes for calcium and vitamin D. http://www.iom.edu/Reports/2010/Dietary-Reference-Intakes-for-Calcium-and-Vitamin-D.aspx (accessed December 1, 2010).

Kamimura, M., Avesani, C., Bazanelli, A., et al. 2011. Are prediction equations reliable for estimating resting energy expenditure in chronic kidney disease patients? *Nephrol Dial Transplant.* 26: 544–550.

Kasiske, B., Lakatua, J., Ma, J., et al. 1998. A meta-analysis of the effects of dietary protein restriction on the rate of decline in renal function. *Am J Kidney Dis.* 31: 954–961.

K/DOQI. 2000. Clinical practice guidelines for nutrition in chronic renal failure. National Kidney Foundation. *Am J Kidney Dis.* 35: S1–S140.

K/DOQI. 2002. Clinical practice guidelines for chronic kidney disease: Evaluation, classification, and stratification. National Kidney Foundation. *Am J Kidney Dis.* 39: S1–S266.

Kent, P. 2005. Integrating clinical nutrition practice guidelines in chronic kidney disease. *Nutr Clin Pract.* 20: 213–217.

Klahr, S., Levey, A., Beck, G., et al. 1994. The effects of dietary protein restriction and blood-pressure control on the progression of chronic renal disease. Modification of Diet in Renal Disease Study Group. *N Engl J Med.* 330: 877–884.

Knight, E., Stampfer, M., Hankinson, S., et al. 2003. The impact of protein intake on renal function decline in women with normal renal function or mild renal insufficiency. *Ann Intern Med.* 138: 460–467.

Kopple, J. 2001. National kidney foundation K/DOQI clinical practice guidelines for nutrition in chronic renal failure. *Am J Kidney Dis.* 37: S66–S70.

Kopple, J. 2010. Obesity and chronic kidney disease. *J Renal Nutr.* 20: S29–S30.

Kris-Etherton, P., Harris, W., Appel, L. 2003. Omega-3 fatty acids and cardiovascular disease: New recommendations from the American Heart Association. *Arterioscler Thromb Vasc Biol.* 23: 151–152.

Levey, A., Eckardt, K., Tsukamoto, Y., et al. 2005. Definition and classification of chronic kidney disease: A position statement from Kidney Disease: Improving Global Outcomes (KDIGO). *Kidney Int.* 67: 2089–2100.

Levey, A., Greene, T., Sarnak, M., et al. 2006. Effect of dietary protein restriction on the progression of kidney disease: Long-term follow-up of the Modification of Diet in Renal Disease (MDRD) Study. *Am J Kidney Dis.* 48: 879–888.

Linden, A., Biuso, T., Butterworth, S.W. 2010. Help patients with chronic kidney disease stave off dialysis. *J Fam Pract.* 59: 212–219.

Mafra, D., Cuppari, L., Favaro, D., et al. 2004. Zinc levels after iron supplementation in patients with chronic kidney disease. *J Ren Nutr.* 14: 164–169.

Marra, M., Boyar, A. 2009. Position of the American Dietetic Association: Nutrient supplementation. *J Am Diet Assoc.* 109: 2073–2085.

Mitch, W., Ikizler, T., eds. 2010. *Handbook of Nutrition and the Kidney*, 6th edn. Philadelphia, PA: Lippincott, Williams & Wilkins.

National Cholesterol Education Program Expert Panel. 2001. Executive summary on detection, evaluation, and treatment of high blood cholesterol in adults (Adult Treatment Panel III). *JAMA.* 285: 2486–2497.

National Kidney Disease Education Program. 2010. http://nkdep.nih.gov/professionals/index.htm (accessed December 1, 2010).

Otten, J., Hellwig, J., Meyers, L., eds. 2006. *Dietary Reference Intakes*, 6th edn. Washington, DC: National Academy of Sciences.

Saran, R., Shahinian, V. 2010. CKD: A pandemic calling for concerted public health action. *Adv Chronic Kidney Dis.* 17: 213–214.

Saran, R., Hedgeman, E., Huseini, M., et al. 2010. Surveillance of chronic kidney disease around the world: Tracking and reining in a global problem. *Adv Chronic Kidney Dis.* 17: 271–281.

Savica, V., Bellinghieri, G., Kopple, J.D. 2010. The effect of nutrition on blood pressure. *Annu Rev Nutr*. 30: 365–401.

Shils, M., Shike, M., Ross, A., et al., ed. 2006. *Modern Nutrition in Health and Disease*, 10th edn. Philadelphia, PA: Lippincott, Williams & Wilkins.

Skeie, G., Braaten, T., Hjartaker, A., et al. 2009. Use of dietary supplements in the European Prospective Investigation into Cancer and Nutrition calibration study. *Eur J Clin Nutr*. 63(Suppl 4): S226–S238.

Slavin, J. 2008. Position of the American Dietetic Association: Health implications of dietary fiber. *J Am Diet Assoc*. 108: 1716–1731.

Stamler, J. 1997. The INTERSALT Study: Background, methods, findings, and implications. *Am J Clin Nutr*. 65: 626S–642S.

Uhlig, K., Berns, J., Kestenbaum, B., et al. 2010. KDOQI US commentary on the 2009 KDIGO Clinical Practice Guideline for the Diagnosis, Evaluation, and Treatment of CKD-Mineral and Bone Disorder (CKD-MBD). *Am J Kidney Dis*. 55: 773–799.

U.S. Department of Agriculture. 2010. Nutrient intakes from food: Mean amounts consumed per individual, by gender and age. What We Eat in America, NHANES 2007–2008. Agricultural Research Service.

Whaley-Connell, A., Sowers, J., Stevens, L., et al. 2008. CKD in the United States: Kidney Early Evaluation Program (KEEP) and National Health and Nutrition Examination Survey (NHANES) 1999–2004. *Am J Kidney Dis*. 51: S13–S20.

Zhang, Q., Rothenbacher, D. 2008. Prevalence of chronic kidney disease in population-based studies: Systematic review. *BMC Public Health*. 8: 117.

9 Nutrition for Chronic Kidney Disease, Stage 4

Ann Grothe
DaVita Peninsula Dialysis

CONTENTS

9.1 INTRODUCTION

Chronic kidney disease Stage 4 (CKD 4) is a transitional stage with significant management challenges due to the wide variation in symptoms, lab values, and overall patient presentation. Nutrition plays a key role not only in the management of progression of the disease but also in minimizing the impact of the comorbidities seen in patients. Nutrition also affects the presentation of symptoms and long-term outcome of treatment of these patients when they undergo renal replacement therapy (RRT). Nutrition management during this critical predialysis stage must be individualized and closely monitored to maximize efficacy and avoid overrestriction of dietary intake.

Standards of care, specifically, with regard to the use of protein restriction remain controversial, requiring the practitioner to balance the competing needs of decreasing the toxin load on the kidneys while limiting protein malnutrition. Goals of nutritional therapy include decreasing uremic toxins, promoting adequate nutritional status, and utilizing dietary strategies to support management of comorbidities. Establishing good self-management skills is vital for the patient to achieve and maintain the necessary behavior and lifestyle changes needed to reach these goals and to ultimately delay the progression to end-stage renal disease (ESRD; Beto and Bansal, 2004).

9.2 BACKGROUND

CKD 4 is historically defined based on an estimated glomerular filtration rate (eGFR) of 15–29 mL/min. However, critics accuse the use of creatinine-based calculation for underestimating the actual function of the kidneys and propose the use of more sensitive equations. The U.S. Renal Data System estimates that about 14.2%–15.2% (depending on which equation is used) of the population is with CKD (U.S. Renal Data System, 2010). In addition, it reports an increasing incidence of diabetes, hyptertension, and cardiovascular disease (CVD) as eGFR decreases. This is significant given that the risk factors for CKD include diabetes, hypertension, obesity, family history, age, and race (U.S. Renal Data System, 2010). Information on stage-specific incidence of CKD has improved since Medicare started using stage-specific ICD-9 codes for tracking and identification of CKD. Based on 2008 Medicare data, 400,000 people were diagnosed with CKD 4 (U.S. Renal Data System, 2010).

Nutrition management for the patients with CKD 4 is highly individual and complex. The goals of nutrition management comprise managing symptoms and comorbidities, delaying progression of the disease, and optimizing nutritional status. CKD 4 is characterized by changes in the lab values and the associated symptoms as the body becomes less able to cope with the failing kidneys. Fluid and electrolyte imbalances become more pronounced, affecting acid–base balance and regulation of sodium and potassium. Patients often present with symptoms such as metabolic acidosis, hyperkalemia, and increased edema. Mineral metabolism with respect to calcium and phosphorus regulation as well as probable deficiency of 25-hydroxy vitamin D should be addressed. Hormonal abnormalities and/or deficiencies in erythropoietin (EPO) and increase in parathyroid hormone (PTH) increase the risk of anemia and secondary hyperparathyroidism in patients. Except for anemia and edema, there are often few symptoms reported with the aforementioned changes in physiology. However, alterations in gastrointestinal (GI) functions, such as anorexia, nausea and vomiting, and altered taste are frequently reported. These symptoms are related to the increase in uremic toxins. Weight changes related to fluid balance as well as decrease in dietary intake may also be seen.

9.3 ASSESSMENT

Nutritional assessment of patients with stage 4 CKD must be comprehensive and include medical and health history, food/nutrition-related history, anthropometrics, and biochemical parameters (ADA, 2010). A thorough review is also important to identify medications such as blood pressure medications, diuretics, or blood thinners, which may affect key lab values in patients with CKD 4. Anthropometrics should include height, weight (edema-free), body mass index (BMI), and recent blood pressure. It is important to note changes in weight that are not related to fluid status and that are related to changes in medications. The National Kidney Foundation Kidney Dialysis Outcome Quality Initiative (NKF-K/DOQI™) recommends incorporating a subjective global assessment (SGA) tool for evaluation and monitoring of nutritional status in the population with CKD 4 (National Kidney Foundation, 2000). Kalantar-Zadeh et al. (2001) developed the Malnutrition Inflammation Complex Syndrome subjective global assessment (MICS SGA) to capture the unique factors associated with malnutrition in predicting morbidity and mortality outcomes in the population with ESRD (Kalantar-Zadeh et al., 2001). This tool combines elements of the conventional SGA with indicators such as BMI, serum albumin, and total iron-binding capacity. It was recently found that morbidity and mortality in patients on renal transplant can be predicted using the tool, and hence the tool should be considered for use in patients with CKD 4 (Molnar et al., 2010).

Tools such as diet recall, food frequency questionnaires, or food diaries can all be utilized to obtain a food- and nutrition-related history but should be geared to renal-specific food groups for assessment of intake of potassium, phosphorus, and protein. Online interactive tools are becoming more prevalent and can be used to complete the assessment from patients' home or office before their medical appointment. In addition, access to appropriate foods should be assessed and taken into account when developing diet recommendations. K/DOQI™ also recommends inclusion of normalized protein nitrogen appearance when assessing dietary intake (National Kidney Foundation, 2000).

The American Dietetic Association (ADA) recently published evidence-based guidelines for CKD, which summarize well the components of a comprehensive assessment. They recommend evaluating not only the nutritional status and evidence of protein-energy malnutrition but also dietary factors related to glycemic control, inflammation, electrolyte disorders, mineral and bone disorders, anemia, dyslipidemia, and, of course, kidney function (ADA, 2010). This approach takes into account the complexity of CKD 4 in patients and the need to minimize the effect of comorbidities and uremic toxins on the kidneys while promoting optimal nutrition.

Assessment and monitoring of renal-specific lab values is essential for appropriate management of patients with CKD 4. K/DOQI Clinical Practice Guidelines for Nutrition in Chronic Renal Failure were published in 2000 and provide specific recommendations for laboratory value targets. Care must be taken when interpreting lab values in patients with CKD 4. Serum albumin is the preferred measurement for visceral protein stores and is found to be predictive of increased risk of mortality in patients with ESRD (National Kidney Foundation, 2000). However, in the population with renal diseases, serum albumin levels are often confounded by fluid status (edema) and chronic inflammation (Fuhrman et al., 2004; Kalantar-Zadeh et al., 2003). Albumin is a negative acute-phase protein that decreases during illness or trauma. In addition, systemic inflammation caused by cytokines and other mediators significantly decreases hepatic proteins such as albumin and prealbumin. This relationship necessitates that in patients with CKD 4, hepatic proteins, specifically albumin, are more appropriately viewed as a prognostic indicator versus a biomarker for nutritional status (Fuhrman et al., 2004). Albumin can be very useful in predicting the severity of the illness and the outcomes in CKD. Consequently, serum albumin alone should not be used to determine the nutritional status but should be used in conjunction with other elements for a comprehensive nutritional assessment.

9.4 NUTRITIONAL RECOMMENDATIONS FOR PATIENTS WITH CKD 4—MACRONUTRIENTS

9.4.1 Protein

K/DOQI Clinical Practice Guidelines for Nutrition in Chronic Renal Failure has become the standard of care for most providers and addresses both macro-and micronutrient needs for patients with CKD. Determining the recommendations for appropriate protein intake for patients with CKD 4 remains the most controversial aspect of care. K/DOQI recommends a low-protein diet (LPD) providing 0.60 g/kg/day for nondialyzed patients with a GFR of <25 mL/min (National Kidney Foundation, 2000). It also recommends a protein level of 0.75 g/kg/day for those patients who are not willing to follow an LPD or are unable to sustain adequate total energy intake on an LPD.

LPDs have been one of the primary interventions initiated for decreasing the workload on the kidneys while reducing uremia and its effects on the rest of the body. Decrease in the intake of phosphorus, potassium, and sodium tends to occur with an LPD, leading to improvements in many of the complications of kidney failure. However, debate remains on the safety of restricting protein intake in patients who are already at the risk of malnutrition. Studies exploring the long-term risks and benefits of an LPD have yielded mixed results. Shortfalls in many of the studies include poor assessment of adherence to prescribed protein intake levels, limited long-term follow-up, and the exclusion of diabetics (Eyre et al., 2008). It should be noted that a spontaneous decrease in protein intake is associated with an eGFR of <25 mL/min secondary to taste changes and GI issues (Ikizler, 2009).

A 2007 Cochrane review looked at protein restriction for diabetics with renal disease and found only small improvements in renal function with protein-restricted diets (Robertson et al., 2007). Interestingly, this review found that the actual protein intake ranged from 0.7 to 1.1 g/kg/day. Cianciaruso et al. (2008) found that in over 400 patients, LPD improved metabolic control without an increased risk of malnutrition (Cianciaruso). In a follow-up study, they concluded that an LPD was not significantly more effective than a moderate-protein diet (0.8 g/kg/day) in decreasing the risk of death or initiation of RRT, and therefore they believe that it has secondary effects on metabolic factors (Cianciaruso et al., 2009). The Modification of Diet in Renal Disease study is considered the definitive study to date on the effect of dietary modifications on CKD outcomes. The study group performed a long-term follow-up of participants in Study B [LPD vs. VLPD (very low protein diet) = 0.28 mg/kg/day plus keto/amino acid supplementation] and concluded that a VLPD had no significant effect on delaying progression of kidney failure but increased the risk of death on long-term use, particularly in those starting dialysis (Menon et al., 2009). Given that restricting protein intake has the potential to preserve renal function and reduce the symptoms of uremia with minimal impact on nutritional status, many feel that this recommendation should be utilized more frequently with close monitoring by a dietitian. Critics believe that the minimal effect of delaying disease progression is far outweighed by the potential for malnutrition and suggest that the focus should be on less risky methods to slow disease progression than on protein restriction (Eyre and Attman, 2008; Kasiski et al., 1998).

While efficacy of the LPD remains questionable, adherence to the diet is a key factor to be considered. Proponents of the LPD emphasize the need to assess a patient's ability to adhere to the recommendations as necessary for the effectiveness of the LPD. Designing a palatable LPD is necessary to promote adherence of the LPD and requires the professional skills of a registered dietitian (RD). Close monitoring is also essential to ensure that the patient does not develop protein-energy malnutrition. Some experts recommend a trial period of 6 months to determine whether use of LPD is an effective strategy for individual patients (Robertson et al., 2007).

The protein source, animal versus vegetable, has also received consideration when determining protein recommendations. There exists a persistent belief that red meat in high amounts accelerates renal failure. A recent review concluded that the absolute amount of protein intake, no matter the source, was associated with renal injury in healthy people and with progression of renal failure in those with CKD (Bersnstein et al., 2007). However, for persons with diabetes, evidence suggests that substituting vegetable or fish protein for animal protein may decrease the amount of protein in the urine. Further study is needed, in this very important area, to make conclusive recommendations, and therefore, the final effective amount of protein intake will need to be based on individual patients and their goals as well as response to medical nutrition therapy (MNT).

9.4.2 Energy

Adequate dietary energy intake is essential to support lower protein recommendations and optimize amino acid utilization. According to K/DOQI Guidelines, an intake of 35 kcal/kg/day is required to maintain nitrogen balance, as well as albumin levels, and weight in nondialyzed patients with a GFR <25 mL/min (National Kidney Foundation, 2000). Patients >60 years or more may require less (30 kcal/kg/day) calories based on lower activity levels. The ADA provides further guidance in its CKD Evidence-Based Guidelines and recommends a range of 22–35 kcal/kg/day factoring in weight status and goals, age, gender, activity level, and other metabolic stressors of patients, such as comorbidities, surgery, or infections (ADA, 2010).

The key to determining the appropriate, individualized recommendation for protein and energy intake rests on the estimated body weight used for the calculations. Actual body weight can reflect fluid overload in the nondialyzed patient and lead to overestimating needs and potential weight gain. Determining the edema-free weight in patients with CKD 4 can be challenging and often necessitates the clinician to use an estimated or desired body weight based on height and weight history. K/DOQI recommends using a standard body weight (SBW) based on National Health and Nutrition Survey (NHANES) II data for age, height, gender, and frame size or an adjusted weight for those who fall below 95% of the SBW or above 115% of the SBW (National Kidney Foundation, 2000). Both under- and overestimation of needs can be detrimental to the patients with CKD 4. Frequent monitoring of adherence to intake recommendations and of the changes in weight and nutritional status is necessary to determine the appropriateness of the recommendations regardless of what method is used. It should also be noted that weight loss might be a necessary goal for patients with CKD 4 to improve overall health, blood pressure, and glycemic control. This goal must be balanced against the risks of malnutrition inherent in restricting both protein and total calories and requires close monitoring by both the physician and the dietitian.

9.5 NUTRITIONAL RECOMMENDATIONS FOR PATIENTS WITH CKD 4—MICRONUTRIENTS

9.5.1 Bone Metabolism and Phosphorus

Phosphorus is an essential mineral for bone structure and a number of physiological processes in the body. Phosphorus is absorbed through the intestines, with the aid of active vitamin D, and is excreted via the kidneys. Consequently, as GFR declines and kidney failure progresses, phosphorus levels in the blood begin to rise. However, owing to the ability of the kidneys to adapt to an increase in phosphorus levels and an increase in PTH and fibroblast growth factor-23, overt hyperphosphatemia does not occur until the onset of CKD 4 (Burke, 2008). It is well established that uncontrolled, chronic high-phosphorus levels contribute to hyperparathyroidism that leads to high-turnover bone disease, promotes vascular calcification, and is associated with increased all-cause mortality (Burke, 2008). The increased incidence of CVD seen in the population with CKD is believed to be related to the arterial calcification mediated by high phosphorus. Hyperphosphatemia is considered an independent risk factor for morbidity and mortality in renal failure (Block et al., 2004). Early and adequate phosphorus control may have long-term implications.

The interplay of phosphorus, calcium, and PTH is very complex as kidney function declines, with common practice standards in the predialysis population focused on addressing the lab values of phosphorus, calcium, and PTH only as they become out of range. Current recommendations, however, suggest preventing high phosphorus levels in patients with CKD 4 by limiting dietary phosphorus intake to 800–1000 mg/day or 10–12 mg/g of protein intake (National Kidney Foundation, 2003; Sigrist et al., 2009). Following an LPD supports this recommendation as most phosphorus comes from protein and dairy sources. Using the protein recommendation guideline as a basis for phosphorus intake minimizes phosphorus sources that have minimal protein content. This is an important consideration when seeking to minimize the risk of malnutrition by overrestricting the diet. As the GFR reaches 15 mL/min, dietary control will often not be adequate to prevent hyperphosphatemia, and phosphate-binding medications may be necessary. Binders may also be a useful tool for patients for whom an LPD is inappropriate.

Dairy products, animal protein, and nuts in the diet have historically been the primary sources of phosphorus, which have been addressed in the diet for patients with CKD. However, phosphorus-containing food additives are frequently being used in food production. They are found in beverages as a stabilizer or in meat products as a preservative and for color enhancement (Murphy-Gutekunst, 2007). Often this additional phosphorus is not captured on food labels, and therefore it is difficult to identify this. In addition, this inorganic phosphorus appears to be more easily absorbed and is estimated to contribute an additional 1000 mg/day of phosphorus in the diet (Uribarri and Calvo, 2003). With ongoing education on these facts, these significant sources of hidden phosphorus must be taken into account for adequate management of phosphorus.

9.5.2 Bone Metabolism and Calcium

Adequate calcium levels are necessary to maintain normal bone turnover. As kidney function declines, the kidney is less able to convert inactive vitamin D (25-OH vitamin D) to active vitamin D (1, 25-OH vitamin D), which stimulates intestinal absorption of calcium. Consequently, calcium levels decrease as GFR decreases. Maintaining serum calcium levels within normal ranges is a key component in preventing hyperparathyroidism (ADA, 2010).

K/DOQI recommends that patients with CKD 4 maintain corrected calcium levels within the normal range of 8.4–10.2 mg/dL (National Kidney Foundation, 2003). It is important to note that calcium should be corrected for albumin levels to avoid underestimating serum levels as serum calcium is bound by albumin. The standard equation is as follows: corrected calcium (cCA) = [(4 - serum albumin) × 0.8] + serum calcium.

Hypocalcemia (<8.4 mg/dL) should be avoided and treated; however, total daily intake of elemental calcium should not exceed 2000 mg/day (National Kidney Foundation, 2003). This is an important consideration when calcium-based phosphorus binders are used to treat hyperphosphatemia. Treatment of hypocalcemia may also include the use of vitamin D sterols (ADA, 2010). Hypercalcemia should be avoided and may necessitate the use of noncalcium-based binders for phosphorus control. Limiting additional calcium to 1500 mg/day is a general rule to avoid this outcome (National Kidney Foundation, 2003). Education on sources of calcium beyond dairy foods is necessary as more common renal friendly products such as juices and cereals are fortified with additional calcium.

9.5.3 Bone Metabolism and PTH

PTH is another parameter that must be monitored and addressed in patients with CKD 4. As previously described, PTH levels are regulated primarily by calcium, phosphorus, and vitamin D. As renal function declines, patients with CKD are at the risk of hyperparathyroidism and subsequent bone diseases. Monitoring and maintaining phosphorus and calcium at recommended levels is essential in reducing the risk of hyperparathyroidism. However, medical management with vitamin D sterols such as doxercalciferol or paricalcitol is often necessary to meet the recommended goal of 70–110 pg/mL for intact PTH. Further discussion on medications used to manage PTH can be found in Chapter 14.

9.6 KEY ELECTROLYTES IN CKD 4

Sodium is a key electrolyte in fluid regulation and balance. The kidney's ability to filter sodium decreases as kidney function declines. Patients with CKD 4 often experience fluid retention and a decrease in urine output, which requires daily use of diuretics. A low-sodium diet that improves the effectiveness of both diuretics and blood pressure-lowering medications is recommended for patients with CKD 4. Sodium recommendations range from 1 to 2 g/day depending on the source. The 2010 Dietary Guidelines for Americans developed by the U.S. Department of Agriculture (USDA) recommend a daily limit of 1500 mg for all people (USDA, 2010). Although this is lower than the standard recommendations for patients with CKD, it should be considered an appropriate goal for most patients with CKD 4. Intake of 1 g or less is difficult to maintain on a long-term basis, and therefore it may not be appropriate for all. Monitoring of fluid status and blood pressure control can be good indications of the intake level that is necessary for each patient.

Potassium is the second key electrolyte that must be monitored in patients with CKD 4. Potassium functions as a regulator of muscle contractions including those of the heart. The body maintains tight regulation of potassium as both hyper and hypo levels are dangerous.

Medications for lowering blood pressure such as an angiotension-converting enzyme inhibitor (ACE-I) can significantly increase potassium levels, whereas some diuretics can decrease blood potassium levels. Other causes of hyperkalemia include uncontrolled diabetes, acidosis, tissue breakdown, and chronic constipation (National Kidney Foundation, 2009). Incidence of hyperkalemia increases in patients with CKD 4; however, it is important to determine the contributing factors before limiting the dietary intake of potassium immediately and further restricting the diet. Intake recommendation for dietary potassium in patients with CKD 4 is <2.4 g/day if they have hyperkalemia. Lower protein intake will support this intake level, but paying attention to intake of fruits and vegetables that are considered high sources of potassium, such as tropical fruits or potatoes, is also important. Reading of food labels is also an important tool, as sodium is increasingly being replaced with potassium in many low-sodium canned and prepackaged foods. Education on appropriate low-sodium alternatives that do not use additional potassium is increasingly necessary for recommendation of appropriate diet to patients with CKD 4.

9.7 VITAMINS AND MINERALS

The diet recommendation for patients with CKD 4 should meet Dietary Reference Intakes (DRIs) for most vitamins; however, supplements that contain minerals such as calcium should be avoided. Many providers recommend a renal-specific vitamin formulation for those with CKD 4 to avoid the accumulation of fat-soluble vitamins as kidney function declines and to discourage the use of megadoses of vitamins found in many over-the-counter products. Oral iron supplementation may also be necessary to address iron-deficient anemia and to provide the additional iron stores needed for effective use of EPO. Education on methods to improve iron absorption with renal-specific foods should be included.

9.7.1 Vitamin D

The body stores vitamin D as 25-OH vitamin D, which must then be activated by the kidney to form 1, 25 OH vitamin D or active vitamin D. Patients with CKD are at increased risk of vitamin D deficiency, which is defined as <30 ng/mL, as a result of limiting dietary phosphorus, chronic illness, age, and renal failure. K/DOQI recommends treating vitamin D deficiency to maintain adequate levels of 25-OH vitamin D (Cuppari and Garcia-Lopes, 2009). Treatment recommendations vary from aggressive treatment of 50,000 IU of ergocalciferol weekly, until levels are >30 ng/mL, to a moderate daily dose of 1000–2000 IU of cholecalciferol (Heaney et al., 2003; National Kidney Foundation, 2003). It should be noted that the current DRI for vitamin D is 600–800 IU/day with an upper limit (UL) of 4000 IU/day (IOM, 2010). Renal-specific vitamin formulations that also contain 1000–2000 IU D3 are available now.

9.7.2 Anemia

Anemia is a common feature in patients with CKD 4, with estimates of >50% of patients in stages 3–5 suffering from anemia. As renal failure progresses, the kidney is unable to produce the hormone EPO, which stimulates red blood cell production. Medical management of anemia in CKD includes the use of recombinant human EPO. In addition, as mentioned earlier, adequate iron stores are necessary to support this treatment. Patients who remain unresponsive to EPO with adequate iron stores should be evaluated for vitamin B_{12} and folic acid deficiency and treated if needed (ADA, 2010). Many continue to recommend vitamin C to enhance the absorption of iron supplements; however, intake of levels above the DRI should be avoided (National Kidney Foundation, 2006).

9.8 COMORBITIES AND CKD 4

Nutrition plays a key role in managing the comorbidities of diabetes, hypertension, hyperlipidemia, and obesity that can profoundly impact the progression of kidney disease.

Often for patients with CKD 4, what began as one chronic illness of hypertension or diabetes then becomes layered with additional chronic issues requiring multiple medications with concomitant diet and/or lifestyle adjustments. Assisting the patients with CKD 4 in balancing priorities and developing goals that are achievable and sustainable is a key role of the renal dietitian. Stressing to the patients the significance of each incremental improvement in the various areas of concern may help them keep their focus and motivation.

9.8.1 Diabetes

Adequate diabetic management can slow the progression of renal failure in patients with CKD 4. Diet management is essential to reach and maintain good glycemic control while avoiding the risks of hypoglycemia. K/DOQI recommends achieving a hemoglobin A1c of <7% or an estimate average glucose of <154 mg/dL to preserve renal function and slow down diabetes-related nephropathy (NKF, 2007). For insulin-dependent diabetics, the risks of hypoglycemia increase as renal failure progresses, and the kidney is less able to clear insulin that then remains longer in the blood stream. Increasing GI issues and poor dietary intake also contribute to more frequent hypoglycemic episodes. Education on renal-specific foods to address hypoglycemia, such as apple juice instead of orange juice, must be included. Often the diet becomes overwhelming for diabetic patients with CKD 4, who must learn to balance carbohydrate, fat, and protein intake while restricting sodium and potassium. RDs who are knowledgeable in renal-specific diet can help the patient with CKD 4 manage this complex diet.

9.8.2 Cardiovascular Disease

CVD is considered the leading cause of death among patients with CKD, and therefore lipid management must be incorporated into the diet of patients with CKD 4. K/DOQI reports that the risk of CVD is particularly high for diabetics with CKD (NKF, 2007). Recommendations follow those of the adult treatment panel III (ATP III) guidelines of the National Cholesterol Education Program for high-risk groups. Therapeutic lifestyle changes such as limiting saturated fat to <10% of total calories and cholesterol to <200 mg/dL are considered standard to reach an low-density lipoprotein (LDL) <100 mg/dL. However, many recommend striving for an LDL <70 mg/dL, which often requires medication in addition to dietary restrictions.

Limiting fat, which is an important source of calories, must be balanced with good diabetic control and adequate protein intake in patients who already have limited options. Evidence also supports the benefits of omega-3 fatty acid for cardioprotection to reduce inflammation and improve lipid profiles in patients with CKD 4 (ADA, 2010). Dietary sources such as cold water fish or flaxseed should be included in the diet of patients with CKD 4, instead of relying on supplements. Weight management can also be an important strategy in reducing the risk of CVD.

9.8.3 Obesity

Obesity and weight management must also be addressed in patients with CKD 4. Obesity plays a critical role in the development and management of diabetes and hypertension as well as CVD. Obesity is also believed to predispose people to renal failure and is an independent risk factor for graft failure and death in posttransplant stage in patients (Kopple, 2010; Meier-Kriesche et al., 2002). However, the goals of weight management must be constantly balanced against preventing protein-energy malnutrition in this at-risk group. As mentioned earlier, LPDs must be supported by adequate energy intake. Therefore, the typical strategy of reduced or low-calorie diets may not be appropriate for patients with CKD 4. Diets that are considered effective in the healthy population, such as low-carbohydrate diets (<35% calories from carbohydrates) or diets high in dairy foods, should be avoided as they often have higher levels of protein, phosphorus, and calcium than that recommended for CKD 4. Research on safe and effective diets for those with CKD is limited. However, a patient who is focused on a high-quality diet that promotes good diabetic and blood pressure control as well as cardiovascular health will likely result in maintaining his/her weight and possibly promoting slow weight loss.

Encouraging increased physical activity (within the physical limitations of the patient) may be an effective tool of weight management in patients with CKD 4, as it also promotes maintenance of lean body mass and improves overall cardiovascular health (ADA, 2010). In addition, physical activity has been shown to improve diabetic control and renal function (Straznicky et al., 2011). The American Diabetes Association and the American College of Sports Medicine have recently released their joint position statement on exercise and type 2 diabetes. They recommend 150 min of moderately vigorous aerobic activity weekly plus 2–3 sessions of resistance training (Colberg et al., 2010). ADA guidelines on adult weight management also recommend the use of multiple behavior strategies for effective weight loss. They include self-monitoring, stress management, stimulus control, problem solving, contingency management, cognitive restructuring, and social support (ADA, 2006). Beyond weight management, these strategies will be necessary for patients with CKD 4 and should be incorporated into the comprehensive plan of care for those patients.

Strategies for improving adherence are also addressed in diabetes and hypertension management in the KDOQ/I guidelines. K/DOQI guidelines emphasize, in the Clinical Practice Recommendations for Diabetics and CKD published in 2007, that effective strategies to effectively manage both diabetes and CKD depend on adequate self-management skills (NKF, 2007). They list six strategies that they believe should comprise the treatment plan for patients with diabetic CKD and that, except for glycemic control, are applicable to all patients with CKD 4. The strategies include the following: monitoring and treatment of blood glucose, blood pressure, nutrition, smoking cessation, exercise, and adherence to medications (NKF, 2007).

Assessment of the patient's ability to adhere to diet and lifestyle recommendations must be done to identify and address potential barriers. The dietitian can provide tools for establishing goals, tracking progress, and problem solving, which can assist patients in managing their complex needs. K/DOQI also stresses the need for education and treatment plans to be culturally and economically sensitive as well as geared to the learning level of the patient. Engaging the support of the family can also be useful when a patient must make significant changes to his diet and lifestyle. A focus on establishing good self-management skills and habits can clearly have an impact on all aspects of care for patients with CKD 4. We must recognize patients with CKD as the central players in the management of their health status and must focus on developing their problem-solving skills so as to address their barriers to adherence of diet/medications and avoid reliance on information-only education.

9.9 MEDICAL NUTRITION THERAPY

MNT is recommended for patients with CKD who are not on dialysis to ensure adequate nutritional status, prevent the progression of renal failure, and delay the need for RRT. The Center for Medicare Services currently provides reimbursement for MNT for patients with an eGFR <60 mL/min for an initial assessment and two follow-ups yearly (3 h of MNT maximum). The RD must obtain a National Provider Number with Medicare in order to be considered qualified to provide these services and bill them. ADA recommends that patients with CKD who are not on dialysis be monitored every 1–3 months if they are stable or more often if they are unstable, with evidence of malnutrition. They report that research on effective MNT suggests that patients with CKD need to spend up to 2 h monthly with a qualified RD for optimal outcomes (ADA, 2006, 2010).

9.10 EDUCATION

Utilizing multiple strategies to improve adherence is essential for successful management of patients with CKD 4. Although education alone is not sufficient, well-designed educational pieces that are patient-specific are a valuable tool for the dietitian. The Internet is a tool that has not been fully utilized. To date, there is limited research on the effectiveness of Web-based nutrition interventions for CKD, diabetes, or hypertension. A review of Web-based weight-loss interventions found those that were dynamic, individualized the process, and utilized self-monitoring tools were more effective and had greater retention (Arem et al., 2010). Currently, large dialysis centers offer such tools free of charge for patients with CKD. However, not all patients have access to the Internet on a daily basis. Effective education pieces should address the amount of sodium, potassium, and phosphorus in basic foods as well include information on reading of food labels to determine the nutrient content of purchased foods. In addition, education that combines components of diabetes management with the above provides patients with a resource that they can apply to their daily life.

9.11 SUMMARY

Nutrition management of patients with CKD 4 requires ongoing collaboration with the patient and the multidisciplinary team to successfully address all the concurrent contributing factors. Nutrition and diet play a key role as many symptoms and disease outcomes are related to dietary intake and can be managed with appropriate adjustments. The comprehensive assessment of patients with CKD 4 should include the following: diet and medication history, knowledge about their disease, behavior and lifestyle assessment, and an understanding about socioeconomic factors that may influence adherence to recommendations. Early and accurate assessment of macro- and micronutrient intake is essential for managing the symptoms related to CKD 4 as well as for slowing down the progression of the disease (Table 9.1). Understanding the role of diet in management of the comorbidities associated with CKD 4 assists in the effectiveness of the medications used to manage both diabetes and hypertension (Grundy et al., 2001; Mitch, 2005). In addition to medical management, behavior and lifestyle changes in weight management, physical activity level, and smoking cessation are needed to support these goals.

TABLE 9.1
Macro and Micronutrient Goals for Patients with CKD 4

Nutrient	Diabetic	Nondiabetic
Energy	22–35 kcal/kg	22–35 kcal/kg
Protein	0.8–1.0 g/kg	0.6–0.8 g/kg
Total fat	25%–35% of total calories	Only if dyslipidemia and/or cardiovascular disease
Saturated and trans fat	<7% of calories	
Cholesterol	<200 mg/day	
Phosphorus	800–100 mg/day (10–12 mg/g protein)	
Calcium	<2000 mg/day includes all sources	
Potassium	<2400 mg if elevated	
Sodium	1500–2300 mg/day (lower end optimal)	
Renal multivitamin intravenous infusion (MVI)		

Data combined from sources: USDA, *Dietary Guidelines for Americans. Dietary Guidelines.gov.* Online: www.cnpp.usda.gov/DGAs2010-DGACReport.htm (accessed September 12, 2010); ADA (American Dietetic Association Evidence Library), *Chronic Kidney Disease Evidence-Based Nutrition Practice Guideline*, 2010. Online: www.adaevidencelibrary.com/topic.cfm?cat=3927 (accessed September 27, 2010); National Kidney Foundation, *Pocket Guide to Nutrition Assessment of the Patient with Chronic Kidney Disease*, 4th ed., National Kidney Foundation, New York, 2009.

However, adherence to behavior and lifestyle changes is particularly challenging for patients with CKD 4 owing to both the complexity and the uniqueness of the diet. The renal dietitian has the opportunity to bring all aspects of disease management together and assist patients in developing strategies to meet their individual goals. The renal dietitian also plays an important role in coordinating care with the various practitioners who comprise the interdisciplinary team for patients with CKD 4. Communicating with the nephrologist on MNT plans and progress can provide an additional layer of reinforcement and accountability for the patient, thereby increasing the likelihood of success of management of CKD. Ultimately, adequate management of CKD 4 will be measured based on the ability to delay the need for RRT and on the nutritional status of patients with CKD 4 when they reach ESRD.

Finally, practice guidelines and standards of care are changing rapidly as organizations such as the National Kidney Foundation continue to evaluate current research on CKD, with frequent updates to the KDOQ/I guidelines. The ADA Evidence Analysis Library produces evidence-based nutrition practice guidelines for specific health problems. Their recently published guideline on CKD is a valuable resource with many useful tools for developing a comprehensive plan for nutrition intervention as well as monitoring and evaluation. It is essential that the dietitians providing MNT to the patient with CKD stay informed. Fortunately, there are multiple tools available to assist them. The following list includes resources that should be checked frequently for the latest recommendations:

ADA Evidence Library	www.adaevidencelibrary.com
NKF KDOQ/I Guidelines	www.kidney.org/professionals/KDOQI/
NKF Council on Renal Nutrition	www.kidney.org/professionals/CRN/
Kidney Disease: Improving Global Outcomes (KDIGO) Guidelines	www.kdigo.org

REFERENCES

ADA. (American Dietetic Association Evidence Library). 2006. *Recommendations Summary Adult Weight Management: Multiple Behavior Therapy Strategies.* May. Online: www.adaevidencelibrary.com/template.cfm?template=guide_summary&key=628 (accessed November 27, 2010).

ADA. (American Dietetic Association Evidence Library). 2010. *Chronic Kidney Disease Evidence-Based Nutrition Practice Guideline.* Online: www.adaevidencelibrary.com/topic.cfm?cat=3927 (accessed September 27, 2010).

Arem, H., and Irwin, M. 2010. Obesity management: A review of web-based weight loss interventions in adults. *Obes Rev.*, August.

Bersnstein, A.,Treyzon, L., Zhaoping, L. 2007. Are high-protein vegetable-based diets safe for kidney function? A review of the literature. *J Am Diet Assoc.* 107 644–650.

Beto, J., and Bansal, V. 2004. Medical nutrition therapy in chronic kidney failure: Integrating clinical practice guidelines. *J Am Diet Assoc.* 104:404–409.

Block, G., Klassen, P., Lazarus, J., et al. 2004. Mineral metabolism, mortality, and morbidity in maintenance hemodialysis. *J Am Soc Nephrol.* 15: 2208–2218.

Burke, S. 2008. Phosphate is a uremic toxin. *J Ren Nutr.* 18(no. 1): 27–32.

Cianciaruso, B., Pota, A., Pisani, A., et al. 2008. Metabolic effects of two low protein diets in chronic kidney disease stage 4–5—A randomized controlled trial. *Nehprol Dial Transplant.* 23: 636–644.

Cianciaruso, B., Pota, A., Bellizzi, V., et al. 2009. Effect of low-versus moderate-protein diet on progression of CKD: Follow-up of a randomized controlled trial. *Am J Kidney Dis.* 54: (no. 61) 1052–1061.

Colberg, S., Sigal, R.J., Fernhall, B., et al. 2010. Exercise and type 2 diabetes: The American College of Sports Medicine and the American Diabetes Association: Joint position statement. *Diabetes Care.* 33:(no. 12) 147–167.

Cuppari, L., and Garcia-Lopes, M. 2009. Hypovitaminosis D in chronic kidney disease patients: Prevalence and treatment. *J Ren Nutr.* 19:(no. 1) 38–43.

Eyre, S., and Attman, P. 2008. Protein restriction and body composition in renal disease. *J Ren Nutr.* 18 (2): 167–186.

Eyre, S., Attman, P., Haraldsson, B. 2008. Positive effects of protein restriction in patients with chronic kidney disease. *J Ren Nutr.* 18: (no. 3) 269–280.

Fuhrman, M., Charney, P., Mueller, C. 2004. Hepatic proteins and nutrition assessment. *J Am Diet Assoc.* 104: (no. 8): 1258–1264.

Grundy, S., Becker, D., Clark, L., et al. 2001. Executive summary of the Third report of the NCEP expert panel on detection, evaluation, and treatment of high blood cholesterol in adults. *JAMA.* 285: 2488–2497.

Heaney, R., Davies, K., Chen, T., et al. 2003. Human serum 25-hydroxycholecalciferol response to extended oral dosing with cholecalciferol. *Am J Clin Nutr.* 77: (no. 1) 204–210.

Ikizler, T. 2009. Dietary protein restriction in CKD: The debate continues. *Am J Kidney Dis.* 53: (no. 2) 208–17.

IOM. 2010. Dietary reference intakes for calcium and vitamin D. *Institute of Medicine Report at a Glance.* Online: www.iom.edu/Reports/2010/Dietarty-Reference-Intakes (accessed December 10, 2010).

Kalantar-Zadeh, K., Kopple, J., Block, G., et al. 2001. A malnutrition-inflammation score is correlated with morbidity and mortality in maintenance hemodialysis patients. *Am J Kidney Dis.* 38: (no. 6) 1251–1263.

Kalantar-Zadeh, K., Stenvinkel, P., Pillon, L., et al. 2003. Inflammation and nutrition in renal insufficiency. *Adv Ren Replace Ther.* 10: (no. 3) 155–169.

Kasiski, B., Lakatua, J., Ma, J., et al. 1998. A meta-analysis of the effects of dietary protein restriction on the rate of decline in renal function. *Am J Kidney Dis.* 31: (no. 6) 954–961.

Kopple, J. 2010. Obesity and chronic kidney disease. *J Ren Nutr.* 20: (no. 5S) S29–S30.

Meier-Kriesche, H., Arndorfer, J., Kaplan, B. 2002. The impact of body mass index on renal transplant outcomes: A significant risk factor for graft failure and patient death. *Transplantation.* 73:70–78.

Menon, V., Kopple, J., Wang, X., et al. 2009. Effect of a very low-protein diet on outcomes: Long-term follow-up of the Modification of Diet in Renal Disease (MDRD) Study. *Am J Kidney Dis.* 53: 208–217.

Mitch, W. 2005. Beneficial responses to modified diets in treating patients with chronic kidney disease. *Kidney Int Suppl.* 94: S133–S135.

Molnar, M., Keszei, A., Czira, M., et al. 2010. Evaluation of the malnutrition-inflammation score in kidney transplant recipients. *Am J Kidney Dis.* 56: (no. 1) 102–111.

Murphy-Gutekunst, L. 2007. Hidden phosphorus: Where do we go from here? *J Ren Nutr.* 17: e31–e36.

National Kidney Foundation. 2000. K/DOQI nutrition guidelines in chronic renal failure. *Am J Kidney Dis.* 35: (no. 6) S56–S63.

National Kidney Foundation. 2003. K/DOQI clinical practice guidelines for bone metabolism and disease in chronic kidney disease. *Am J Kidney Dis.* 42: (no. 4) S1-S201.

National Kidney Foundation. 2006. K/DOQI clinical practice guidelines and clinical practice recommendations for anemia in chronic kidney disease. *NKF KDOQ/I Guidelines.* Online: www.kidney.org/professionals/KDOQI/guidelines_anemia/index.htm (accessed Nov 14, 2010).

National Kidney Foundation. 2007. Clinical practice guidelines and clinical practice recommendations for diabetes and chronic kidney disease. *NKF KDOQI Guidelines.* Online: www.eatright.org/kdoqi/guideline_diabetes (accessed October 15, 2010).

National Kidney Foundation. 2009. *Pocket Guide to Nutrition Assessment of the Patient with Chronic Kidney Disease.* 4th. ed. New York: National Kidney Foundation.

Robertson, L., Waugh, N., Robertson, A. 2007. Protein restriction for diabetic renal disease. *Cochrane Database Syst Rev* 4.

Sigrist, M., Chiarelli, G., Lim, L., et al. 2009. Early initiation of phosphate lowering dietary therapy in non-dialysis chronic kidney disease: A critical review. *J Ren Care.* 35: Suppl 71–78.

Straznicky, N., Grima, M.T., Lambert, E.A., et al. 2011. Exercise augments weight loss induced improvement in renal function in obese metabolic syndrome individuals. *J Hypertens.* 29: (no. 3) 553–564.

U.S. Renal Data System. 2010. *USRDS 2010 Annual Data Report: Atlas of Chronic Kidney Disease and End-Stage Renal Disease in the United States.* Bethesda, MD: National Institute of Health, National Institute of Diabetes and Digestive and Kidney Diseases.

Uribarri, J. and Calvo, M. 2003. Hidden sources of phosphorus in the typical American diet: Does it matter in nephrology? *Semin Dial.* 16(no. 3): 186–188.

USDA. 2010. Dietary Guidelines for Americans. *Dietary Guidelines.gov.* June. Online: www.cnpp.usda.gov/DGAs2010-DGACReport.htm (accessed September 12, 2010).

10 Nutrition for Chronic Kidney Disease, Stage 5

Lesley McPhatter
University of Virginia

CONTENTS

10.1 INTRODUCTION

Just as nutrition is a cornerstone of treatment for many diseases, including diabetes and obesity, diet is paramount in the treatment of all stages of chronic kidney disease (CKD). When the glomerular filtration rate is 10% or less than the normal rate (90–120 mL/min/1.73m^2), a patient is considered to be in end-stage renal disease (ESRD; KDOQI™ Guidelines, 2002). Dialysis is needed to replace diminished kidney function. Some patients in end-stage renal failure receive kidney transplants. This restores kidney function, and the patient is able to return to a more normal diet (Figure 10.1).

The diet for dialysis patients is complicated, multifaceted, and must be individualized to each patient's needs. Maximizing intake with adequate protein and calories while limiting fluid, sodium, potassium, and phosphorus for a chronic disease requires diligence and a patient-centered team approach for the best overall patient outcome.

Mortality rates for patients with CKD on dialysis (CKD—Stage 5) in the United States are higher than the general population. Among dialysis patients aged 20–44 and 45–64, mortality rates in 2008 reached 83 and 174 deaths per 1000 patient years, respectively—both figures are eight times greater than those seen in the general population. Rates among transplant patients are closest to those of non-ESRD patients, ranging from 1.2 times greater in those aged 20–44 to 1.6 times higher among the patients above 65 years of age (USRDS, 2010).

Malnutrition affects 40%–70% of all dialysis patients and significantly increases mortality risk. There are many reasons for these alarming malnutrition statistics in dialysis patients. These include the complications from kidney failure: uremia, fatigue, weakness, nausea, and vomiting. Studies also show that patients do not eat secondary to poor appetite, dietary monotony, and lack of physical/financial support (Sundell, 2007). Complications from various comorbid conditions such

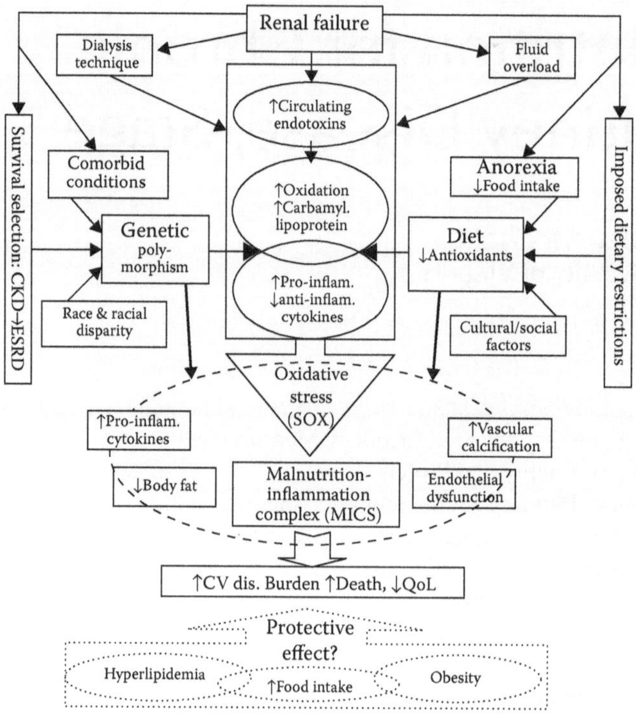

FIGURE 10.1 Schematic representation of the pathophysiology of kidney disease wasting in maintenance hemodialysis patients. (Reproduced from Kalantar-Zadeh, K. and Balakrishnan, V, *Hemodial Int.*, 10, 315–325, 2006. With permission from Blackwell Publishing.)

as diabetes mellitus and cardiovascular disease also affect dietary intake. Thirty-seven percent of dialysis patients have diabetes mellitus, 82% have hypertension, and 63% have cardiovascular disease (USRDS, 2008).

Yet another reason for the development of malnutrition is poor intake related to inadequate dialysis. Under dialyzed patients experience decreased taste acuity and anorexia resulting in insufficient dietary energy and protein intake. In patients who are adequately dialyzed, dietary restrictions and fluid limitations may impair oral intake. Appetite stimulants (megace, prednisone) and antidepressants with an appetite enhancing side effect (remeron) may be used in some settings. Use is controversial and clinical trials predicting long-term positive outcomes are limited. Use should be monitored closely and dosing should be adjusted and tapered carefully to avoid negative side effects.

10.2 DIALYSIS TREATMENT OPTIONS AND ADEQUACY MEASUREMENTS

Conventional hemodialysis (CHD) accounts for 92% of all dialysis in the United States. Patients typically undergo a 3–5-h treatment three times per week in a dialysis facility. Six percent of patients perform peritoneal dialysis (PD) at home 6 days per week. The remaining 2% of patients perform hemodialysis at home as CHD, nocturnal home hemodialysis (NHD), or short daily dialysis (SDD). The latter two types of home hemodialysis require more dialysis treatment time than CHD. Therefore, most of those patients eat better, feel better, and have an increased quality of life; recent data also suggest that these patients have an improved mortality outcome compared to their CHD or PD counterparts (Friedman et al., 2002; Kjellstrand and Ing, 1998; Mohr et al., 2001; Raj et al., 2000).

The dialysis prescription is individualized within a range. Patients typically run at a specified blood flow rate (BFR), dialysate flow rate (DFR), and against a specific dialysis bath with a prescribed artificial kidney called the dialyzer. The composition range of the dialysis bath is outlined as follows:

- Sodium (Na): 137–140 mEq/L or mmol/L
- Potassium (K): 2–3 mEq/L or mmol/L
- Bicarbonate($HCO3$): 28–35 mEq/L or mmol/L
- Calcium (Ca): 2–3 mEq/L or 1–1.5 mmol/L

Variations depend on the facility standard, individual patient parameters, and tolerance for the dialysis treatment. Machine choice is facility preference, but machines have a variety of specifics to maximize the treatment for that patient with the best BFR, DFR, adjustments for bicarbonate and sodium parameters, and the ability to monitor achievement of the adequacy goals for that patient throughout the treatment. The artificial kidney or dialyzer is chosen based on patient's needs and biocompatibility parameters (Locatelli et al., 2004; Palmer, 2001).

Dialysis adequacy is calculated using the urea reduction ratio, which determines the decrease in blood urea over the course of the treatment. Pre- and post-dialysis-treatment blood samples of blood urea nitrogen (BUN) are drawn, and the following formula is used to calculate the results: (Pre BUN – post BUN)/pre BUN× 100.

A goal of ≥65% is the current objective for CHD. In 2011, the Centers for Medicare and Medicaid Services (CMS) began to require facilities to achieve this goal in at least 96% of their patients who dialyze in the clinic. Most CHD patients should reach this goal after their first 6 months on dialysis (Federal Register, 2008). Eventually, all dialysis patients adequacy will be evaluated using the KT/V, a more complex measure of adequacy that includes an residual renal function and is an adequacy marker that is calculated for PD. The goal for KT/V is >1.2.

10.3 DIET PRESCRIPTION: ENERGY AND PROTEIN

In the United States, the age of new dialysis patients continues to climb. Patients are older, with more comorbidities, and are often malnourished at the beginning of treatment. The diet for any CKD patient on hemodialysis is individualized to the patient's dietary needs, preferences, and other medical problems. A good starting place is daily energy needs.

The current energy recommendations are generally 30–35 calories/kg actual or adjusted body weight based on the current K/DOQI guidelines for any hemodialysis patient (KDOQI, 2000; McCann, 2009). There is debate over the use of adjusted body weight. Though formulas for calculating adjusted body weight are no longer used in most disease states, the renal community has not reached a consensus on weight calculations for assessing nutrient needs. The most current references are the updated Chronic Kidney Disease guidelines updated in July 2010 from the Evidence Analysis Library of the American Dietetic Association. The recommendations suggest that the registered dietitian use clinical judgment to maximize the most effective individualized goals for all CKD patients including Stage 5 patients with dialysis. Adjustments in total energy recommendations plus macronutrient percentages are based on age, body composition, weight loss or gain, and the presence of comorbid conditions (ADA, 2011). Calorie guidelines based on the established weight range from 30 to 35 calories/kg/day for CHD and 25–35 cal/kg/day for PD. PD calories should include calories absorbed from the dialysis solutions. The amount will vary depending on the specific characteristics of the patient's membrane, the type of PD, and the dextrose concentrations of the solutions the patient uses each day. Average daily calories absorbed from peritoneal dialysate are approximately 350 (Burkart, 2004).

Once the energy goal is established, an intake of approximately 1.2 g/protein/kg per day is recommended for hemodialysis patients according to current K/DOQI guidelines. Protein needs for PD patients may be slightly higher because of increased protein losses ranging from 1.2 to 1.3 g/kg/day. PD patients are encouraged to maintain or increase protein intake to maintain serum albumin within the higher limit of normal range (KDOQI, 2000). Since 2008, the CMS has recommended a goal albumin for all dialysis patients of 4 g/dL. Amino acid losses are estimated at 8–12 g per CHD treatment (Federal Register, 2008). Tables 10.1 and 10.2 contain summary energy and nutrient data for hemodialysis and PD.

10.4 DIET PRESCRIPTION: FLUIDS, SODIUM, AND POTASSIUM

Fluid restriction varies with the type of dialysis. Typically, CHD dialysis goals are <3% of dry or target weight between treatments. Many patients just starting CHD have residual urine output that allows for a more liberal fluid prescription. The usual fluid restriction is 1000 mL/day plus urine output. Included in the fluid restriction are all foods or beverages that are liquid at room temperature. Dialysis patients who are diabetic appear to have greater thirst. Suspected causes include poor glucose control, sodium shifts associated with the dialysis treatment, or high dietary intake of sodium. Educating patients about all sources of fluid, including ice chewing, is paramount to controlling fluid weight gain between treatments. Cardiomyopathy and other cardiovascular diseases may make it hard for some patients to tolerate even small amounts of fluid removal. Fluid intake will need to be adjusted to accommodate patients' individual needs. Fluid weight-removal goals are individualized based on the patient's intake and dialysis prescription. Patient education and follow-up are needed to ensure that the patient understands the risk of ongoing fluid overload. There is significant cardiovascular stress created from attempting to remove excessive fluid in a defined treatment time of 3–5 h for CHD. For the more-frequent dialysis modalities PD, SDD, and NHD, it

TABLE 10.1
Daily Nutrient and Fluid Needs for Adults Undergoing Conventional Hemodialysis

Nutrients	Recommendations
Energy	30–35 kcal/kg
Protein	≥ 1.2 g/kg
Sodium	1500–2400 g
Potassium	2–3 g
Fluids	Urine output plus 1000 mL
Calcium	≤2 g including binder load
Phosphorus	10–12 mg/g/protein
Ascorbic acid	60–100 mg
Pyridoxine	5–10 mg
B12	3 μg
Folic acid	1–5 mg
No A or K	
Zinc	15 mg
Riboflavin	1.8–2.0 mg
Niacin	20 mg
Thiamin	1.5–2.0 mg
Biotin	20–30 μg
Vitamin E	10–15 IU
Pantothenic acid	10 mg
Iron	Individualized
Active vitamin D	As needed to treat mineral bone disorder (MBD)
Nutritional vitamin D	Replete to normal lab value for D3

TABLE 10.2
Daily Nutrient and Fluid Needs for Adults Undergoing Peritoneal Dialysis

Nutrient	Recommendations
Energy[a]	30–35 kcal/kg
Protein	1.2–1.3 g/kg
Sodium	1500–2400 g
Potassium	3–4 g
Fluids	As tolerated
Calcium	≤ 2 g including binder load
Phosphorus	10–12 mg/g/protein
Ascorbic acid	60–100 mg
Pyridoxine	5–10 mg
B12	3 μg
Folic acid	1–5 mg
No A or K	
Zinc	15 mg
Riboflavin	1.8–2.0 mg
Niacin	20 mg
Thiamin	1.5–2.0 mg
Biotin	20–30 μg
Vitamin E	10–15 IU
Pantothenic acid	10 mg
Iron	Individualized
Active vitamin D	As needed to treat MBD
Nutritional vitamin D	Replete to normal lab value for D3

[a] Includes kcal from dialysate (3.4 kcal/g).

is not always necessary to restrict fluid intake unless it exceeds the maximum that can be removed during the treatment regimen.

Sodium restriction is determined by the patient's fluid and hypertensive state. Hypotensive patients may benefit from additional dietary sodium, and normotensive patients may need only a healthy dietary limitation of 2400 mg/day (KDOQI, 2000). The 2010 U.S. Dietary Reference Intake guidelines recommend further limiting Na to <1500 mg/day for people with chronic diseases such as diabetes, hypertension, and kidney disease (IOM, 2010). The feasibility of this and the long-term benefit for CKD Stage 5 patients will require further study. Convenience foods, table salt, fast foods, enhanced meats, canned vegetables, and other highly processed foods are the greatest sources of sodium for dialysis patients.

Potassium (K) intake for patients on CHD is usually restricted to 2–3 g/day. Patients on the more-frequent dialysis modalities may not require restriction or may only need to restrict K on their days off dialysis. Patients with low-normal serum levels may not need to limit K. Patients who have low potassium levels should be encouraged to increase potassium intake to avoid symptoms such as muscle cramping.

Monthly laboratory test results can guide decisions on optimal K intake. Some patients may need to restrict more during their longest interdialytic period and may eat more freely during the week. The sources of hidden potassium in processed foods continue to grow as lower sodium goals are embraced. Unfortunately, in most cases, potassium is not listed on a product's nutrition label. Patients and families should be provided with a list of the potassium content of common foods. They should also be aware that reduced sodium products such as salt substitutes, low sodium soups, popcorn, and frozen entrees often replace sodium with potassium chloride (KCl).

The goal for K, as noted earlier, varies with laboratory reference range values, but is typically 3.5–6 mEq/L for CKD patients. Hyperkalemia may present as general muscle weakness, difficult ambulation, or bradycardia and can be life threatening; however, many patients are asymptomatic. Treatment goals include determining the cause of hyperkalemia. Nondietary causes include hemolysis of lab sample, inadequate dialysis, high K concentration in dialysate, catabolism, hyperglycemia, insulin deficiency in diabetics, acidosis, and interactions with drugs including angiotensin-converting enzyme inhibitors and beta blockers. Dietary sources of high potassium are potatoes, tomatoes, oranges, nuts, and any products containing KCl. One teaspoon of salt substitute as NOSalt contains 664 mg potassium. See Table 10.3 for an expanded list of foods that are high in potassium (USDA, 2011).

Potatoes and other tuberous root vegetables (e.g., yucca, batata, eddo, yampi, and yams) are a significant part of the diet for many persons. The potassium content of these vegetables can be reduced by double cooking. The vegetables should be peeled and sliced, covered in water, brought to a boil, cooked 5–10 min, and then drained. Fresh water should be added to the cooking pot, brought to a boil for the second time, and the vegetable cooked until it is soft and tender (Burrowes and Ramer, 2008; Figure 10.2).

TABLE 10.3
Higher Potassium Foods

Food	Portion	Amount of Potassium (mg)
Baked beans	1 cup	653
Banana	1 medium	422
Beet greens	1 cup	1309
Cantaloupe	1 c pieces	427
Honeydew melon	1 c pieces	388
Lima (butter) beans	½ cup	445
Milk, reduced fat, 2%	1 cup	366
Milk shake, chocolate	11 oz	672
Orange juice, fresh	1 cup	443
Peaches	1 medium	285
Prunes, dried, stewed	½ cup	494
Peanuts, oil roasted	½ cup	573
Potato with skin, baked	1 medium	751
Potato fries	10 strips	334
Raisins	½ cup	543
Sweet potato, baked	1 medium	542
Spinach, cooked from raw	½ cup	418
Tomato	1 medium	292

Source: USDA Nutrient Database for Standard Reference. http://www.nal.usda.gov/fnic/foodcomp/search (accessed March 22, 2011).

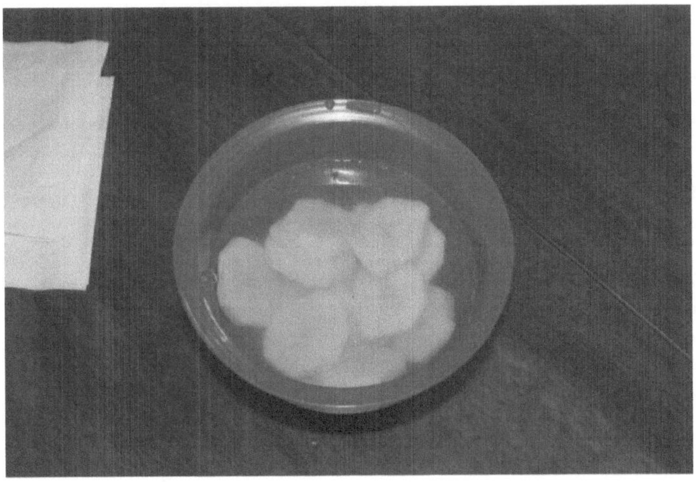

FIGURE 10.2 Soaking potatoes to reduce potassium.

10.5 VITAMINS AND MINERALS

In hemodialysis, vitamin needs are increased because of the loss of B vitamins. All patients should be on a renal multivitamin to ensure adequate vitamin replacement in addition to dietary intake. Table 10.4 contains a sampling of current supplement formulations. Vitamin replacement is typically one renal vitamin per day after dialysis. Patients doing more frequent hemodialysis may need additional supplementation due to higher losses with increased dialysis time, and therefore, removal of water-soluble vitamins (Kopple, 2010). Over-the-counter multivitamins are contraindicated in CKD Stage 5 because of the risk of toxicity from excessive fat-soluble vitamins, particularly vitamin A. Vitamin C should not be supplemented beyond the reference daily intake (RDI) due the risk of oxalic stone development. Newer renal vitamins contain zinc and/or nutritional vitamin D and may be appropriate for use in some patients. Use of herbal supplements and over-the-counter nutritional supplements should be evaluated closely. There is little data on the risks associated with supplementation in CKD patients. Since vitamins, minerals and herbs are cleared through the kidney, it is reasonable to recommend limiting or avoiding use of supplementation when kidney function is impaired.

Calcium intake should be limited to <2000 mg of elemental calcium/day from all sources: dialysate, calcium-based phosphate binders, calcium supplements, and diet. Dairy products can be consumed in small amounts depending on the patient's dietary prescription. Consumption of calcium-fortified foods should be limited. Calcium blood levels should be maintained within the normal range (KDIGO™, 2009).

Phosphorus intake is limited in conjunction with recommended protein intake. Typical restriction is 10–12 mg/g of protein or 800–1000 mg/day; however, the use of daily dialysis liberalizes any restrictions (Sullivan, 2010). Historically, organic phosphorus was the greatest concern and source of phosphate intake. In 1990, inorganic phosphorus made up approximately 400 mg of dietary phosphorus intake/day. Although there are no comprehensive study results available, inorganic phosphorus intake is now estimated to approach 1500–2000 mg/day. Inorganic phosphorus is not attached to protein and is therefore absorbed at 100% versus approximately 60% for organic phosphorus. Inorganic phosphorus is a food additive, enhancer, and preservative (Sarathy et al., 2008). There are no labeling guidelines and the amounts may vary significantly. The use of convenience or enhanced foods leads to a much higher phosphorus intake than is recommended for CKD. Table 10.5 contains a list of high-phosphorus foods that should be used in moderation by dialysis patients.

TABLE 10.4
General Vitamin and Mineral Renal Formulations

Vitamin	Recommended Amount/Day	Vitamin	Recommended Amount/Day
Vitamin C	60–100 mg	Thiamin (B1)	1.5 mg
Riboflavin (B2)	1.7 mg	Niacin	20 mg (as niacinamide)
Pyridoxine (B6)	10 mg	Cobalamin (B12)	6 mcg
Folic acid	1 mg	Pantothenic acid	5–10 mg
Biotin	150 mcg	Zinc	12.5 mg

TABLE 10.5
Higher Phosphorus Foods

Food	Portion	Amount of Phosphorus (mg)
Almonds	22	133
Baked beans	1 cup	258
Black-eyed peas, frozen, boiled	1 cup	208
Bran cereal, 100%	½ cup	344
Cheese sauce	½ cup	278
Couscous	1 cup	294
Ice cream, chocolate	1 cup	170
Ice cream, vanilla	1 cup	138
Lima (butter) beans, boiled	½ cup	110
Milk, 2%	1 cup	229
Peanuts, oil roasted	1 cup	572
Peanut butter, creamy smooth	2 Tbsp	115
Split peas, boiled	1 cup	194
Sunflower seeds	1 oz	322
Taco	1 large	313
Trail mix with chocolate, nuts, and seeds	½ cup	283
Whole wheat bread	1 slice	59
Yogurt, low-fat-fruit flavor	8 oz	270

Source: USDA Nutrient Database for Standard Reference. http://www.nal.usda.gov/fnic/foodcomp/search (accessed March 22, 2011).

Phosphorus levels are difficult to control in ESRD through dietary restrictions only. Phosphate binders are necessary to maintain acceptable blood serum levels. Typical binders include calcium carbonate, calcium acetate, magnesium carbonate, lanthanum carbonate, and sevelamer carbonate. Aluminum hydroxide is a very effective binder, but it is rarely used because of the potential for aluminum toxicity.

Iron deficiency is a frequent concern in patients receiving dialysis. Causal factors include gastrointestinal loss, blood draws, bleeding at the dialysis access site, and blood collection in the hemodialyzer membrane. There is also increased demand for iron during erythropoietin therapy. Some patients are able to maintain adequate serum levels through diet and oral supplements; however, the majority of patients require parenteral iron therapy.

10.6 SPECIAL CONSIDERATIONS

10.6.1 Cardiovascular Disease

Many patients reach CKD Stage 5 secondary to complications from cardiovascular disease. It is the most common cause of death in the CKD population (USRDS, 2010). Sodium and fluid restrictions help to control blood pressure in patients in all stages and on all types of dialysis, but the prevention of dyslipidemia is not always targeted. Elevated serum levels of low-density lipoprotein (LDL) cholesterol and triglycerides are associated with increased risk of atherosclerotic cardiovascular disease. The most common serum lipid irregularities in patients with CKD are elevated triglycerides and very low-density lipoproteins. In addition, high-density lipoprotein (HDL) levels are often low. Normal or elevated levels of HDL cholesterol seem to protect against the development of cardiovascular disease.

The diet recommended by the National Institutes of Health (NIH) is restricted in the amount of cholesterol, type and amount of fat, and calories. Dyslipidemias (Tables 10.6 through 10.9) are dealt with through the use of medication and therapeutic lifestyle modifications as suggested by the NIH, the American Heart Association, and the KDOQI Clinical Practice Guidelines (AHA, 2010; KDOQI, 2003; Mathes, 2010; NIH, 2011). Physical activity is recommended. Alcohol is to be used only in moderation and tobacco use is not advised.

Plant sterols and stanols have been shown to block the absorption of dietary cholesterol and may be used within CKD dietary guidelines. Unabsorbed dietary cholesterol is then excreted in the stool. For example: an intake of 2–3 g plant sterols/day has been shown to lower LDL by 6%–15% (KDOQI, 2003).

The use of viscous fiber in the diet can also help reduce total cholesterol and LDL cholesterol. Achieving optimal amounts in the Stage 5 CKD diet can be difficult, especially for the anuric hemodialysis patient receiving treatment three times per week. The renal dietitian can help maximize viscous fiber intake while not compromising serum potassium and phosphorus values. It is especially important that patients read the nutritional labels on packaged foods. Bran cereals vary widely in fiber, potassium, and phosphorus content. Consumption of high-fiber fruits and vegetables can also add to the patient's overall fiber intake (Table 10.10).

L-Carnitine (a transport molecule used in the oxidation of free fatty acids) supplementation has been shown to enhance cardiac function in dialysis patients. The literature suggests that treatment results in lower inflammation levels and improved lipid metabolism in some cases (Pertosa et al., 2005; Tabibi et al., 2011). No clear guidelines for the use of L-carnitine supplementation have been approved at this time.

TABLE 10.6
The National Cholesterol Education Program (2010) Uses the Following Heart Disease Risk Classifications

Total Cholesterol	mg/dL	mmol/L	HDL-CHOL	mg/dL	mmol/L
Desirable	< 200	< 5.2	High	≥ 60	≥ 1.6
Borderline high	200–239	5.2–6.2	Low	< 40	< 1.0
High	> 240	≥ 6.2			
LDL-CHOL	**mg/dL**	**mmol/L**	**Triglycerides**	**mg/dL**	**mmol/L**
Optimal	< 100	< 2.6	Normal	≥ 150	≥ 1.7
Near optimal	100–129	2.6–3.3	Borderline	150–197	1.7–2.2
Borderline high	130–159	3.4–4.1	High	200–499	2.3–5.6
High	160–189	4.1–4.9	Very high	> 500	≥ 5.7
Very high	≥ 190	≥ 5.0			

TABLE 10.7
American Heart Association Diet and Lifestyle Recommendations for Cardiovascular Disease Risk Reduction

- Balance kilocalorie intake and physical activity to achieve or maintain a healthy body weight.
- Consume a diet rich in vegetables and fruits.
- Choose whole-grain, high-fiber foods.
- Consume fish at least twice per week.
- Limit your intake of saturated fat to < 7% of energy, *trans* fat to < 1% of energy, and CHOL to < 300 mg/day.
- Minimize your intake of sugary beverages and foods. Added sugar should be limited to no more than 100 kcal for women and 150 kcal for men each day.
- Choose and prepare foods with little or no salt.
- If you consume alcohol (ETOH), do so in moderation.

The *Dash Diet* is a well researched low fat diet that is very popular for use in prevention of cardiac disease. It is especially helpful for reduction of elevated blood pressures.

DASH Food Categories	Daily Servings Based on a 2000 kcal Diet
Breads, cereals, and other grain products (three servings should be whole grain)	6–8
Vegetables	4–5
Fruits	4–5
Low-fat-dairy products	2–3
Lean meat, seafood, and poultry	6 ozs or less
Fats and sweets	limit
Nuts, seeds, and legumes	4–5 per week

TABLE 10.8
Therapeutic Lifestyle Diet

Guidelines for Adults	NCEP Guidelines for Patients with High CHOL
Total fat	Up to 35% total calories if mostly monounsaturated
Saturated	< 7%
Cholesterol	200 mg/day
Total calories	Maintain desirable weight
Soluble fiber	10–25 g/day
Plant stanols/sterols	2 g/day
Physical activity	As recommended

10.6.2 Dialysis Patients with HIV/AIDS

It is difficult for many patients with HIV/AIDS to maintain an adequate nutritional status. Gastrointestinal effects such as malabsorption and diarrhea are frequent. When HIV/AIDS nephropathy leads to dialysis, the patient is often severely malnourished before treatment begins. Improving and then maintaining nutrition status are special challenges in this population.

Daily nutrient recommendations start with 35–45 calories/kg/actual weight. Protein is increased to 1.5–2.5 g/kg actual weight. Fat recommendations (amount and type) are adjusted based on tolerance. When diarrhea is a factor, sodium and fluid restrictions are relaxed. Vitamin and mineral supplements are increased to twice the suggested amounts during times of malabsorption (Plourd, 1995).

TABLE 10.9
American Heart Association Recommendations for Lowering Elevated Blood Lipid Levels in Adults

Prudent Diet Guidelines	Step 1% Total Calories	Step 2 % Total Calories
Total fat	< 30	< 30
Saturated	< 10	< 7
Trans	< 1	< 1
Monounsaturated	10–15	10–15
Polyunsaturated	10	10
Carbohydrates	50–60	50–60
Protein	15–20	15–20
Cholesterol	< 300 mg/day	< 200 mg/day

TABLE 10.10
Dialysis Friendly High Fiber Fruits and Vegetables

Item	Serving Size	Fiber (g)	Potassium (mg)	Phosphorus (mg)
Apple	1 medium	3.3	148	15
Blackberries raw	1 cup	7.6	233	32
Blueberries raw	1 cup	3.5	112	17
Carrot raw	1 medium	2.0	230	25
Cauliflower boiled	1 cup	4.9	250	43
Collards boiled	1 cup	5.3	220	57
Dates dried	4	206	210	20
Frozen mixed vegetables boiled	1 cup	8.0	308	93
Green snap beans boiled	1 cup	4.0	182	36
Peaches canned	1 cup	3.1	206	22
Pears canned	1 cup	3.9	129	17
Pineapple raw	1 cup	2.2	169	12
Raspberries frozen	1 cup	11.0	285	42
Winter squash	1 cup baked	2.2	181	22

Source: USDA Nutrient Database for Standard Reference. http://www.nal.usda.gov/fnic/foodcomp/search (accessed April 25, 2011).

The use of protease inhibitors and/or nucleoside reverse transcriptase inhibitors can exhibit symptoms of fat redistribution and peripheral lipodystrophy. Clinical signs are elevated blood lipids, insulin resistance, and enlarged truncal girth. A diet that avoids simple carbohydrates, is higher in fiber and lower in saturated fats, with necessary adjustments for kidney disease, is generally recommended (American Dietetic Association, 2010).

10.6.3 Older Adults with CKD

More than 50% of patients receiving kidney replacement treatments are older than 65 years (USRDS, 2010). Older adults with Stage 5 CKD often experience sensory, gastrointestinal, and musculoskeletal changes that can increase the risk of inadequate nutritional status. CKD is also known to impair taste perception.

Dry mouth, or xerostomia, is quite common in older adults, and the usual fluid restriction required for dialysis patients serves to exacerbate the problem. Therapies can include sucking on sugarless candy or chewing sugarless gum, using mouth sprays, avoiding tobacco and alcohol use, and limiting salty foods. At home, the use of a humidifier can help to moisten the air. If possible, medications that contribute to dry mouth should be changed.

Taste perception and olfaction decline with aging. Salt and sugar tastes are the last strong sensations. The older patient's diet should contain some of these strong flavors to enhance appetite (NIH Senior Health, 2011).

Poor dentition and periodontal disease also plague older adults. Five percent of seniors older than 65 years have no teeth, and 23% have untreated decay (NIDCR, 2011). Dietary modifications, such as recommending canned fruits instead of fresh, can help increase overall food intake.

As aging reduces the pleasure of eating, anorexia and weight loss may occur. Poor intake along with impaired digestion and absorption of nutrients leads to malnutrition.

Patient dietary education should emphasize frequent small meals and snacks. For patients with mobility problems, approved ready-to-eat meals and easy-to-prepare recipes are very helpful. Nutritional supplements, either canned or homemade, are an easy way to add protein and calories to the diet.

Education materials should be in large print, sans serif type, with high contrast between the words and background, and should be at the appropriate reading level for the patient. Patients' families and caregivers should always be included in the educational counseling experience (Thomas et al., 2001).

10.6.4 Disaster Planning and Emergency Diet

Stage 5 CKD patients are dependent on dialysis to sustain life. Emergencies such as earthquakes, hurricanes, tornadoes, or floods may limit or delay access to dialysis. The patient must then follow a diet restricted in fluids, protein, and electrolytes to survive until dialysis is once again available. Table 10.11 lists guidelines for use in the event of a disaster or emergency. The ESRD network provides disaster planning. Materials can be accessed online at http://www.esrdnetwork.org/disaster-planning/index.asp.

10.7 SUMMARY

Maintaining proper nutrition in the dialysis patient requires a patient-centered team approach. Socioeconomic status, mental and physical cognitive levels, and comorbid conditions all play a role in the maintenance of a patient's nutritional status. To determine the best course of action for each patient, an individualized care plan must be established along with measurable goals as soon as CKD is recognized. Interventions can include dietary nutritional supplementation and appetite stimulants. Use of appetite stimulants is controversial and clinical trials predicting long-term positive outcomes are limited. Use should be monitored closely and dosing should be adjusted and tapered carefully to avoid negative side effects (Bossola et al., 2009, 2010). They can improve nutrition outcomes quickly. In extreme cases of malnutrition, patients may require short- or long-term use of intradialytic parenteral nutrition or home total parenteral nutrition. The correction of social and/or economic barriers through assistance programs such as Meals On Wheels or home health care providers can be beneficial. In some cases, placing the patient in assisted living or nursing facilities will provide the best outcome. Regardless, a patient who is failing nutritionally will not survive if not treated aggressively and correctly. Focusing on the total nutrition picture, prioritizing goals and helping the patient and family understand the need for changes to the diet will ultimately prove the most valuable to the dialysis patient.

TABLE 10.11
Emergency Shopping List for the Adult Dialysis Patient

Food stored in the refrigerator and/or freezer should be used first. Limit fluid intake as much as possible.
(Food for 2–3 days)
Bottled water: allow 5 gallons
(~2–3 L) for hygiene purposes plus usual fluid restriction
Boxed juices
Powdered milk, boxed milk, or small cans of evaporated milk
Loaf of white bread
Dry cereal: corn flakes, rice flakes, cheerios, puffed wheat and rice, or shredded wheat
Box of vanilla wafers or other plain cookies
Box of graham crackers
Box of unsalted crackers
Granulated sugar
Small jars of mayonnaise (open one each day)
Small cans/packets of canned meats and fish (open, eat, and then throw away leftovers. Do not try to save without refrigeration)
Peanut butter
Hard candy in different flavors
Canned fruit: peaches, fruit cocktail, pears, pineapple, mandarin oranges, and applesauce
Fresh apples, lemons, carrots, if available
Jellies: apple, grape, strawberry, blueberry, blackberry
Marshmallows
Plastic dinnerware and utensils, paper towels, napkins, and a nonelectrical can opener.

REFERENCES

American Dietetic Association. 2010. Position paper: Nutrition intervention and human immunodeficiency virus infection. *J Am Diet Assoc.* 110: 1105–1119.

American Dietetic Association. 2011. *Evidence-Based Nutrition Practice Guidelines on CKD.* Available at: http://www.adaevidencelibrary.com/category.cfm (accessed July, 2011).

American Heart Association. 2010. www.heart.org, accessed July 8, 2010.

Bossola, M., Tazza, L., Luciani, G. 2009. Mechanisms and treatment of anorexia in end-stage renal disease patients on hemodialysis. *J Renal Nutr.* 19(1): 2–9.

Bossola, M., Tazza, L., Giungi, S., et al. 2010. Artificial nutritional support in chronic hemodialysis patients: A narrative review. *J Renal Nutr.* 20(4): 213–223.

Burkart, J. 2004. Metabolic consequences of peritoneal dialysis. *Semin Dial.* 17(6): 498–504.

Burrowes, J. and Ramer, N. 2008. Changes in potassium content of different potato varieties after cooking. *J Renal Nutr.* 18(6): 530–534.

Federal Register. 2008. Conditions for coverage for end stage renal disease facilities interpretive guidelines, final rule. *Federal Register*, 73(73),Tuesday, April 15.

Institutes of Medicine. 2010. Dietary reference intakes: Electrolytes and water. Available at: http://www.iom.edu/Global/News%20Announcements/~/media/442A08B899F44DF9AAD083D86164C75B.ashx

Friedman, A., Boston, A., Levey, A., et al. 2002. Plasma total homocysteine levels in patients undergoing nocturnal versus standard hemodialysis. *J Am Soc Nephrol.* 13: 265–268.

Kalantar-Zadeh, K. and Balakrishnan, V. 2006. The kidney disease wasting: Inflammation, oxidative stress, and diet-gene interaction. *Hemodial Int.* 10: 315–325.

KDIGO Guidelines for CKD Mineral bone disorder. 2009. *J Int Soc Nephrol.* 76: Supplement 113.

KDOQI Bone Disease Work Group. 2003. K/DOQI clinical practice guidelines for bone metabolism and disease in chronic kidney disease. Serum calcium and calcium–phosphorus product. *Am J Kidney Dis.* 42: S77–S83.

KDOQI Clinical Practice Guidelines for Chronic Kidney Disease. 2002. Guideline 1: Definition and Stages of Chronic Kidney Disease. National Kidney Foundation. www.kidney.org (accessed March 24, 2011).

KDOQI Nutrition Work Group. 2000. K/DOQI clinical practice guidelines for nutrition in renal failure. Management of protein and energy intake. *Am J Kidney Dis.* 35:S40–S45.

Kjellstrand, C. and Ing, T. 1998. Daily hemodialysis—History and revival of superior dialysis method and literature review. *ASAIO J.* 44:117–122.

Kopple, J. 2010 Trace elements and vitamins. In Mitch, W. and Ikizler, T. (Eds.), *Handbook of Nutrition and the Kidney*. Wolters Kluwer, Philadelphia, PA, 163–176.

Locatelli, F., Covic, A., Chazot, C., et al. 2004. Optimal composition of the dialysate with emphasis on its influence on blood pressure. *Nephrol Dial Transplant.* April 19: 785–796.

Mathes, H. 2010. Management of cardiovascular disease in patients with impaired renal function. *Renal Nutrition Forum.* Summer 29(3): 6–8.

McCann, L. ed. 2009. *Pocket Guide to Nutrition Assessment of the Patient with Chronic Kidney Disease*, 4th ed. New York: National Kidney Foundation.

Mohr, P., Nuemann, P., Franco, S., et al. 2001. The case for daily dialysis: Its impact on costs and quality of life. *Am J Kidney Dis.* 37(4):777–789.

National Cholesterol Education Program. 2010. http://www.nhlbi.nih.gov/guidelines/cholesterol/atglance.htm (accessed March 29, 2011).

National Institutes of Dental and Craniofacial Research. 2011. http://www.nidcr.nih.gov/DataStatistics/ (accessed April 1, 2011).

National Institutes of Health (NIH). 2011. http://nihseniorhealth.gov/problemswithtaste/toc.html (accessed March 31, 2011).

Palmer, B. 2001. Individualizing the dialysate for hemodialysis patients. *Semin Dialysis*. Jan–Feb 14 (1): 41–49.

Pertosa, G., Grandaliano, G., Simone, S., et al. 2005. Inflammation and carnitine in hemodialysis patients. *J Renal Nutr.* 15(1): 8–12.

Plourd, D. 1995. Nutritional management of the dialysis patient with AIDS. *J Renal Nutr.* 5(4): 182–193.

Raj, D., Ouwendyk, M., Francoeur, R., et al. 2000. Beta 2-microglobulin kinetics in nocturnal hemodialysis. *Nephrol Dial Transpl.* 15: 58–64.

Sarathy, S., Sullivan, C., Leon, J., et al. 2008. Fast food, phosphorus-containing additives and the renal diet. *J Renal Nutr.* 18(5): 466–470.

Sullivan, J. 2010. Effect of short daily hemodialysis and nightly home hemodialysis on phosphorus status. *Renal Nutrition Forum.* Summer 29(3): 1–5.

Sundell, M. 2007. Actual intake vs. prescribed diet in a hemodialysis population: Comparison using a two day dietary recall. *Renal Nutrition Forum.* 26(3): 8–12.

Tabibi, H., Hakeshzadeh, F., Hedayati, M., et al. 2011. Effects of L-carnitine supplement on serum amyloid A and vascular inflammation markers in hemodialysis patients: A randomized controlled trial. *J Renal Nutr.* 21(6): 485–491.

Thomas, L., Michels, P., Richter, D., et al. 2001. Identification of the factors associated with compliance to therapeutic diets in older adults with end stage renal disease. *J Renal Nutr.* 11(2): 80–89.

USDA. 2011. Nutrient database for standard reference. http://www.nal.usda.gov/fnic/foodcomp/search (accessed March 22, 2011).

US Renal Data System, USRDS. 2008. *Diabetes and Digestive and Kidney Diseases*, Bethesda, MD, 2008.

US Renal Data System, USRDS. 2010. *Annual Data Report: Atlas of Chronic Kidney Disease and End-Stage Renal Disease in the United States*, National Institutes of Health, National Institute of Diabetes and Digestive and Kidney Diseases, Bethesda, MD.

11 Nutrition for Children and Adolescents with Chronic Kidney Disease

Peggy Solan
Seattle Children's Hospital

CONTENTS

11.1 ETIOLOGIES OF CHRONIC KIDNEY DISEASE IN CHILDREN

Congenital abnormalities account for the majority of cases of chronic kidney disease (CKD) in children. The leading causes of CKD in children listed by the North American Pediatric Renal Trials and Collaborative Studies database are renal aplasia/hypoplasia/dysplasia, 16%; obstructive uropathy, 15%; focal segmental glomerulosclerosis, 12%; reflux nephropathy, 5%; chronic glomerulonephritis, 3%; and polycystic kidney disease, 3%.

Less common causes of CKD in children include genetic disorders such as cystinosis, oxalosis, and Alport's syndrome. Other causes include hemolytic-uremic syndrome, prune belly syndrome, and interstitial nephritis. In contrast to adult causes of CKD, diabetic nephropathy and hypertension are rare causes of pediatric CKD (NAPRTCS, 2010).

11.2 EPIDEMIOLOGY OF CKD IN CHILDREN

Kidney disease is uncommon in children. The incidence of kidney disease in children is estimated at 75 per million in the age-related population for all stages of CKD (Kher et al., 2007). The incidence of pediatric end-stage renal disease in the United States, reflected by those starting on dialysis, is approximately 15 per million population (U.S. Renal Data System, 2010).

11.3 STAGING OF CKD IN CHILDREN

The National Kidney Foundation (NKF) Kidney Diseases Quality Outcome Initiative (KDOQI™) staging system for CKD applies to individuals ≥ 2 years of age. The stages are estimated based on height and serum creatinine level as defined by an estimated glomerular filtration rate (GFR). Table 11.1 provides a description of the five stages. The following equation is used to estimate GFR in pediatric patients (Schwartz et al., 2009):

$$\text{GFR (mL/min/1.73 m}^2\text{)} = (0.413 \times \text{height [cm]})/\text{Serum creatinine (mg/dL)}$$

For example, a 6-year-old boy with a height of 120 cm and creatinine of 3 mg/dL would have a GFR of 20. He would be classified as having stage 4 CKD and may be nearing the need for kidney replacement therapy (Hogg et al., 2003).

11.4 PEDIATRIC NUTRITION ASSESSMENT

Assessment of the infant, child, or adolescent with CKD is fraught with potential errors associated with manifestations of the disease that affect weight and length or height. Also, classic markers of nutritional status may not be useful because of fluid status and inflammation.

Nutrition assessment of children with CKD is needed more frequently than assessments for normal children. KDOQI guidelines suggest monitoring children with CKD at least twice as frequently as normal children. Infants and toddlers require the most frequent assessments. Infants may require

TABLE 11.1
Stages of Chronic Kidney Disease

CKD Stage	1	2	3	4	5 or 5D
GFR (mL/min/1.73 m²)	≥90	60–89	30–59	15–29	<15
Stage description of kidney damage	With normal or increased GFR	Mild reduction of GFR	Moderate reduction of GFR	Severe reduction of GFR	Kidney failure
Nutrition treatment	Ensure adequate nutrition for growth, treat comorbidites, and monitor CVD risk	Modify diet as necessary for growth and estimate CKD progression	Modify diet as necessary for growth; evaluate and treat complications	Continue to further modify diet; prepare for kidney replacement therapy	Modify diet dependent on dialysis treatment

Sources: Hogg, et al., *Pediatrics*, 111, 1416–1421, 2003; Heilbron, et al., *Pediatr. Nephrol.*, 5, 5–11, 1991; NKF K/DOQI, *Am. J. Kidney Dis.*, 35, S1–S140, 2000; NKF K/DOQI, *Am. J. Kidney Dis.*, 53, S16–S123, 2009.
Abbreviations: CKD, chronic heart disease; CVD, cardiovascular disease; GFR, glomerular filtration rate.

weekly outpatient follow-up until a stable pattern of growth is established. Toddlers will likely require monthly follow-up at least.

Recommended assessment components include dietary intake, height- or length-for-age percentile or standard deviation score (SDS); height or length velocity-for-age percentile or SDS; estimated dry weight and weight-for-age percentile or SDS; head circumference until age 3, and normalized protein catabolic rate (nPCR). See Table 11.2 for recommended monitoring schedule (National Kidney Foundation's Kidney Disease Outcomes Quality Initiative, 2009).

Malnutrition is common in children with CKD. It is related to inadequate intake and is associated with anorexia, taste changes and a multitude of other gastrointestinal issues, including reflux, especially in infants, and constipation, especially in those with polyuria.

The best markers of nutritional status are problematic with kidney disease. For example, fluid overload makes it difficult to estimate lean body mass. Also, the child may appear to have adequate weight for length or weight for height according to the growth grid but may be cachexic upon visual exam. Arm anthropometry may be useful to document malnutrition in this child.

Protein malnutrition is common, related to inadequate intake associated with anorexia and the taste changes reported by some with kidney disease. Here, the commonly used marker of albumin may not be useful because albumin may be normal in the setting of starvation and depressed

TABLE 11.2
Frequency of Nutritional Assessment for Children with CKD Stages 2 to 5 and 5 Dialysis

	Minimum Interval in Months										
	Age 0 to <1 years			Age 1–3 years			Age >3 years				
Measure	CKD 2–3	CKD 4–5	CKD 5D	CKD 2–3	CKD 4–5	CKD 5D	CKD 2	CKD 3	CKD 4–5	CKD 5D
Dietary intake	0.5–3	0.5–3	0.5–2	1–3	1–3	1–3	6–12	3–4	3–4	3–4
Height or length-for age percentile or SDS	0.5–1.5	0.5–1.5	0.5–1	1–3	1–2	1	3–6	6–12	1–3	1–3
Height or length velocity-for-age percentile or SDS	05–2	0.5–2	0.5–1	1–6	1–3	1–2	6	6	6	6
Estimated dry weight and weight-for-age percentile or SDS	0.5–1.5	0.5–1.5	0.25–1	1–3	1–2	0.5–1	3–6	3–6	1–3	1–3
BMI-for-height-age percentile or SDS	0.5–1.5	0.5–1.5	0.5–1	1–3	1–2	1	3–6	3–6	1–3	1–3
Head circumference-for-age percentile or SDS	0.5–1.5	0.5–1.5	0.5–1	1–3	1–2	1	N/A	N/A	N/A	N/A
nPCR	N/A	N/A	N/A	N/A	N/A	N/A	N/A	N/A	N/A	1[a]

Abbreviation: BMI, body mass index; CKD, chronic heart disease; N/A, not applicable; nPCR, normalized protein catabolic rate; SDS, standard deviation score.

[a] Only applies to adolescents receiving HD.

Source: National Kidney Foundation. *Am. J. Kidney Dis.*, 53, S1–S124, 2009 (suppl 2). With permission.

in the setting of volume overload and inflammation. Hypoalbuminemia has been associated with increased mortality in children as well as adults (Wong et al., 2002).

Pre-albumin is not typically used in the assessment of pediatric patients with CKD because levels increase due to decreased clearance of the molecule with kidney disease.

Food records may supply valuable information for the nutrition assessment of a child. However, the common problems of accurate completion and avoidance of recording foods not recommended may yield false results.

Growth retardation is a common concern in children with CKD. Short stature has been associated with increases in morbidity and mortality (Wong et al., 2000). Adequate growth may continue until significant wasting occurs (Behrman and Kliegman, 1996). Use of the SDS or z score is an alternate method of expressing percentiles. For example, an SDS of −2 correlates with the second percentile. An SDS of >−2.5 has been associated with increased risk of death and increased hospitalization time (Wong et al., 2000).

Adequate intake of calories and protein is especially important for optimal growth. Growth and development deficits acquired during infancy may never fully recover (Foster and Leonard, 2004).

11.5 NUTRIENT NEEDS

11.5.1 Energy Needs

Infants and children with CKD are thought to have the same energy needs as normal children of the same age. See Table 11.3 for energy estimation equations. The use of standard methods for estimating energy requirements based on age and sex is the recommended starting point. Physical activity coefficients are included in the equations (Intakes, 2002). Children newly diagnosed with CKD may be cachexic and thus may benefit from additional energy for catch-up growth. As in other conditions, individual evaluation and revision of goals is needed to maintain optimal caloric intake (U.S. Department of Agriculture and U.S. Department of Health and Human Services, 2010).

Calorie supplementation in the form of formulas and modular components (single macronutrient products that provide extra carbohydrates, proteins, or fats) and manipulation of the diet to include high-calorie choices and to increase caloric density are frequently necessary. Conversely, children with excess body fat may require diet manipulation to decrease calories. Children treated with steroids for various medical conditions may also have a body mass index suggesting overweight or obesity. Also, the infant or child on peritoneal dialysis (PD) may gain excess weight associated with caloric absorption from dextrose dialysate. The child and family may benefit from counseling about lifestyle changes regarding intake and activity (Figure 11.1).

TABLE 11.3
Estimated Daily Calorie Needs Children at Healthy Weights

Age (Years)	Inactive	Moderate Activity	Active
2–3 either gender	1000–1200	1000–1400	1000–1400
4–8	1200–1400	1400–1600	1600–2000 Male 1400–1800 Female
9–13	1400–1600 Male 1600–2000 Female	1800–2200 Male 1600–2000 Female	2000–2600 Male 1800–2200 Female
14–18	2000–2400 Male 1800 Female	2400–2800 Male 2000 Female	2800–3200 Male 2400 Female

Source: U.S. Department of Agriculture and U.S. Department of Health and Human Services. *Dietary Guidelines for Americans, 2010*, U.S. Government Printing Office, December 2010, Washington, DC.

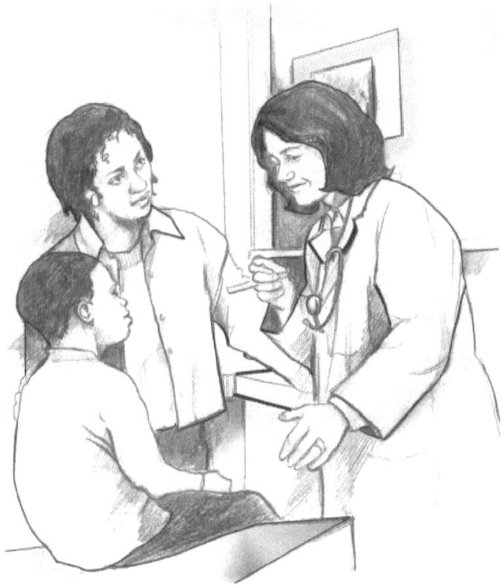

FIGURE 11.1 Counseling session. (Courtesy of the National Institute of Diabetes and Digestive and Kidney Diseases, National Institutes of Health.)

11.5.2 Protein

Protein intake is an important part of all children's diets for general health reasons, such as prevention of infection and illness, as well as optimal growth. The healthy child typically exceeds the recommended daily allowance for protein. The young child takes in 3–5 times the estimated average requirement (Fulgoni, 2008). Although there are data suggesting that restricting protein intake limits progression of kidney disease in adults, whether this is also true in pediatrics is controversial and may be problematic (Chaturvedi and Jones, 2007). Limiting protein intake to recommended daily needs may be helpful in reducing uremia and its side effects. However, it is important that the child maintains adequate caloric intake for growth. Depending upon the family situation, limiting protein may contribute to failure to thrive. Nutrition counseling is indicated to determine feasibility of this therapy with each family (Figure 11.2).

The latest KDOQI pediatric guidelines decreased the recommended protein needs for pediatric patients with CKD (Table 11.4). This resulted in lower protein recommendations for children on dialysis than for adults on dialysis on a per-kilogram basis. For example, the recommendation for an adolescent on hemodialysis is 0.95 g protein/kg, whereas the adult recommendation is 1.2 g protein/kg (National Kidney Foundation's Kidney Disease Outcomes Quality Initiative, 2009).

Individualization of protein goals remains important. Protein intake may be suboptimal due to anorexia and preference for foods other than protein sources. Creative methods to increase protein intake may be successful, including use of special recipes, modular supplements, protein-containing bars, and special shakes or smoothies.

Children on peritoneal dialysis have the highest estimated protein needs per kilogram. Dialysis-related protein losses are variable. The risk for kwashiorkor exists if protein intake does not meet needs, whereas energy needs can be partly met by the dextrose absorbed from dialysate.

Typical protein losses from peritoneal dialysis are reported as 0.28 g/kg in the first year of life decreasing to less than 0.1 g/kg in adolescents (Quan and Baum, 1996). Additional protein requirements range from 0.15 to 0.35 mg/kg, depending on age. Table 11.4 presents recommended protein intake. High peritoneal transporters may need increased dietary protein. Studies on aminoacid and protein loss have not been quantified on children. It is estimated that adding 0.1 g/kg/day of protein will meet needs

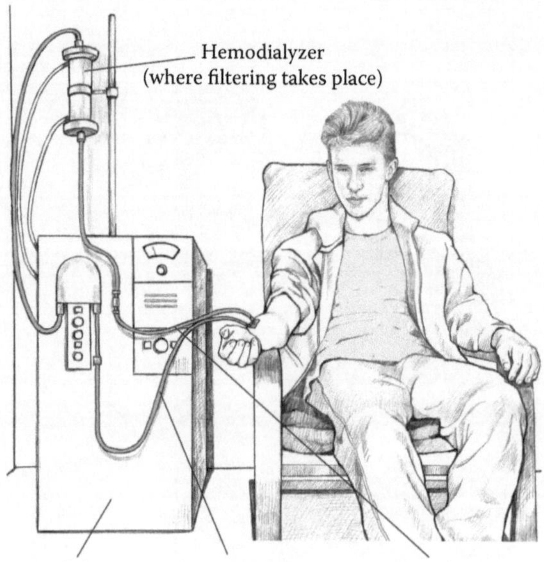

FIGURE 11.2 Teenager on dialysis. (Courtesy of the National Institute of Diabetes and Digestive and Kidney Diseases, National Institutes of Health.)

TABLE 11.4
Recommended Dietary Protein Intake in Children with CKD Stages 3–5 and 5 Dialysis

Age	Daily Reference Intake (DRI) (g/kg/day)	Recommended for CKD Stage 3 (g/kg/day) (100%–140% DRI)	Recommended for CKD Stages 4–5 (g/kg/day) (100%–120% DRI)	Recommended for HD (g/kg/day)[a]	Recommended for PD (g/kg/day)[b]
0–6 months	1.5	1.5–2.1	1.5–1.8	1.6	1.8
7–12 months	1.2	1.2–1.7	1.2–1.5	1.3	1.5
1–3 years	1.05	1.05–1.5	1.05–1.25	1.15	1.3
4–13 years	0.95	0.95–1.35	0.95–1.15	1.05	1.1
14–18 years	0.85	0.85–1.2	0.85–1.05	0.95	1.0

Source: National Kidney Foundation, *Am. J. Kidney Dis.*, 53, S1–S124, 2009. With permission.
Abbreviations: CKD, chronic kidney disease; DRI, dietary reference intake.
[a] DRI + 0.1 g/kg/d to compensate for dialysis losses.
[b] DRI + 0.15–0.3 g/kg/d depending on patient's age to compensate for peritoneal losses.

for children dialyzing 3 days per week. Increased protein needs would be expected with more frequent dialysis (National Kidney Foundation's Kidney Disease Outcomes Quality Initiative, 2009).

11.5.3 Fluid

Fluid goals are variable and dependent on the child's diagnosis, urine output, and other losses. The infant with polyuria may require up to 240 mL fluid per kilogram, whereas the child with polyuria may require several liters of fluid per day.

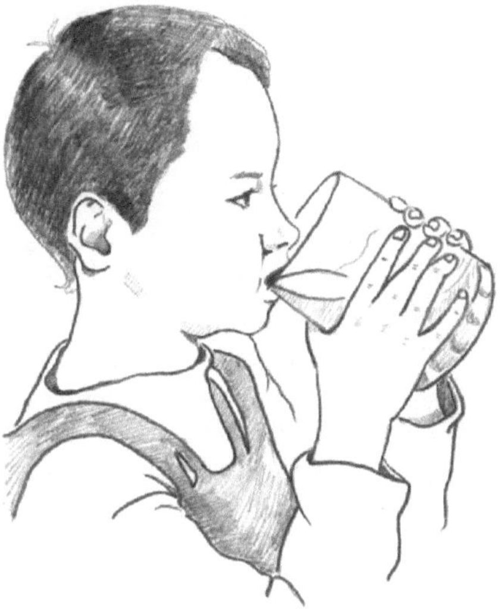

FIGURE 11.3 Fluids. (Courtesy of the National Institute of Diabetes and Digestive and Kidney Diseases, National Institutes of Health.)

Urine output commonly decreases on dialysis. Limiting fluid input to urine output plus insensible losses is generally recommended. This may require use of very concentrated formulations to meet the needs of those primarily fed by liquid formulas. For example, a typical infant formula contains 20 calories per ounce. To meet caloric needs of a child with CKD and a fluid restriction, formula may need to be gradually concentrated to greater than 40 calories per ounce.

Children on hemodialysis (HD) often require a very restricted fluid intake for optimal dialysis runs. It may be necessary to dialyze an infant daily to meet caloric needs until the transition to a concentrated formula is tolerated. It is important to provide adequate nutrition for growth. Increasing frequency of dialysis to allow adequate nutritional intake may not be popular with family or staff but may be necessary for growth. Transitioning to peritoneal dialysis may result in a liberalization of fluid restriction (Figure 11.3).

11.5.4 Sodium

Infants or children with kidney disease may need increased sodium intake for optimal growth or may need to limit sodium intake owing to problems with fluid retention and/or hypertension. Limiting sodium intake is a major challenge for families used to eating and cooking with processed foods and eating out. Involving the entire family in the new lower sodium diet is recommended. The American Heart Association recommends that all Americans decrease their sodium intake to less than 1500 mg/day (Lloyd-Jones et al., 2010). The entire family may benefit from the sodium reduction, and the child will likely better meet recommendations if the whole family transitions to a low-sodium diet. Given that the typical American consumes 3400 mg sodium per day, reducing sodium intake to the recommended levels may be a drastic change, and adaptation will take time. Children with nephrotic syndrome are placed on a low-sodium diet at diagnosis, and it is recommended that it be continued during remissions due to the difficulty of readjusting to a low-sodium diet during disease flares.

Conversely, infants and children with polyuria may benefit from sodium supplementation for optimal growth. A study of infants and toddlers found that sodium supplementation in the form of chloride and/or bicarbonate at doses of 2–4 mEq/100 ml fluid intake and a fluid intake of 180–240 ml/kg resulted in improvements in linear growth without the aid of growth hormone (Parekh et al., 2001).

Medications such as sodium phosphate, sodium bicarbonate, sodium chloride, and sodium polystyrene sulfonate administered to treat other renal-related abnormalities may add to the sodium intake.

11.5.5 Potassium

Potassium typically needs to be limited as disease progresses to Stage 5. Infants may be placed on breast milk treated with sodium polystyrene sulfonate or on a low-potassium infant formula. Standard progression for infant feeding is followed utilizing low-potassium fruits and vegetables. Rather than advance to regular milk at 1 year of age as per usual pediatric guidelines, a low-potassium infant formula is often continued to help control both potassium and phosphorus intake.

Potassium control may be easier than sodium control for many children. Learning to choose low-potassium beverages and to limit high-potassium fruits and vegetables becomes second nature for most children and they seem to easily transition back to the limitation if needed temporarily during the post-transplant period and if the transplanted kidney fails.

11.5.6 Iron

Iron supplementation becomes an important part of the life of the infant or child with kidney disease. Maintaining iron stores is important to help maintain energy for the normal activities of childhood and to prevent anemia-related learning problems. The healthy infant typically requires iron supplementation during the first year of life to ensure normal levels and prevent failure to thrive and learning issues. In addition, the infant or child with kidney disease frequently receives erythropoietic-stimulating agents to help achieve optimal iron status.

Parents often note the effects of iron supplementation such as black stools and constipation. Stool softeners may be included in the daily regimen in order to prevent problems such as the anorexia, abdominal pain, and vomiting experienced with severe constipation.

11.6 BONE HEALTH

Kidney disease may have an impact on the bone health of infants and children. Delay in advancement to walking may be seen if renal osteodystrophy develops. Older children may develop intense bone pain. The result of failure to control bone-related parameters in childhood is a grave one given the child's lifelong need to deal with kidney disease and its related side effects.

11.6.1 Calcium

Hypercalcemia and hypocalcemia are seen in infants and children with kidney disease. It is recommended that the dietary reference intake (DRI) for calcium be the goal, adjusted as needed based on clinical status. The 2011 DRIs for calcium include the selected expansion of the upper levels of intake, especially during the teenage years. At this time, there is no evidence that these parameters will be acceptable for children with CKD. Table 11.5 shows the new data.

Hypocalcemia is commonly seen in the child with newly diagnosed end-stage disease. Calcium supplementation between meals can help to normalize labs and if taken with meals provides phosphorus binding. Calcium in liquid form is available and is especially useful with infant and toddlers and in older children with swallowing issues.

Calcium intake varies with age, but one should ensure that the the upper limits of calcium intake are not exceeded once the hypocalcemic period resolves. The risk of mineral deposits throughout the body increases with an elevated calcium and phosphorus product (serum calcium times serum phosphorus). The calcium phosphorus product should be less than 65 for young children and less than 55 for those older than 12 years (National Kidney Foundation's Kidney Disease Outcomes Quality Initiative, 2005).

TABLE 11.5
Recommended Calcium Intake for Children with CKD Stages 2–5 and 5 Dialysis

Age	DRI	Upper Limit (for Healthy Children)	New 2011 Upper Limit Changes[a]	Upper Limit for CKD Stages 2–5, 5D (Dietary + Phosphate Binders)
0–6 months	210	ND	1000	≤420
7–12 months	270	ND	1500	≤540
1–3 years	500	2500	No change	≤1000
4–8 years	800	2500	No change	≤1600
9–18 years	1300	2500	3000	≤2500

Source: Some data in the table reproduced from National Kidney Foundation, *Am. J. Kidney Dis.*, 53, S1–S124, 2009. With permission.

Abbreviations: CKD, chronic kidney disease, DRI, dietary reference intake; ND, not determined.

[a] Column insert from the Institute of Medicine, National Academies, DRIs for Calcium, 2011.

Hypercalcemia may be associated with calcium supplements and vitamin D therapies of the active form, and less frequently, the inactive form. Also, hypercalcemia may be seen in vitamin A toxicities associated with kidney disease. Treatment involves discontinuing supplements or adjusting formula and diet to decrease vitamin A and calcium intake. Avoiding use of topical agents containing vitamins A and D is also recommended (National Kidney Foundation's Kidney Disease Outcomes Quality Initiative, 2009).

11.6.2 Phosphorus

Finding the balance between adequate but not excessive phosphorus intake is a challenge in managing most infants and children with kidney disease and is exacerbated as the older child and adolescent become more independent. As with calcium, maintaining normal phosphorus levels is recommended to promote optimal bone health and prevent mineral deposits throughout the body.

The infant may need phosphorus supplementation. Intravenous products, such as sodium phosphate for injection, may be used enterally if the infant is too young to tolerate other methods of increasing phosphorus intake.

Limiting dietary phosphorus and including phosphorus-binding agents in the diet are important components of the nutrition plan for children with kidney disease. The official guideline is to limit phosphorus intake to varying percentages of the DRI. Helping families understand that limiting dairy products and finding alternatives is a first step in phosphorus control education. Low-mineral infant formulas and specially designed adult renal formulas may help control phosphorus intake while maintaining adequate nutritional intake.

Phosphorus binders taken with meals and snacks along with a low-phosphorus diet can control phosphorus levels. Hyperphosphatemia may be seen in a child who is not eating, so caution is advised before assuming nonadherence. If calcium-based binders are needed at levels that exceed upper limits of calcium, the use of noncalcium–containing binders is recommended. Variations of the sevelamer product are frequently used. The powdered form can be used by those infants and children who are unable to take the pill form.

11.6.3 Vitamin D

The promotion of optimal vitamin D levels for the prevention of various diseases has caught the attention of the general press. Children with CKD, like healthy children, may require supplementation to achieve normal levels. Guidelines for monitoring of 25-hydroxy vitamin D levels and

TABLE 11.6
Recommended Supplementation for Vitamin D Deficiency/Insufficiency in Children with CKD

Serum 25 (OH) D (ng/mL)	Definition	Ergocalciferol (Vitamin D2) or Cholecalciferol (Vitamin D3) Dosing	Duration (months)
<5	Severe vitamin D deficiency	8000 IU/day orally or enterally × 4 weeks or (50,000 IU twice per month for 2 months) × 2 months	3
5–15	Mild vitamin D deficiency	4000 IU/day orally or enterally × 12 weeks or (50,000 IU every other week, for 12 weeks)	3
16–30	Vitamin D insufficiency	2000 IU/day or (50,000 IU every 4 weeks)	3

Source: National Kidney Foundation, *Am. J. Kidney Dis*., 53, S1–S124, 2009. With permission.
Abbreviation: CKD, chronic kidney disease.

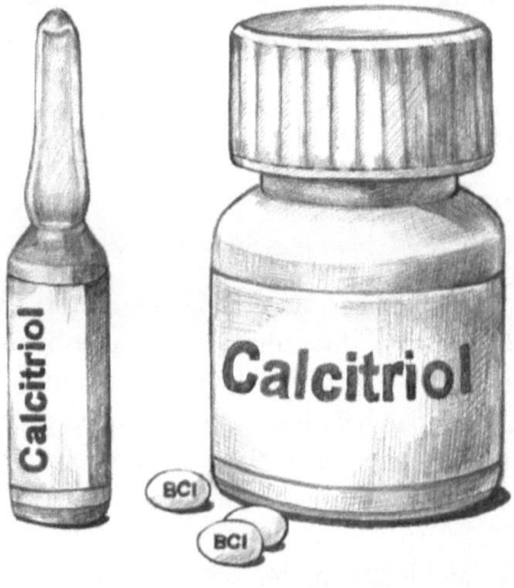

FIGURE 11.4 Calcitriol. (Courtesy of the National Institute of Diabetes and Digestive and Kidney Diseases, National Institutes of Health.)

supplementation are provided by the pediatric KDOQI guidelines (Table 11.6). Provision of both the inactive and active forms of vitamin D may be needed by children with kidney disease. The inactive form of vitamin D can be given on a weekly or monthly basis if the daily pill burden from other medications is limiting adherence to the medication regimen (National Kidney Foundation's Kidney Disease Outcomes Quality Initiative, 2009).

Hypercalcemia while the child is on active vitamin D may be treated by discontinuing or decreasing active vitamin D or by initiating a trial of an alternate vitamin D analog that may cause less hypercalcemia. A review of the child's diet and supplements for excess calcium and vitamin A intake is also indicated (Figure 11.4).

11.6.4 Parathyroid Hormone

The parathyroid hormone (PTH) level is monitored frequently in the child with CKD. Control of PTH levels is critical in managing renal osteodystrophy and has other implications such as the

TABLE 11.7
Recommended Frequency of Measurement for Bone Disease Markers

Stage	GFR	Calcium, Phosphorus, Total CO_2	PTH and Alkaline Phosphatase
3	30–59	Semi-annually	Semi-annually
4	15–29	Quarterly	Quarterly
5	<15	Monthly	Quarterly

Abbreviations: GFR, glomerular filtration rate; PTH, parathyroid hormone.

relation to the effectiveness of erythropoiesis-stimulating agents. Vitamin D 25-hydroxy and/or vitamin D analogus are used to treat elevated PTH levels. Target ranges for serum PTH are set by CKD stage. The Stage 3 (GFR 30–59) target is 35–70 pg/mL. Stage 4 (GFR 15–29) target is 70–110 pg/mL. Stage 5, including dialysis (GFR less than 15), is 200–300 pg/mL (NKF K/DOQI, 2005).

Monitoring of both PTH and 25-hydroxy vitamin D is recommended by KDOQI guidelines. The frequency of monitoring of the bone-related markers calcium, phosphorus, total CO_2, PTH, and alkaline phosphatase is based on the stage of disease. Controlling PTH levels can be difficult in those fed by tube given the adherence of the medication to plastic. Intravenous forms of active vitamin D are frequently provided to children on hemodialysis.

Hyperphosphatemia and hypercalcemia may drive up PTH levels, and active vitamin D may be withheld for high levels of calcium and phosphorus (National Kidney Foundation's Kidney Disease Outcomes Quality Initiative, 2005).

Use of cinacalcet to lower PTH levels has not been approved for pediatrics. A liquid version is not currently available, limiting potential usefulness in the pediatric population (Table 11.7; National Kidney Foundation's Kidney Disease Outcomes Quality Initiative, 2005).

11.7 VITAMIN AND MINERAL SUPPLEMENTS

Vitamin and trace element needs are thought to be the same as those for children without kidney disease. However, whereas the normal child may be able to tolerate excessive amounts of vitamins, the child with advanced kidney disease is at risk for hypervitaminosis A due to the kidneys' limited ability to clear vitamin A. Families should be advised to avoid supplements and foods fortified with vitamin A that contribute to a daily intake that exceeds the recommended daily allowance.

Renal vitamin supplements formulated for adults can be used for children on dialysis to replace the water-soluble vitamin losses that occur with dialysis. A liquid renal vitamin is available. A decreased dose as compared to adult dosing can be used to avoid excessive intake.

Given the increased use of processed foods and the trend to fortify more foods, the family should be instructed to read labels and watch for foods fortified with the nutrients of concern for that child. Potassium is listed on many baby foods but not on other products. Also, phosphorus may not be clearly labeled. Ongoing monitoring of intake and education about nutrient content of various foods remains useful.

11.8 GROWTH HORMONE

Use of growth hormone has aided children who are failing to maintain normal growth velocity. Children with renal disease do not have inadequate growth hormone; instead, they are unable to utilize their natural growth hormone. Children must be receiving adequate nutritional intake before growth hormone is initiated. Correction of acidosis, hyperphosphatemia, and hyperparathyroidism should have occurred prior to growth hormone initiation. Administration typically begins after the first year of life and is most effective in toddlers started on it before the age of two. Growth hormone is most effective in the first year of use. Growth hormone administration usually involves a daily injection. One study reported height increases of 10.7 ± 3.1 cm/year versus 6.5 ± 2.6 cm/year for the first year and 7.8 ± 2.1 cm/year versus 5.5 ± 1.9 for the second year of growth hormone (Mahan et al., 2006).

Growth velocity should be monitored, with the expectation that height velocity will reach above average levels so that catch-up height may be achieved. Calculations for mid-parental height can provide an indication of expected genetic height potential for the child. Paternal height (cm) plus maternal height (cm) plus 13 cm/2 is predictive for boys. For girls, add together paternal and maternal heights (cm) and then subtract 13 cm/2 (Abitbol et al., 1996).

11.9 NUTRITION SUPPORT

Children with kidney disease are frequently unable to meet their nutritional needs on their own. Nutrition support is indicated if diet manipulation and formula supplements do not result in adequate growth.

11.9.1 Enteral Nutrition

Inadequate nutritional intake may be supplemented by enteral nutrition, which has been shown to reverse weight loss and growth retardation in children with CKD. Achievement of significant catch-up growth is seen if started before 2 years of age (Ledermann et al., 1999).

Enteral choices for infants include breast milk or infant formula treated to reduce potassium load, as needed. Standard formulas may be appropriate in the early stages of CKD, transitioning to low-mineral infant or adult renal formulas as needed. There is no pediatric renal formula. The chosen formula base can be adjusted to provide the appropriate amount of nutrient of concern and combined with modulars to the caloric density needed to meet goals. Feeding tubes are often needed by infants to meet calorie goals as well as the high-fluid needs associated with polyuria. Once the child reaches toddlerhood, growth hormone supplementation may be required to maintain normal growth velocity owing to the child's inability to utilize naturally occurring growth hormone.

Enteral feedings via nasogastric tube can be used for temporary needs; however, the need for frequent replacement may limit actual administration of formula and may result in food aversions. Gastrostomy tubes placed for nutrition support may also prove to be useful in the initial post transplant phase to help with the administration of medications and fluids. However, families may need support to understand the benefit to the child. Families may experience reduced stress because they no longer feel obligated to spend most of their day ensuring the child takes in adequate nutrition by mouth. Using a gastrostomy tube to provide part or all of the child's nutrition needs may help normalize family life.

11.9.2 Parenteral Nutrition

Parenteral nutrition is used less frequently than enteral feedings in children with CKD, but comorbid conditions may require parenteral nutrition support. Complications such as pancreatitis or diseases such as acute-phase hemolytic-uremic syndrome may warrant use of parenteral nutrition. Guidelines for nutrition support in renal disease can be found in the American Society of Parenteral and Nutrition guidelines (Nutrition, 2002).

Parenteral nutrition during hemodialysis, known as intradialytic parenteral nutrition (IDPN), has a controversial history. This form of nutrition support will provide supplemental calories and protein. Because dialysis time is limited, concentration of the parenteral nutrition solution is limited and thus does not provide all nutrition needs. Therefore, calorie and protein needs will need to be met by a combination of parenteral, oral, and/or enteral support. Criteria for third-party coverage include evidence of energy or protein malnutrition and inadequate dietary protein and/or energy intake. Reports in children and adolescents are few. Studies report improvements in weight, albumin levels, and nPCR. IDPN was not found to be effective in correcting malnutrition associated with psychological issues (Orellana et al., 2005).

11.10 SUMMARY

The child with CKD faces many challenges as does the team providing care. As the stage of CKD progresses, the child will require frequent monitoring in order to optimize nutritional status and growth. Diets for children with CKD are as individualized and as liberal as possible to promote adequate intake. Families will require frequent, ongoing education and support as their child grows and they transition through the stages of CKD with their child. A multidisciplinary team consisting of a pediatric dietitian along with other pediatric specialists including nurses, social workers, therapists, and nephrologists will help the child achieve optimal growth and nutritional status.

REFERENCES

Abitbol, C., Chan, J., Trachtman, H., et al. 1996. Growth in children with moderate renal insufficiency: Measurement, evaluation, and treatment. *J Pediatr* 129(2):S3–S8.

Behrman, R. and Kliegman, R. 1996. *Nelson Textbook of Pediatrics*. Edited by R.E.K. Behrman, Robert; Nelson, Waldo E. 15th edition. Philadelphia, PA: WB Saunders.

Chaturvedi, S. and Jones, C. 2007. Protein restriction for children with chronic renal failure. *Cochrane Database Syst Rev* (4):CD006863.

Foster, B. and Leonard, M. 2004. Measuring nutritional status in children with chronic kidney disease. *Am J Clin Nutr* 80(4):801–814.

Fulgoni, V. 2008. Current protein intake in America: Analysis of the National Health and Nutrition Examination Survey, 2003–2004. *Am J Clin Nutr* 87(5):1554S–1557S.

Heilbron, D., Holliday, M., Al-Dahwi, A., et al. 1991. Expressing glomerular filtration rate in children. *Pediatr Nephrol* 5(10):5–11.

Hogg, R., Furth, S., Lemley, K., et al. 2003. National Kidney Foundation's Kidney Disease Outcomes Quality Initiative clinical practice guidelines for chronic kidney disease in children and adolescents: Evaluation, classification, and stratification. *Pediatrics* 111 (6 Pt 1):1416–1421.

Intakes, Subcommittees on Upper Reference Levels of Nutrients and Interpretation and Uses of Dietary Reference Intakes; Standing Committee on the Scientific Evaluation of Dietary Reference. 2002. *Dietary Reference Intakes for Energy, Carbohydrate, Fiber, Fat, Fatty Acids, Cholesterol, Protein, and Amino Acids (Macronutrients)*. Washington, D.C.: National Academies.

Kher, K., Schnaper, H., and Makker, S. 2007. *Clinical Pediatric Nephrology*. Edited by K. K. Kher, H. W. Schnaper and S. P. Makker. 2nd ed. London: Informa Healthcare.

Ledermann, S., Shaw, V., and Trompeter, R. 1999. Long-term enteral nutrition in infants and young children with chronic renal failure. *Pediatr Nephrol* 13(9):870–875.

Lloyd-Jones, D., Hong, Y., Labarthe, D., et al. 2010. Defining and setting national goals for cardiovascular health promotion and disease reduction: The American Heart Association's strategic Impact Goal through 2020 and beyond. *Circulation* 121(4):586–613.

Mahan, J., Warady, B., and Committee Consensus. 2006. Assessment and treatment of short stature in pediatric patients with chronic kidney disease: A consensus statement. *Pediatr Nephrol* 21(7):917–930.

NAPRTCS (North American Pediatric Renal Trials and Collaborative Studies). 2010. Annual Transplant Report.

National Kidney Foundation's Kidney Disease Outcomes Quality Initiative. 2005. Clinical practice guidelines for bone metabolism and disease in children with chronic kidney disease. *Am J Kidney Dis* 46 (4, Suppl 1):S1–S122.

National Kidney Foundation's Kidney Disease Outcomes Quality Initiative. 2009. KDOQI clinical practice guideline for nutrition in childrens with CKD: 2008 Update. *Am J Kidney Dis* 53 (3, Suppl 2):S16–S123.

Nutrition, The American Society for Parenteral and Enteral. 2002. Guidelines for the use of parenteral and enteral nutrition in adult and pediatric patients. *J Parent Ent Nutrit* 26(1):1SA–138SA.

Orellana, P., Juarez-Congelosi, M., and Goldstein, S. 2005. Intradialytic parenteral nutrition treatment and biochemical marker assessment for malnutrition in adolescent maintenance hemodialysis patients. *J Ren Nutr* 15(3):312–317.

Parekh, R., Flynn, J., Smoyer, W., et al. 2001. Improved growth in young children with severe chronic renal insufficiency who use specified nutritional therapy. *J Am Soc Nephrol* 12(11):2418–2426.

Quan, A. and Baum, M. 1996. Protein losses in children on continuous cycler peritoneal dialysis. *Pediatr Nephrol* 10(6):728–731.

Schwartz, G., Munoz, A., Schneider, M., et al. 2009. New equations to estimate GFR in children with CKD. *J Am Soc Nephrol* 20 (3):629–637.

U.S. Department of Agriculture and U.S. Department of Health and Human Services. December 2010. *Dietary Guidelines for Americans, 2010.* 7thEd., Washington, DC: U.S. Government Printing Office.

U.S. Renal Data System. 2010. *USRDS 2010 Annual Data Report: Atlas of Chronic Kidney Disease and End-Stage Renal Disease in the United States*. Bethesda, MD: National Institutes of Health, National Institute of Diabetes and Digestive and Kidney Diseases.

Wong, C., Gipson, D., Gillen, D., et al. 2000. Anthropometric measures and risk of death in children with end-stage renal disease. *Am J Kidney Dis* 36 (4):811–819.

Wong, C., Hingorani, S., Gillen, D., et al. 2002. Hypoalbuminemia and risk of death in pediatric patients with end-stage renal disease. Kidney Int 61 (2):630–637.

12 Pregnancy and Kidney Disease

Jeannine C. Lawrence
University of Alabama

CONTENTS

12.1 BACKGROUND

Pregnancy in women with kidney disease or renal failure is an infrequent occurrence. Generally, more severe kidney dysfunction along with a higher number of associated comorbidities, means it is more likely that a woman's fertility will be impaired and that an ensuing pregnancy will be more complicated (Piccoli et al., 2010a; Vidaeff et al., 2008). It is estimated that the pregnancy rate of women of childbearing age with renal disease ranges from 0.03% to 7% (Fink et al., 1998; Holley and Reddy, 2003), which is well below the estimated pregnancy rate of 10.3% in the general U.S. population (CDC, 2009). Causes for the reduction in pregnancy rates in women with renal disease are not completely understood; however, it is known that there is a marked reduction in presence of menses and/or ovulation in women undergoing dialysis (Holley et al., 1997; Piccoli et al., 2010b). Once pregnancy has begun, it is considered to be high risk and requires complex and intensive management by the health-care team (Figure 12.1).

In case of pregnancy in women with mild kidney disease, the pregnancy itself does not result in a chronic decrease in kidney function but may result in alternative damaging effects, such as development of proteinuria, preeclampsia, and/or initiation or exacerbation of preexisting hypertension (Fischer, 2007). However, as the severity of the maternal kidney disease increases to moderate or severe, a concomitant decline in kidney function during pregnancy can be seen (Fischer, 2007). Accordingly, the effects of maternal kidney disease on fetal outcomes vary based on the severity

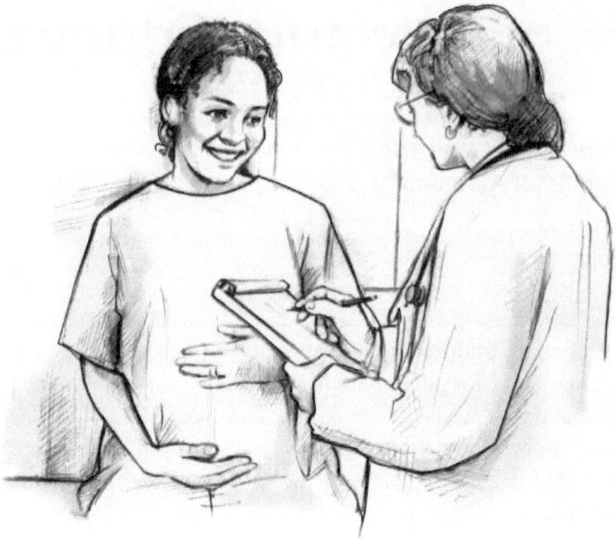

FIGURE 12.1 Prenatal care. (Courtesy of National Institute of Diabetes and Digestive and Kidney Diseases, National Institutes of Health.)

of the disease. In cases of mild maternal kidney disease, successful pregnancy outcomes have been described in 68%–98% of observed pregnancies, with no obstetrical or fetal complications reported in approximately 65% of these pregnancies (Bar et al., 2000; Chapman et al., 1994; Holley et al., 1996). These data contrast markedly with fetal outcomes in women with severe kidney disease. In this group, pregnancy is extremely rare and, when it does occur, typically it results in preterm delivery, intrauterine growth retardation, or fetal death (Fischer, 2007). Dialysis, especially daily dialysis treatments, can be an important therapeutic tool in improving maternal and fetal outcomes in maternal kidney disease (Piccoli et al., 2010b). The goal of nutritional intervention in maternal kidney disease is to find the appropriate balance between minimizing the intake of nutrients detrimental to kidney function and reducing toxemia while still providing appropriate nutrition for the developing fetus.

Conversely, in postrenal transplant patients, pregnancy is relatively common, and medical management is more focused on management of risks associated with immunosuppressive medications. The goal of nutritional intervention in postrenal transplant patients during pregnancy is typically oriented toward maintaining an appropriate rate of weight gain and monitoring the development of potential comorbidities including, most notably, type 2 diabetes mellitus.

12.2 PHYSIOLOGY IN PREGNANCY AND RENAL DISEASE

It is known that hormonal changes in pregnancy, beginning soon after conception, result in an increased blood volume of 30%–50% with an associated increase in renal blood flow and glomerular filtration rate (Maynard and Thadhani, 2009). This hyperfiltration increases through the second trimester of pregnancy and remains elevated up to 3 months postpartum (Lindheimer and Katz, 1992, 2001; Sturgiss et al., 1994). Pregnancy is also associated with increases in blood pressure and the potential for progressive insulin resistance. Both these comorbidities could accelerate the progression of preexisting renal disease (Hou, 1999).

The dialysis regimen of a pregnant woman with end-stage renal disease (ESRD) will change to better accommodate the needs of both the fetus and the changing physiology of the mother. A patient receiving hemodialysis (HD) three times per week before pregnancy will often transition to a more frequent, or even daily, HD regimen during pregnancy (Piccoli et al., 2010b). A patient who undergoes a peritoneal dialysis (PD) regimen with daily dialysate exchanges may become uncomfortable using her prepregnancy exchange volumes in later pregnancy. To accommodate the decreased availability of abdominal space, the clinician may prescribe a reduced exchange volume with a higher number of exchanges performed daily (Hou, 1999). These alterations in dialysis prescription will necessarily affect the nutrition prescription.

12.3 ASSESSMENT/EVALUATION OF PREGNANT PATIENT WITH CKD

12.3.1 Clinical Data

As pregnancy results in profound alterations in blood volume and renal filtration, the standard measures of serum creatinine or use of creatinine- or weight-based formulas for estimating kidney function become less appropriate in maternal kidney disease. Therefore, a 24-h urinary creatinine clearance test is considered the most appropriate measurement method for monitoring renal function in these patients (Maynard and Thadhani, 2009). In addition, nutrition-related values that should be monitored regularly throughout pregnancy include blood pressure, blood urea nitrogen (BUN), albumin, casual plasma glucose, HgA1c (in patients with concomitant diabetes mellitus), and serum cholesterol (Wiggins, et al. 2002; Williams and Davison, 2008). Specific serum nutrients that should be monitored include potassium, phosphorus, calcium, sodium, and iron (as serum ferritin and transferrin saturation; Wiggins and Harvey, 2002). Anthropometrics that should be evaluated regularly include weight, fluid retention status, and intradialytic fluid gains (HD).

12.3.2 Medical History/Medications

Upon initial evaluation, a complete medical history should be collected. This data should include current comorbidities, surgeries, medications and dosage schedules, and allergies.

12.3.3 Dietary Intake

Evaluation of dietary intake data is invaluable in helping the nutrition professional develop a realistic, individualized nutrition prescription for pregnant women with renal disease. Ideally, dietary intake data should be received and analyzed before consultation to optimize the consultation time. The data can be collected in the form of food records or multiple, 24-h recalls, and this should be done weekly throughout the pregnancy. These data will be of particular importance in evaluating protein status, as serum albumin levels normally decrease by up to 1 g/dL secondary to plasma volume dilution as pregnancy progresses (Hyten, 1988; Figure 12.2).

12.3.4 Physical Activity

In the absence of contraindications, such as uncontrolled hypertension or severe anemia, and following medical evaluation, moderate-intensity exercise is recommended throughout pregnancy to improve overall maternal and fetal health and to decrease the risk of developing gestational diabetes (ACOG Committee, 2002; Artal and O'Toole, 2003). Assessment of current physical activity should be performed in order to maintain the balance between energy intake and energy expenditure.

12.4 NUTRITION PRESCRIPTION

12.4.1 Weight Gain

Recommendations for weight gain in patients with maternal kidney disease or postrenal transplantation do not differ from the recommendations for the general population and are based on the

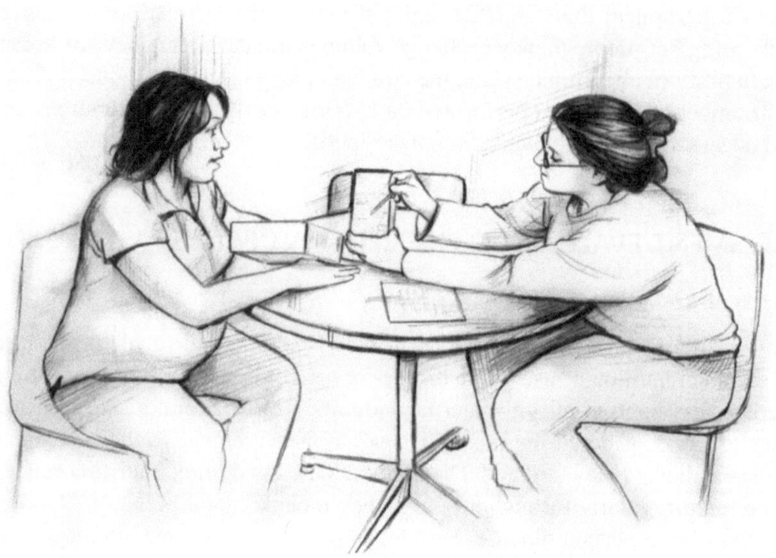

FIGURE 12.2 Dietary counseling. (Courtesy of National Institute of Diabetes and Digestive and Kidney Diseases, National Institutes of Health.)

TABLE 12.1
Recommendations for Weight Gain during Pregnancy

	Total Weight Gain Range	
Prepregnancy Body Mass Index (kg/m²)	**Single Pregnancy (kg/lbs)**	**Twin Pregnancy (kg/lbs)**
<18.5 (Underweight)	12.5–18/28–40	Insufficient data available to set guidelines
18.5–24.9 (Normal weight)	11.5–16/25–35	17–25/37–54
25.0–29.9 (Overweight)	7–11.5/15–25	14–23/31–50
≥30.0 (Obese)	5–9/11–20	11–19/25–42

mother's pregravid body mass index (BMI; Rasmussen et al., 2009). In patients receiving dialysis, dry weight should be used for BMI calculation (Table 12.1).

12.4.2 Macronutrients

Once the total energy and protein needs have been established, the remaining calories can be distributed between fat and carbohydrate sources. As coronary heart disease is the leading cause of death in patients undergoing HD, PD, or kidney transplantation (Kasiske et al., 2004), recommendations for dietary fat intake are modified based on the absence or presence of hyperlipidemia. In the absence of hyperlipidemia, minimize cardiovascular disease (CVD) risk by implementing the American Heart Association guidelines, including limiting saturated fat (<7% of energy), trans fats (<1%), and cholesterol intake (<300 mg/day). In the presence of hyperlipidemia, implement the Therapeutic Lifestyle Changes dietary goals for fat intake, including a total fat intake of 25%–35% of calories, with a saturated fat intake of <7% of calories and the remaining bulk of fat calories (up to 20%) distributed primarily toward monounsaturated fats and secondarily toward polyunsaturated fats and cholesterol of <200 mg/day (NCEP Panel, 2002). Remaining calorie requirements are to be met with carbohydrate sources.

12.4.3 Micronutrients

Patients in stages 1–3 of chronic kidney disease (CKD) or postrenal transplantation are advised to take a standard prenatal vitamin daily. However, patients in later stages of CKD or in ESRD are typically prescribed a standard, water-soluble renal vitamin dosage that is double the typical, nonpregnancy dosage. In cases of dialysis, the recommendations for folic acid intake are increased due to increased losses during dialysis. In these patients, ≥1.8 mg of folic acid is recommended daily (Hou, 1999; Stover, 2007). In addition, micronutrients that may require supplementation if they are not provided in adequate amounts in the standard multivitamin dosage prescribed during pregnancy include vitamin D, calcium, iron, and zinc (15 mg/dL; Stover, 2007) (Table 12.2).

12.5 MEDICATIONS WITH NUTRITIONAL IMPLICATIONS

12.5.1 Hypertension

The use of diuretics and angiotensin-converting enzyme inhibitors is contraindicated during pregnancy due to the adverse effects on fetal outcomes (Hou, 1999). When possible, hypertension in pregnant women with kidney disease should be managed by dietary control of fluid intake and fluid removal during dialysis. If these techniques prove ineffective, some medications that have been shown to be safer during pregnancy, including β-blockers, labetalol, and α-methyldopa, can be used (Hou, 1999; Stover, 2008).

12.5.2 Anemia

Anemia is a common complication during pregnancy and is even more frequently observed in pregnant patients receiving HD. Oral iron supplements may be used to treat milder cases of anemia. However, intravenous (IV) iron, in the forms of iron sucrose or iron gluconate, may be used if oral supplements prove ineffective (Vidal et al., 1998). It should be noted that the use of IV iron preparations may result in increased absorption by the fetus with subsequent acute iron toxicity (Hou and Firanek, 1998). Therefore, this route of administration is to be used conservatively and monitored carefully.

12.5.3 Electrolyte and Acid–Base Disturbances

Alterations in the frequency and/or volume of dialysis regimens may require adjustments to the composition of the dialysate bath to minimize occurrences of hypokalemia, hypercalcemia, or alkalosis from excessive bicarbonate accumulation (Hou, 1999).

12.5.4 Transplantation

Maternal immune suppression is essential during pregnancy; therefore, the effects of certain immunosuppressive agents at this lifecycle stage are well studied. The primary agents used for immune suppression in this population are prednisone, azathioprine, cyclosporine, and tacrolimus (Vidaeff et al., 2008). Although each has demonstrated potential risks to fetal development, these risks are outweighed by the potential costs of insufficient immune suppression to both the mother and the fetus. Nutrition considerations during pregnancy, which are related to the use of these drugs, include osteopenia (prednisone); exacerbation of diabetes or increased risk of development of gestational diabetes (prednisone, cyclosporine, and tacrolimus); hypertension (prednisone and cyclosporine); and elevated creatinine levels (cyclosporine) (American College of Rheumatology Ad Hoc Committee on Clinical Guidelines, 2006; Kitridou, 1997; Kainz et al., 2000).

TABLE 12.2
Nutritional Guideline for Pregnant Patients with CKD and for Patients on Dialysis or Postrenal Transplant

Energy	
CKD/HD/PD	First trimester: BEE × activity factor (1.2–1.4) or 35 kcal/kg prepregnancy IBW[a]; second and third trimesters: add 300 kcal/dL[b]
Posttransplantation	First trimester: BEE × activity factor (1.2–1.4) or 25–35 kcal/kg prepregnancy IBW; second and third trimesters: add 300 kcal/dL
Protein	
CKD	Stages 1–3: 0.8 g/kg + 10 g/day Stages 4–5 without dialysis: 0.6 g/kg + 10 g/day[c]
HD	1.1–1.4 g/kg prepregnancy IBW + 10 g/day
PD	1.2–1.5 g/kg prepregnancy IBW + 10 g/day
Posttransplantation	1.0–1.2 g/kg prepregnancy IBW + 10 g/day
Fluid	
CKD	Unrestricted unless fluid retention is present
HD	1000–2000 mL/interdialytic interval, not to exceed 2 kg interdialytic fluid weight gain
PD	Sufficient to maintain fluid balance. Monitor fluid retention status
Posttransplantation	Unrestricted unless fluid retention is present
Calcium	
CKD	1000 mg/day
HD/PD	Individualized—evaluate serum Ca^{++}, phosphorus, and PTH values; ~1000–1200 mg/day. Evaluate calcium concentration of dialysate and phosphate binder dosage
Posttransplantation	1200–1500 mg/day
Phosphorus	
CKD/HD/PD	Individualized per serum values; ~1200 mg/day
Posttransplantation	1200 mg/day
Potassium	
CKD	Unrestricted unless hyperkalemic, then 2–4 g/day
HD	Individualized per serum values; ~40 mg/kg prepregnancy IBW
PD	Individualized per serum values, may not require restriction
Posttransplantation	Unrestricted unless hyperkalemic, then 2–4 g/day
Sodium	
CKD	Individualized—evaluate serum values, blood pressure, and fluid retention status; ~2–4 g/day
HD	Individualized—evaluate serum values, blood pressure, and fluid retention status; ~2–3 g/day
PD	Individualized—evaluate serum values, blood pressure, and fluid retention status; ~2–4 g/day
Posttransplantation	Individualized; ~2–4 g/day

Source: Hou, S., *Am. J. Kidney Dis.*, 33, 235–252, 1999; Stover, J., *Adv. Chronic Kidney Dis.*, 14, 212–214, 2007; and Wiggins, K. and Harvey, K., *J. Ren. Nutr.*, 12, 190–196, 2002.

Abbreviations: CKD, chronic kidney disease; HD, hemodialysis; PD, peritoneal dialysis; PTH, parathyroid hormone.

[a] IBW = Ideal Body Weight

[b] When calculating energy prescription for women receiving PD, be certain to factor in glucose calories received from the dialysate solution.

[c] Recognize that while this protein goal is recommended to minimize the deterioration of kidney function, it may not be achievable given the increased total energy needs required during pregnancy.

12.6 MANAGING COMORBIDITIES

Common comorbid conditions associated with kidney disease include diabetes mellitus, hypertension, and/or CVD. Dietary management of the pregnant patient with kidney disease will need to incorporate the appropriate dietary guidelines for these conditions into the nutrition prescription. In addition, specific conditions associated with pregnancy itself may warrant adaptations to the nutrition prescription. Intractable hyperemesis gravidarum may result in inadequate dietary intake to support a healthy pregnancy. In addition to the standard medications used to reduce nausea and nutrition techniques used to increase intake (supplements, etc.), intradialytic parenteral nutrition has been used successfully in some situations to improve the medical outcomes in acutely ill patients on HD, and it may also be useful in improving weight gain and pregnancy outcomes (Brookhyser, 1989; Korzets et al., 2008; Tuot et al., 2010).

12.7 POSTPREGNANCY AND BREASTFEEDING

The physiologic changes associated with pregnancy may take up to 3 months to resolve, requiring continued monitoring of the postpartum patient with kidney disease (Williams and Davison, 2008). The choice to breastfeed is ultimately up to the mother, and it is the role of the health-care provider to provide her with the information required to make an informed decision. There are no contraindications to breastfeeding for women with CKD, provided their health is otherwise stable (Williams and Davison, 2008). Postrenal transplant recipients should be made aware that some immunosuppressive agents do appear in varying levels in breast milk (Josephson and McKay 2007). The American Academy of Pediatrics has established limited recommendations for this population, supporting breastfeeding by women taking prednisone but warning against breastfeeding by women taking cyclosporine (American Academy of Pediatrics Committee on Drugs, 1994). The Academy currently does not have established recommendations regarding the usage of azathioprine or tacrolimus during breastfeeding. Should a mother choose to breastfeed, her calorie requirements during lactation would be approximately 330 kcal higher than the weight-maintenance needs of her nonpregnant counterpart during the first 6 months postpartum and approximately 400 kcal higher during the second 6 months postpartum (Erick, 2008). Fluid intake should be appropriate to support milk production; however, in this population, careful monitoring of fluid retention status is required.

REFERENCES

ACOG Committee. 2002. Opinion no. 267: Exercise during pregnancy and the postpartum period. *Obstet Gynecol.* 99:171–173.

American Academy of Pediatrics Committee on Drugs. 1994. The transfer of drugs and other chemicals into human milk. *Pediatrics.* 93:137–150.

American College of Rheumatology Ad Hoc Committee on Clinical Guidelines. 1996. Guidelines for monitoring drug therapy in rheumatoid arthritis. *Arthritis Rheum.* 39:723–731.

Artal, R. and O'Toole, M. 2003. Guidelines of the American College of obstetricians and gynecologists for exercise during pregnancy and the postpartum period. *Br J Sports Med.* 37: 6–12.

Bar, J., Ben-Rafael, Z., Padoa, A., et al. 2000. Prediction of pregnancy outcome in subgroups of women with renal disease. *Clin Nephrol.* 53(6):437–444.

Brookhyser, J. 1989. The use of parenteral nutrition supplementation in pregnancy complicated by end-stage renal disease. *J Am Diet Assoc.* 89(1):93–94.

Centers for Disease Control (CDC). October 14, 2009. Estimated pregnancy rates for the United States, 1990–2005: An update. *Natl Vital Stat Rep.* 58(4):2.

Chapman, A., Johnson, A. and Gabow, P. 1994. Pregnancy outcome and its relationship to progression of renal failure in autosomal dominant polycystic kidney disease. *J Am Soc Nephrol.* 5(5):1178–185.

Erick, M. 2008. Nutrition during pregnancy and lactation. In Mahan, L.K., and Escott-Stump, S. eds. *Krause's Food and Nutrition Therapy*. St. Louis, MO: Saunders Elsevier, 187.

Fink, J., Schwartz, S., Benedetti, T., et al. 1998. Increased risk of adverse maternal and infant outcomes among women with renal disease. *Paediatr Perinat Epidemiol.* 12(3):277–287.

Fischer, M. 2007. Chronic kidney disease and pregnancy: Maternal and fetal outcomes. *Adv Chronic Kidney Dis.* 14(2):132–145.

Holley, J., Bernardini, J., Quadri, K., et al. 1996. Pregnancy outcomes in a prospective matched control study of pregnancy and renal disease. *Clin Nephrol.* 45(2):77–82.

Holley, J. and Reddy, S. 2003. Pregnancy in dialysis patients: A review of outcomes, complications, and management. *Semin Dial.* 16(5):384–388.

Holley, J., Schmidt, R., Bender, F., et al. 1997. Gynecologic and reproductive issues in women on dialysis. *Am J Kidney Dis.* 29(5):685–690.

Hou, S. 1999. Pregnancy in chronic renal insufficiency and end-stage renal disease. *Am J Kidney Dis.* 33(2):235–252.

Hou, S. and Firanek, C. 1998. Management of the pregnant dialysis patient. *Adv Ren Replace Ther.* 5(1):24–30.

Hyten, F. 1988. Nutrition and metabolism. In: Hyten, F., ed., *Clinical Physiology in Obstetrics*. Oxford, England: Blackwell Scientific Publications, 177.

Josephson, M. and McKay, D. 2007. Considerations in the medical management of pregnancy in transplant recipients. *Adv Chronic Kidney Dis.* 14(2):156–167.

Kainz, A., Harabacz, I., Cowlrick, I., et al. 2000. Review of the course and outcome of 100 pregnancies in 84 women treated with tacrolimus. *Transplantation.* 27; 70(12):1718–1721.

Kasiske, B., Cosio, F., Beto, J., et al. 2004. National Kidney Foundation. Clinical practice guidelines for managing dyslipidemias in kidney transplant patients: A report from the managing dyslipidemias in Chronic Kidney Disease Work Group of the National Kidney Foundation Kidney Disease Outcomes Quality Initiative. *Am J Transplant.* 4(S7):13–53.

Kitridou, R. 1997. The mother in systemic lupus erythematosus. In Wallace, D.J. and Hahn, B.H. *Dubois' Lupus Erythematosus* 5th ed., Baltimore, MD: Williams & Wilkins, 967–1002.

Korzets, A., Azoulay, O., Ori, Y., et al. 2008. The use of intradialytic parenteral nutrition in acutely ill haemodialysed patients. *J Ren Care.* 34(1):14–8.

Lindheimer, M. and Katz, A. 1992. Renal physiology and disease in pregnancy. In Seldin, D.W. and Giebisch, G. eds. *The Kidney: Physiology and Pathophysiology*, 2nd ed., New York: Raven Press, 3371–3405.

Lindheimer, M. and Katz, A. 2001. The normal and diseased kidney in pregnancy. In Schrier, R.W., ed. *Diseases of the Kidney and Urinary Tract*, 7th ed., Philadelphia, PA: Lippincott Williams and Wilkins, 2129–2165.

Maynard, S. and Thadhani, R. 2009. Pregnancy and the kidney. *J Am Soc Nephrol.* 20(1):14–22.

National Cholesterol Education Program (NCEP) Expert Panel on Detection, Evaluation, and Treatment of High Blood Cholesterol in Adults (Adult Treatment Panel III). 2002. Third Report of the National Cholesterol Education Program (NCEP) expert panel on detection, evaluation, and treatment of high blood cholesterol in adults (Adult Treatment Panel III) final report. *Circulation.* 106(25):3143–3421.

Piccoli, G., Attini, R., Vasario, E. et al. 2010a. Pregnancy and chronic kidney disease: A challenge in all CKD stages. *Clin J Am Soc Nephrol.* 5(5):844–855.

Piccoli, G., Conijn, A., Consiglio, V. et al. 2010b. Pregnancy in dialysis patients: is the evidence strong enough to lead us to change our counseling policy? *Clin J Am Soc Nephrol.* 5(1):62–71.

Rasmussen, K., Yaktine, A., eds. Committee to Reexamine IOM Pregnancy Weight Guidelines; Institute of Medicine; National Research Council. 2009. Weight gain during pregnancy: Reexamining the guidelines. Online: http://www.nap.edu/catalog/12584.html (accessed January 1, 2011).

Stover, J. 2007. Nutritional management of pregnancy in chronic kidney disease. *Adv Chronic Kidney Dis.* 14(2):212–214.

Stover, J. 2008. Pregnancy. In: Byham-Gray, L., Burrowes, J. and Chertow, G. eds. *Nutrition and Health: Nutrition in Kidney Disease*. Totowa, NJ: Humana Press, 419–329.

Sturgiss, S., Dunlop, W. and Davison, J. 1994. Renal haemodynamics and tubular function in human pregnancy. *Baillieres Clin Obstet Gynaecol.* 8(2):209–234.

Tuot, D., Gibson, S., Caughey, A., et al. 2010. Intradialytic hyperalimentation as adjuvant support in pregnant hemodialysis patients: Case report and review of the literature. *Int Urol Nephrol.* 42(1):233–237.

Vidal, M., Ursu, M., Martinez, A., et al. 1998. Nutritional control of pregnant women on chronic hemodialysis. *J Ren Nutr.* 8(3):150–156.

Vidaeff, A., Yeomans, E. and Ramin, S. 2008. Pregnancy in women with renal disease. Part I: General principles. *Am J Perinatol.* 25(7):385–397.

Wiggins, K. and Harvey, K. 2002. A review of guidelines for nutrition care of renal patients. *J Ren Nutr.* 12(3):190–196.

Williams, D. and Davison, J. 2008. Chronic kidney disease in pregnancy. *BMJ.* 26; 336(7637):211–215.

13 Obesity and Physical Activity

Tanis Vye Mihalynuk
Acadia University

CONTENTS

13.1 INTRODUCTION

Obesity increases the risk of several chronic diseases, such as type 2 diabetes, hypertension, cardiovascular disease (CVD), inflammatory disorders, common cancers, depression, and chronic kidney disease (CKD). Although the global incidence of CKD is on the rise, it is termed a "silent epidemic" (Stenvinkel, 2010). Pandemic trends in overweight and obesity may be largely responsible for eclipsing this public health problem. Although there are various causes of CKD, there is a growing evidence that obesity is a risk factor—independent of conditions such as diabetes and CVD (Eknoyan, 2006; Ting et al., 2009). A Swedish case-control study of over 900 cases and matched controls with chronic renal failure (CRF) showed a threefold increase in CRF among cases who were overweight at the age of 20 (Ejerblad et al., 2006). Moreover, a recent systematic review and meta-analysis estimated that in the United States, about one-fourth and one-third of cases with kidney disease among men and women, respectively, could be attributed to overweight and obesity (Wang et al., 2008).

It has been established that kidney damage leads to discharge of protein into the urine (albuminuria and proteinuria) and subsequent muscle wasting and anemia as well as higher blood pressure. Several mechanisms by which excess body weight further alters renal physiology, including insulin resistance, increase in oxidative, endoplasmic reticulum, and proinflammatory stresses, impairment of fibrinolysis, dysregulation of the renin–angiotensin–aldosterone system, and compensatory hyperinsulinemia (Lastra et al., 2006), have been proposed. More recent ones include lipid accumulation in the kidney (Corpeleijn et al., 2009) and secretion of adverse signaling molecules, including adipokines (Axelsson, 2008; Mathew, 2011) (leptin, adiponectin, and retinol-binding protein) and cytokines (resistin, visfatin, interleukin 6, and tumor necrosis factor), by the adipose tissue.

As with most chronic diseases, demographic variables such as age, sex, ethnicity, and socioeconomic status may affect the incidence and prevalence of CKD (Kiberd, 2006). A study by Hallan et al. (2006) of over 30,000 men and women each showed that although obesity, smoking, and physical activity (PA) were associated with CKD, men were less susceptible than women to these risk factors. However, Krol et al. (2010) recently reported, in a cohort study of over 2500 participants, that increasing age and comorbidities are more detrimental to men than to women. In the classical, multigenerational Framingham prospective study of over 2500 participants (Fox, 2004), at about 19-years follow-up it was found that cardiovascular risk factors combined with obesity and use of tobacco were the predictors of new-onset CKD. Further investigation is needed to elucidate demographic determinants of CKD and related comorbidities such as obesity.

13.2 ENERGY BALANCE

It has been postulated that poor diet, particularly excessive consumption of cheap, energy-dense, sugar- and fat-laden substances, and physical inactivity will soon supersede the use of tobacco as the leading cause of modifiable deaths in the United States—primarily due to the increase in numbers of people who are overweight and obese (Mokdad, 2004). Excessive fat accumulates in the body, from the cellular level to the organ system level, when the calories consumed are greater than the energy expended over time. Energy sources of calories include calorie-providing macronutrients—proteins, carbohydrates, and fats—and alcohol, which supply 4, 4, 9, and 7 cal/g, respectively.

PA is the most variable component of energy expenditure, which also encompasses basal and resting metabolic rate and the thermic effect of food—the energy required to digest, absorb, and metabolize food. This simplified view of energy balance in relation to body weight regulation is confounded by a myriad of factors affecting both sides of the energy balance equation (energy in/out). Multiple effects of nutrition and PA patterns, and their intricate relationships, are detailed in the United Kingdom's Foresight frameworks (UK Foresight Project, 2010). Although one can assume that energy expenditure in patients with CKD is low, this is not necessarily so (Monteon et al., 1986). Therefore, the role of energy balance in the management of CKD and other chronic diseases calls for public health and integrative medical approaches for preventing and treating obesity and related comorbidities (Heber, 2010).

13.3 PHYSICAL ACTIVITY

In the literature on CKD, PA, exercise, physical exercise, and related terms are often used synonymously. Unless otherwise indicated, these terms are used as such in this chapter also. PA refers to any body movement that works one's muscles and uses energy over and above that expended in the resting state. Exercise, such as weight lifting and sports, is a planned and structured subset of PA. PA can be further classified as aerobic or cardiovascular (requiring oxygen) and anaerobic. Aerobic activities (e.g., walking, running, swimming, dancing, and yoga) put large muscle groups to use for extended periods of time, whereas anaerobic activities (e.g., strength and circuit training, short walks, and stretching) are generally characterized by short bursts of activity. Flexibility activities, which may be aerobic and/or anaerobic, are increasingly being recommended for both general and subpopulations. Examples include gentle reaching, bending, and stretching to enhance the relaxation of muscles and the mobility of joints. Examples of endurance, flexibility, and strength activities can be found in Canada's Physical Activity Guide for Healthy Living (Canada's Physical Activity Guide, 2010). Notably, CKD is not yet listed as a chronic condition in this guide.

PA has many benefits for general and subpopulations. The 2008 United States Department of Health and Human Services Guidelines (USDHHS, 2010) recommends PA for both healthy individuals and those with chronic diseases, who are under the supervision of a health care provider. It outlines the physical, mental, and physiological benefits of PA, along with recommendations for including cardiovascular and resistance activity for at least 150 min a week. Overwhelming scientific evidence also supports regular PA for patients with CKD, who tend to be even less active than persons without CKD. A recent National Health and Nutrition Examination Survey (NHANES) report of more than 15,000 adults (Beddu et al., 2009) observed that, compared to participants without CKD, twice as many participants with CKD reported inactivity (28% vs. 13.5%). Furthermore, for both groups, physical inactivity was associated with increased mortality.

Although exercise programs for those with CKD had been reportedly introduced 30 years ago (Goldberg et al., 1979), an ongoing concern regarding those with CKD and other chronic conditions is the lack of regular PA. This is of particular concern with those on regular hemodialysis (HD), given the added time burden associated with the procedure. An innovative means of surmounting CKD, a lifestyle hurdle, is the inclusion of PA during HD treatment, otherwise known as intradialytic exercise (Figure 13.1), which is considered safe and beneficial (Davis and Holcombe, 2011). Several questionnaires have been used to estimate the role of PA in CKD (Johansen et al., 2001), with the Human Activity Profile correlating best with three-dimensional accelerometers compared with the Physical Activity Scale for the Elderly and the Medical Outcomes Study Short Form. Gait length and speed, stair-climbing time and chair-raising time, and overall physical and physiological functioning (e.g., V02 Max) are examples of various parameters studied in individuals with CKD.

Exercise can contribute to reduced blood pressure and enhanced physical capacity, as recently observed by Henrique et al. (2010). In this study, 14 patients with CKD who were undergoing HD were assessed before and after 12 weeks of PA. In a systematic review of 29 clinical trials (Cheema and Fiatarone Singh, 2005), physical and physiological improvements were noted following aerobic training in patients with CKD, who were undergoing HD. Moreover, in a 12-month study of 10 patients on HD, who were free from severe comorbidities, it was noted that moderate exercise improved aerobic capacity, overall physical functioning, and quality of life (QoL) (Capitanini et al., 2008). Similar benefits have also been observed in those on peritoneal dialysis (Beasley et al., 1986).

As with nutrition, PA as part of a lifestyle intervention should be individualized (Kutner, 2007) and promoted as early as possible, as a progressive decline in PA may occur as a consequence of anemia and skeletal muscle dysfunction. It has been documented that patients on HD may experience a decline of over 3% in PA each month after dialysis (Johansen et al., 2003). Fatigue can be a chief complaint of patients with CKD because of anemia and muscle wasting. Therefore, it is imperative to impress upon them that PA will not aggravate these symptoms but promote health and well-being. Brunier and Graydon, (1993) looked at the effect of anemia, nonspecific symptoms, and PA on the fatigue level of 43 patients with end-stage renal disease, who were on dialysis. He found that the degree of anemia

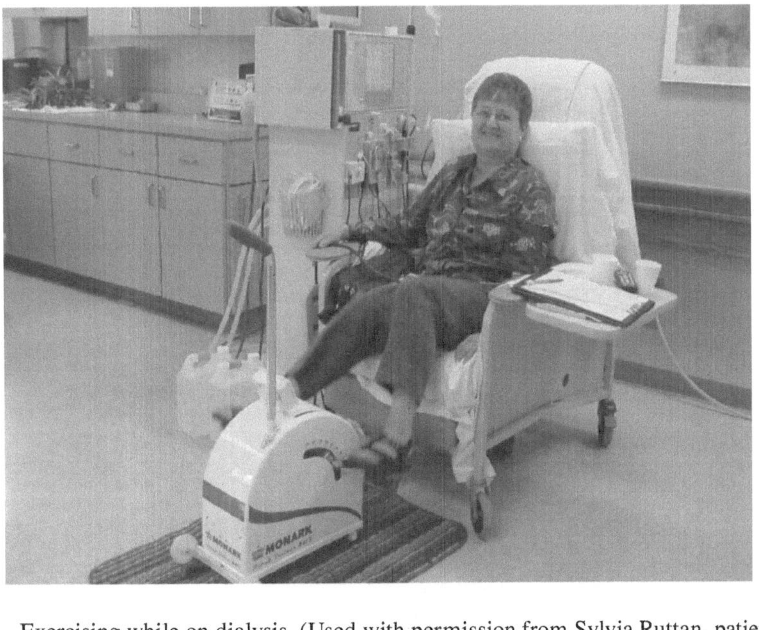

FIGURE 13.1 Exercising while on dialysis. (Used with permission from Sylvia Ruttan, patient at Kingston General Hospital Satellite Dialysis Unit, and Cheryl King-Van Vlack, PhD, associate professor and lead study investigator on the effects of intradialytic exercise on physical function, dialysis efficacy, and cardiovascular function, School of Rehabilitation Therapy, Queen's University, Ontario.)

was not related to fatigue and that inactivity contributed more to fatigue than the symptoms. Even in patients with CKD who are on a protein-restricted diet, resistance training has been observed to build muscle mass and strength (Castaneda et al., 2001). Further, in a cross-sectional study of over 90 men and women each on HD (median age = 59 years), it was found that factors associated with PA included age, serum albumin concentration, and physical function (Li and Fan, 2010).

Among the recommended forms of PA, a combination of endurance, flexibility, and strength training is often encouraged. Bed bicycle ergometers are frequently used in inpatient HD programs that include a PA component (Kosmadakis et al., 2010). It is believed that exercise programs combined with dialysis may have higher participation rates than outpatient programs, given the habitual, structured nature of HD. Moreover, no adverse events were reported in a study of exercisers in 200 German dialysis centers, from 1994 to 2004 (Daul et al., 2004). In this study, nearly all participants were able to do some form of PA. The program included low-intensity endurance activities, training with a bed bicycle ergometer, gymnastics to increase muscular strength, coordination, and flexibility, and relaxation techniques. Headley et al. (2002) found that more than 12 weeks of resistance training improved the strength and functional capacity of patients with CKD who were on HD. Other PA recommendations for patients with CKD include community-based walking programs, tai chi, yoga, swimming and/or water exercises, and physical therapy, which can be adopted to meet appropriate strength-training needs when necessary. Patients undergoing peritoneal dialysis should not swim in ponds or lakes where catheter-exit infections are possible (Figures 13.2 through 13.5).

To avoid injury and excessive risks associated with PA, it is recommended that patients with CKD build on activity patterns slowly (Knap et al., 2005). Ten minutes of walking or household chores is a start. Patients using wheelchairs can try stretching exercises (Figure 13.6). Health care providers should keep a watch on fluid restrictions and medications. In a recent review of indications and contraindications of PA in patients with CKD, the authors concluded as follows: "While there

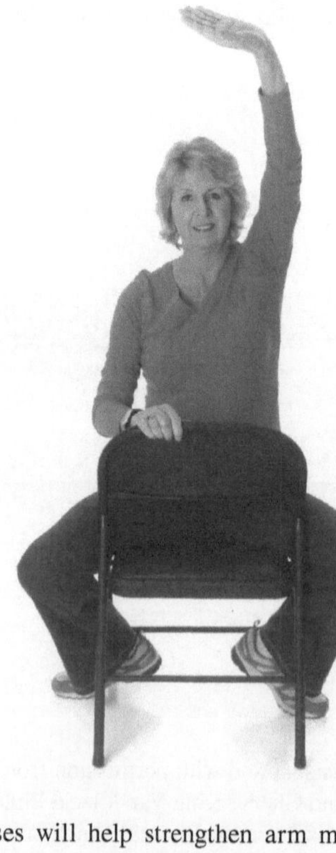

FIGURE 13.2 Stretching exercises will help strengthen arm muscles. (From Waxart/Dreamstime.com, Dreamstime USA Headquarters, Brentwood, TN. With permission.)

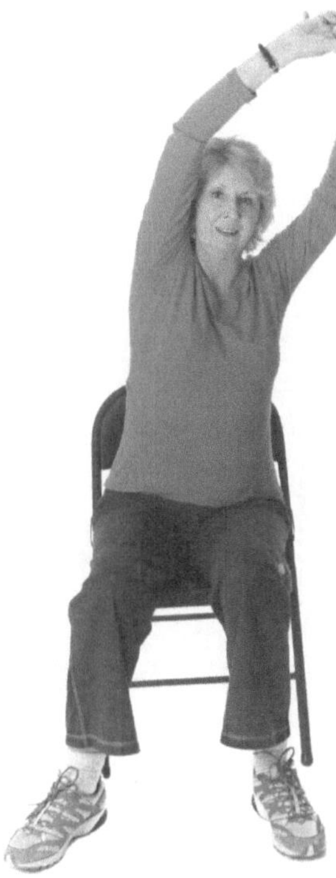

FIGURE 13.3 Stretching exercises will improve flexibility. (From Waxart/Dreamstime.com, Dreamstime USA Headquarters, Brentwood, TN. With permission.)

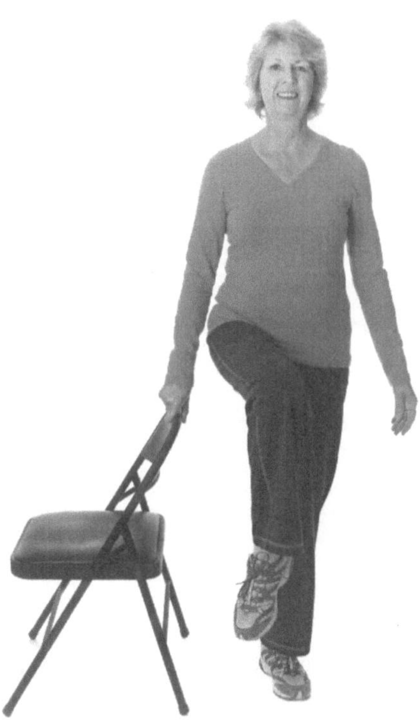

FIGURE 13.4 Exercise that will help improve balance. (From Waxart/Dreamstime.com, Dreamstime USA Headquarters, Brentwood, TN. With permission.)

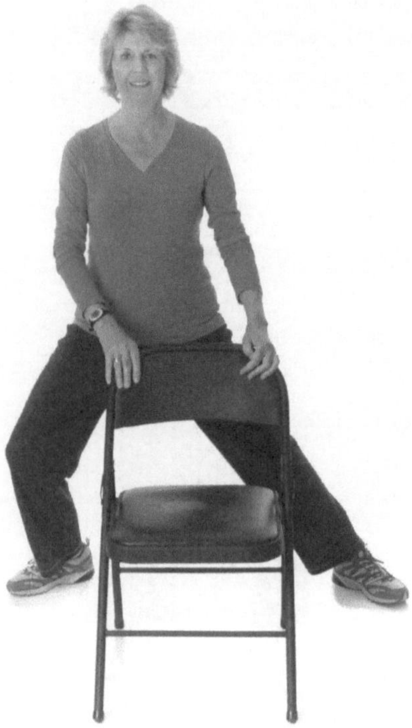

FIGURE 13.5 Exercise that will help strengthen hips and thighs and will also improve balance. (From Waxart/Dreamstime.com, Dreamstime USA Headquarters, Brentwood, TN. With permission.)

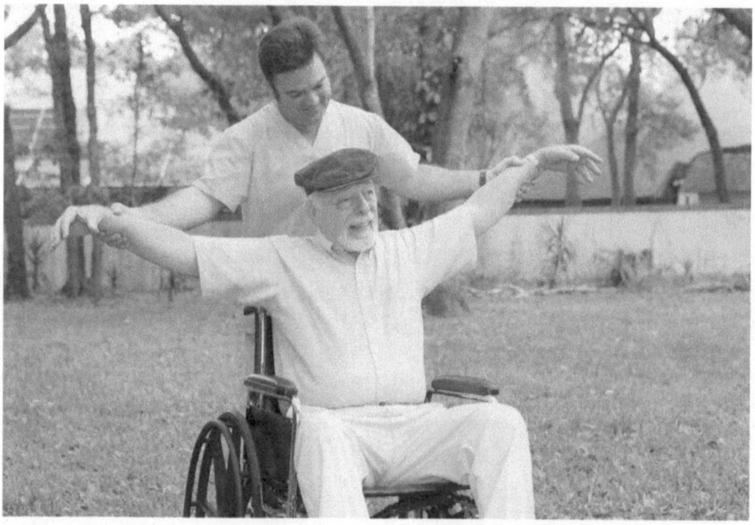

FIGURE 13.6 Flexibility exercises recommended for everyone. (From Lisa F. Young/Dreamstime.com, Dreamstime USA Headquarters, Brentwood, TN. With permission.)

are still no large randomized controlled trials evaluating the survival benefits of exercise, the evidence reviewed justifies regular use of exercise programmes in patients with advanced chronic kidney disease" (Kosmadakis et al., 2010). Although data regarding indications and contraindications are primarily observational and epidemiological, one can conclude with a high degree of certainty that the potential benefits of regular PA to patients and to the society at large are vast, including better physical and physiological functioning and mobility, improved QoL, and savings in health care cost. Rare complications of PA have been reported in this population, the most common being low blood pressure during HD, as per a meta-analysis (Cheema and Fiatarone Singh, 2005). Yet, surprisingly, PA has not been adopted as a routine component of patient-care programs. In a report on nephrologists' views on exercise for CKD, 95% of the 45 physicians surveyed included physical inactivity as a risk factor for CKD, over 75% wanted nephrologists to provide counseling on PA, and 74% sought written guidance on PA for their patients (Krause, 2004).

The key message for individuals with chronic conditions is the importance of medical approval and supervision before making significant changes in PA. Clearly, the more comorbid the condition, the likelihood of medical risks is higher, and hence the need for close supervision is greater. A simple "talk test" can be recommended to patients with CKD to ensure that they are not exercising too vigorously; particularly during lengthy aerobic activities, patients should be able to carry on a regular conversation. This basic test was closely correlated with VO2, heart rate, and ventilator threshold on both treadmill and cycle ergometer, in 16 healthy participants (Persinger et al., 2004). Finally, a lifestyle change that includes PA is highly recommended for patients with CKD.

13.4 PA AND QOL

QoL measures are increasingly being considered key markers of individual and population-based health status, including that in the context of CKD. Soni et al. (2010) highlighted the growing evidence on the impact of CKD and related comorbidities on diminished QoL. Reduced QoL measures may be due to the side effects of hypertension medications, frailty secondary to anemia, reduced muscle mass, and depression. Furthermore, in a study of 19 patients on HD, Hsieh et al. (2007) reported that QoL is lowered with increasing body mass index (BMI).

Research on the impact of PA on QoL has yielded positive results. In a study of 2264 new patients on HD in the United States, Stack and Murthy (2008) observed that a majority of them were exercising less than once a week. Kutner et al. (2000) looked at factors associated with QoL in individuals early in treatment and concluded that the most significant and independent predictor of QoL was participants' usual level of exercise. In a study of 19 patients on HD, it was found that the group with high energy expenditure had significantly higher QoL and physical functioning scores (Brenner and Brohart, 2008). Increased QoL scores have also been reported for physically active patients on peritoneal dialysis (Brodin et al., 2001). QoL may be impaired by increasing age (McClellan et al., 2010) in patients with CKD, further highlighting the importance of early and ongoing adoption of PA by these patients. Self-reported depression symptoms may also be reduced by including PA in CKD treatment (Kouldi et al., 1997; Ouzoni et al., 2009). Further research on the type and overall effectiveness of QoL measures in CKD treatment is recommended before routine assessments of QoL are integrated into patient-care programs.

13.5 OBESITY AND WEIGHT MANAGEMENT

As in the case of patients with many chronic diseases, weight management is often the main treatment for improved mental, physical, psychological, and physiological functioning in patients with CKD. In a systematic review and meta-analysis of weight loss interventions in patients with CKD (n = 13), nonsurgical weight loss was found to be associated with a reduction in BMI, proteinuria, and systolic blood pressure; in morbidly obese individuals, surgical interventions were associated with a reduction in BMI, glomerular filtration rate, albuminuria, and systolic blood pressure (Navaneethan et al., 2009). The authors concluded that larger and long-term trials are necessary to confirm these relationships—and as with the general population, further focus on long-term weight management is warranted. Moreover, a community-based microalbuminuria-screening program in the United Kingdom (Bello et al., 2010) found that the main determinants of microalbuminuria were diabetes, advanced age, hypertension, and obesity. It also found that obesity was a more robust correlate of microalbuminuria than diabetes and hypertension.

In patients with CKD stages 1–4, weight loss is generally recommended, as it reduces proteinuria and glomerular hyperfiltration (Teta, 2010). Notably, urinary albumin excretion is a predictor of both CKD and CVD. PA can be a protection against discharge of protein into urine, given its role in enhancing endothelial function. Several treatment pathways may be adapted from the guidelines on obesity treatment and prevention, put forth by Lau (2007), based on the degree of overweight and comorbidities. Notably, lifestyle modifications, such as diet, PA, and psychological/emotional supports, are vital to CKD treatment. PA should be emphasized to increase muscle mass, decrease body weight, and enhance the overall emotional, physical, and physiological well-being of patients. For nutrition, total macronutrient energy intake over protein restriction should be encouraged, whenever possible. Studies of patients who have undergone gastric bypass surgery for morbid obesity have shown a significant reduction in mortality, owing to major weight loss of the patients (Adams et al., 2007; Cook et al., 2008). This includes evidence from a long-term trial (Sjostrom et al., 2007) in which after over 7 years, a reduction of 40% for all-cause mortality, 56% for heart disease, 60% for cancer, and 92% for diabetes was observed. As focal-segmental glomeruli-sclerosis is related to obesity, particularly abdominal obesity, bariatric surgery is emerging as a highly effective, long-term treatment (Alexander et al., 2009).

Several tools are available to assess the potential risks of CKD and other chronic diseases due to excess body weight. BMI provides a measure of body weight in relation to height—for most people, the number correlates with direct measures of body fat, including underwater weighing and dual-energy x-ray absorptiometry (Garrow et al., 1985; Mei et al., 2002). At BMIs less than 18.5 and greater than 24.9, a robust association with increased mortality exists, as illustrated by a U- or J-shaped mortality curve (Allison et al., 1997). An adult with a BMI of 30 or more is considered obese. The National Heart, Lung and Blood Institute has further classified obesity into types I–III, with type III being an indicator of morbid obesity (BMI > 40) (NHLBI, 2010) (Table 13.1). Online BMI calculators are available to simplify BMI calculations for patients with CKD and their health care providers (CDC, 2010).

Waist circumference (WC) is rapidly emerging as the preferred weight-related indicator of CKD. Although ethnic variation has been reported for WC cut-off values, measures of 35 and 40 in. for

TABLE 13.1

Classification of Overweight and Obesity by BMI, Waist Circumference, and Associated Disease Risks

			Disease Risks[a] Relative to Normal Weight and Waist Circumference	
	BMI (kg/m²)	Obesity Class	Men ≤ 102 cm (≤ 40 in.) Women ≤ 88 cm (≤ 35 in.)	Men > 102 cm (> 40 in.) Women > 88 cm (> 35 in.)
Underweight	18.5	—	—	—
Normal[b]	18.5–24.9	—	—	—
Overweight	25.0–29.9	—	Increased	High
Obesity	30.0–34.9	I	High	Very high
	35.0–39.9	II	Very high	Very high
Morbid obesity	≥40	III	Extremely high	Extremely high

Source: National Heart, Lung, and Blood Institute's Obesity Education Initiative: Guidelines on overweight and obesity.
Abbreviations: BMI, body mass index; CVD, cardiovascular disease; CKD, chronic kidney disease.
[a] Disease risks for type 2 diabetes, hypertension, CVD, and CKD.
[b] Increased waist circumference can also be a marker for increased risk even in persons of normal weight.

women and men, respectively, seem to pose increased risks of chronic diseases. Central or abdominal fat tissue is generally more metabolically active and readily mobilized to cells, tissues, and organ systems in which accumulation can cause damage, such as oxidative stress, proinflammation, and atherosclerotic lesions (Beydoun and Wang, 2007).

As with type 2 diabetes, most of the deaths due to CKD in the United States (Chen et al., 2004) and, presumably, in other countries are due to CVD, with atherosclerosis being the primary form of CVD. A robust association exists between metabolic syndrome and type 2 diabetes, which is often a precursor to CKD (USRDS, 2003). Metabolic syndrome includes a cluster of cardiometabolic conditions, including dyslipidemia, insulin resistance, hypertension, hyperglycemia, and abdominal obesity. Nearly one-fourth of Americans over 20 years have this syndrome—excess weight being the main cause of these symptoms (Wassink et al., 2008). It was found that WC was a better prognostic marker for mortality than BMI in a prospective cohort of 993 kidney transplant recipients (Kovesdy et al., 2010). Moreover, in a representative sample of over 3000 participants, Noori et al. (2009) concluded that WC was a more important determinant of CKD in adults than waist-to-hip ratio and BMI.

Regarding physiological implications, the U.S. NHANES findings from 1998 to 1994 (Guarnieri et al., 2010) revealed that participants with 3, 4, and 5 aspects of the metabolic syndrome had increased odds of 1.62, 2.45, and 3.19, respectively, for microalbuminuria—compared to those with 0 or 1 aspects. These associations were independent of sex, age, race, or ethnicity. This creates a vicious cycle because increased renal damage may aggravate features of the metabolic syndrome, including insulin resistance and hypertension. Therefore, addressing the interactions between CKD, obesity, and metabolic syndrome is of utmost importance.

As physiological benefits are evident with as little as 5%–10% reduction in on total body weight, long-term weight management is crucial for CKD. The challenge is to address long-term weight management in the treatment of chronic diseases. Innovative means of increasing PA are warranted. The overwhelming population-based evidence of the benefit of the use of the pedometer in weight management (Bravata et al., 2007) also appears relevant to the population with CKD. The practice goal of 10,000 steps a day provides a ready, teachable concept in patient care. Nowicki et al. (2010) observed a decrease in BMI and blood pressure in patients with CKD with an increase in the use of the pedometer. Zamojska et al. (2006) further noted that simple pedometer use can correlate with key clinical and biochemical parameters in this population. In this instance, the less physically active participants had lower concentrations of albumin and increased anemia.

13.6 OBESITY PARADOX

Several well-designed studies have noted an inverse association between overweight, obesity, and CKD, particularly in those on long-term dialysis (Stolic, 2010). Obermayr et al. (2009) recently concluded that individuals with proteinuric CKD should not be provided counseling for weight loss, as increased BMI markedly reduced mortality in a U-shaped manner. Other investigators are recommending further examination of the components of body composition as they relate to survival of patients with CKD. For example, Agarwal et al. (2010) recently suggested examination of anthropometric measures, including skin-fold thickness and bioelectrical impedance, to better assess the role of body composition in morbidity and mortality due to CKD. Kalantar-Zadeh et al. (2010) found that higher BMI with increased muscle mass was associated with increased survival. This finding highlights the importance of both cardiovascular and resistance training in increasing muscle mass in patients with CKD. Further investigation of the role of body composition and related indices in CKD (e.g., skin-fold measures, muscle:fat ratio, and computed tomography scans) is recommended.

13.7 CONCLUSIONS

It is highly likely that PA contributes to reduced morbidity and mortality and increased QoL in patients with CKD, with weight management being central to these health benefits. PA guidelines

TABLE 13.2
Online Resources

Physical Activity Guidelines, U.S. Department of Health and Human Services (HHS) (http://www.health.gov/paguidelines)	National Kidney Foundation: Staying Fit with Kidney Disease (www.Kidney.org/atoz/content/stayfit.cfm)
Life Options (www.lifeoptions.org)	healthfinder®: A Guide to Reliable Health Information on Physical Activity and Other Topics, HHS (http://www.healthfinder.gov)
Office of Disease Prevention and Health Promotion, HHS (http://odphp.osophs.dhhs.gov)	Centers for Disease Control and Prevention (CDC), HHS (http://www.cdc.gov/physicalactivity)
Food and Nutrition Service, USDA (http://www.fns.usda.gov/fns)	CDC Information about Preventing Falls in Older Adults, HHS (http://www.cdc.gov/ncipc/factsheets/adultfalls.htm)
U.S. Department of Health and Human Services Online (www.health.gov/PAGuidelines)	National Institute on Aging Exercise Guide, HHS (http://www.nia.nih.gov/HealthInformation/Publications/ExerciseGuide/chapter01.htm)

for patients with CKD are generally congruent with those for the general population, with an important caution about starting and progressing PA slowly and requiring patients to be under the supervision of a health care provider. As with other robust behavior change modalities, it is essential to provide small, measurable, and realistic recommendations of PA and weight management for patients with CKD. Multidisciplinary care (Cueto-Manzano et al., 2010; Johansen, 2005)—including primary care physicians, dietitians, nurses, and social workers—along with self-help/support groups is recommended, for which there are many online resources available (Table 13.2).

In a recent article, Painter (2009) commented, "although there is robust evidence that these [CKD] patients benefit from regular exercise training and/or increasing physical activity, the nephrology community has not adopted recommendations and encouragement for physical activity as a part of the routine care plan." Given the high likelihood of comorbid conditions, national PA guidelines that ideally align with those for other chronic diseases are warranted. Moreover, a multidimensional approach for treatment and prevention of chronic diseases is recommended. Qualitative (Jennette et al., 2010) and quantitative (Nikolas et al., 2004) data support the heightened need for increased knowledge and awareness of risk factors associated with CKD, including type 2 diabetes, family history, and hypertension. Further focus is needed on innovations in this area and on community-based initiatives such as education and health screening, improved measures of body composition and energy expenditure, and better understanding of the mechanisms underlying the relationship between CKD and obesity.

REFERENCES

Adams, T., Gess, R., Smith, S., et al. 2007. Long-term mortality after gastric bypass surgery. *N Engl J Med.* 357(8):753–761.

Agarwal, R., Bills, J., Light, R. 2010. Diagnosing obesity by body mass index in chronic kidney disease: An explanation of the "obesity paradox"? *Hypertension* 56(5):893–900. Epub 2010 September 27.

Alexander, J., Coodman, H., Hawver, L., et al. 2009. Improvement and stabilization of chronic kidney disease after gastric bypass. *Surg Obes Relat Dis.* 5(2):237–241. Epub 2008 August 27.

Allison, D., Myles, S., Moonseong, H., et al. 1997. Hypothesis concerning the U-shaped relation between body mass index and mortality. *Am J Epidem.* 146:339–349.

Axelsson, J. 2008. Obesity in chronic kidney disease: Good or bad? *Blood Purif.* 26(1):23–29. Epub 2008 January 10.

Beasley, C., Smith, D., Neale, T. 1986. Exercise capacity in chronic renal failure patients managed by continuous ambulatory peritoneal dialysis. *Aust NZ J Med.* 16:5–10.

Beddu, S, Baird, B., Zitterkoph, J., et al. 2009. Physical activity and mortality in chronic kidney disease (NHANES III). *Clin J Am Soc Nephrol.* 4:1901–1906.
Bello, A., Peters, J., Wight, J., et al. 2010. The kidney evaluation and awareness program in Sheffield (KEAPS): A community-based screening for microalbuminuria in a British population. *Nephron Clin Pract.* 116(2):c95–c103. Epub 2010 May 21.
Beydoun, M. and Wang, Y. 2007. Gender-ethnic disparity in BMI and waist circumference shifts in US adults. *Obesity* 17(1):169–176.
Bravata, D., Smith-Spangler, C., Sundaram, V., et al. 2007. Using pedometers to increase physical activity and improve health: A systematic review. *JAMA* 21;298(19):2296–304.
Brenner, I. and Brohart, K. 2008. Weekly energy expenditure and quality of life in hemodialysis patients. *CANNT J.* 18(4):36–40.
Brodin, E., Ljungman, S., Hedberg, M., et al. 2001. Physical activity, muscle performance and quality of life in patients treated with peritoneal dialysis. *Scan J Urol Nephrol.* 35(1):71–78.
Brunier, G. and Graydon, J. 1993. The influence of PA on fatigue in pts with ESRD on dialysis. *ANNA J.* 20(4):457–461. Discussion 462, 521.
Canada's Physical Activity Guide for Healthy Living. 2010. Public Health Agency of Canada and Canadian Society for Exercise Physiology. Online: www.paguide.com (accessed December 2010).
Capitanini, A., Cupisti, A., Mochi, N., et al. 2008. Effects of exercise training on exercise aerobic capacity and quality of life in hemodialysis patients. *J Nephrol.* 21(5):738–743.
Castaneda, C., Gordon, P., Uhlin, K., et al. 2001. Resistance training to counteract the catabolism of a low-protein diet in patients with chronic renal insufficiency. *Ann Intern Med.* 135:965–976.
CDC. 2010. Online ref for BMI calculator. Online: www.cdc.gov/healthyweight/assessing/bmi/adult_bmi/english_bmi_calculator/bmi_calculator.html (accessed December 2010).
Cheema, B. and Fiatarone Singh, M. 2005. Exercise training in patients receiving maintenance hemodialysis: A systematic review of clinical trials. *Am J Nephrol.* 25:352–364.
Chen, J., Muntner, P., Hamm, L., et al. 2004. The metabolic syndrome and chronic kidney disease in US adults. *Ann Intern Med.* 140:167–174.
Cook, S., MacLaughlin, H., Macdougall, I. 2008. A structured weight management programme can achieve improved functional ability and significant weight loss in obese patients with chronic kidney disease. *Nephrol Dial Transplant.* 23:263–268.
Corpeleijn, E., Bakker, S., Stolk, R. 2009. Obesity and impaired renal function: Potential for lifestyle intervention? *Eur J Epidemiol.* 24(6):275–280. Epub 2009 May 7.
Cueto-Manzano, A., Martinez-Ramirez, H., Cortes-Sanabria, L. 2010. Management of chronic kidney disease: Primary health-care setting, self-care and multidisciplinary approach. *Clin Nephrol.* Sup;74(S1):99–104.
Daul, A., Schafers, R., Daul, K., et al. 2004. Exercise during hemodialysis. *Clin Nephrol.* 61(Suppl1): S26–S30.
Davis, J. and Holcombe, J. 2011. Intradialytic exercise: A pilot program. *Dialysis Transplant.* 40(6):258–260.
Ejerblad, E., Fored, C., Lindblad, P., et al. 2006. Obesity and risk for chronic renal failure. *J Am Soc Nephrol.* 17:1695–1702.
Eknoyan, G. 2006. A history of obesity, or how what was good became ugly and then bad. *Adv Chronic Kidney Dis.* 13(4):421–427.
Fox, C., Larson, M., Leip, E., et al. 2004. Predictors of new-onset kidney disease in a community-based population. *JAMA* 291:844–850.
Garrow, J. and Webster, J. 1985. Quetelet's index (W/H2) as a measure of fatness. *Int J Obes.* 9:147–153.
Goldberg, A., Hagberg, J., Delmez, J., et al. 1979. Exercise training improves abnormal lipid and carbohydrate metabolism in hemodialysis patients. *Trans Am Soc Artif Intern Organs.* 25:431–437.
Guarnieri, G., Zanetti, M., Vinci, P., et al. 2010. Metabolic syndrome and chronic kidney disease. *J Ren Nutr.* 20(5 Suppl):S19–S23.
Hallan, S., de Mutsert, R., Carlsen, S., et al. 2006. Obesity, smoking and physical inactivity as risk factors for CKD: Are men more vulnerable? *Am J Kidney Dis.* 47(3):396–405.
Headley, S., Germain, M., Mailloux, P., et al. 2002. Resistance training improves strength and functional measures in patients with end-stage renal disease. *Am J Kidney Dis.* 40(2):355–364.
Heber, D. 2010. An integrative view of obesity. *Am J Clin Nutr.* 9(suppl):280S–283S.
Henrique, D., Reboredo Mde, M., Chaoubah, A., et al. 2010. Aerobic exercise improves physical capacity in patients under chronic hemodialysis. *Arq Bras Cardiol.* 94(6):823–828.
Hsieh, R., Lee, W., Huang, H., et al. 2007. Quality of life and its correlates in ambulatory hemodialysis patients. *J Nephrol.* 20:731–738.

Jennette, C., Vupputuri, S., Hogan, S., et al. 2010. Community perspectives on kidney disease and health promotion from at-risk populations in rural North Carolina, USA. *Rural Remote Health.* 10:1388. Online: www.rrh.org.au

Johansen, K., Kaysen, G., Young, B., et al. 2003. Longitudinal study of nutritional status, body composition and physical function in hemodialysis patients. *Am J Clin Nutr.* 77:842–846.

Johansen, K., Painter, P., Kent-Braun, J,. et al. 2001. Validation of questionnaires to estimate physical activity and functioning in end-stage renal disease. *Kidney Int.* 59(3):1121–1127.

Johansen, K. 2005. Exercise and CKD: Current recommendations. *Sports Med.* 35(6):485–499.

Kalantar-Zadeh, K., Streja, E., Kovedsky, C., et al. 2010. The obesity paradox and mortality associated with surrogates of body size and muscle mass in patients receiving hemodialysis. *Mayo Clin Proc.* 85(11):991–1001.

Kiberd, B. 2006. The chronic kidney disease epidemic: Stepping back and looking forward. *J Am Soc Nephrol.* 17:2967–2973.

Knap, B., Butorvic-Ponikvar, J., Ponikvar, R., et al. 2005. Regular exercise as part of treatment for patients with end-stage renal disease. *Ther Apher Dial.* 9(3):211–213.

Kosmadakis, G., Bevington, A., Smith, A., et al. 2010. Physical exercise in patients with severe kidney disease. *Nephron Clin Pract.* 115:c7–c16.

Kouldi, E., Lacovides, A., Iordanidis, P. 1997. Exercise renal rehabilitation program: Psychosocial effects. *Nephron.* 77:152–158.

Kovesdy, C., Czira, M., Rudas, A., et al. 2010. Body mass index, waist circumference and mortality in kidney transplant recipients. *Am J Transplant.* 10(12):2644–2651. Epub 2010 November 18.

Krause, R. 2004. WGRR-European Working Group on Renal Rehabilitation and Exercise Physiology. Nephrologists' view on exercise training in chronic kidney disease (results of the questionnaire at the WCN 2003). *Clin Nephrol.* 61(Suppl 1):S2–S4.

Krol, E., Rutkowski, B., Czarniak, P., et al. 2010. Aging or comorbid conditions—what is the main cause of kidney damage? *J Nephrol.* 23(4):444–452.

Kutner, N., Zhang, R., Mclellan, W. 2000. Patient-reported quality of life early in dialysis treatment: Effects associated with usual exercise activity. *Nephrol Nurs J.* 27(4):357–367.

Kutner, N. 2007. How can exercise be incorporated into the routine care of patients on dialysis? *Int Urol Nephrol.* 39(4):1281–1285.

Lastra, G., Manrique, C., Sowers, J. 2006. Obesity, cardiometabolic syndrome and chronic kidney disease: The weight of the evidence. *Adv Chronic Kidney Dis.* 13(4):365–373.

Lau, D. 2007. Obesity Canada Clinical Practice Guidelines Steering Committee and Expert Panel. Synopsis of the 2006 Canadian clinical practice guidelines on the management and prevention of obesity in adults and children. *CMAJ* April 10;176(8):1103–1106.

Li, M. and Fan, X. 2010. Patients having hemodialysis: Physical activity and associated factors. *J Adv Nurs.* 66(6):1338–1345. Epub 2010 April 1.

Mathew, A., Okada, S., Sharma, K. 2011. Obesity related kidney disease. *Curr Diabetes Rev.* 7(1):41–49.

McClellan, W., Abramson, J., Newsome, B., et al. 2010. Physical and psychological burden of CKD among older adults. *Am J Nephrol.* 31(4):309–317. Epub 2010 February 13.

Mei, Z., Grummer-Strawn, L., Pietrobelli, A., et al. 2002. Validity of body mass index compared with other body-composition screening indexes for the assessment of body fatness in children and adolescents. *Am J Clin Nutr.* 75(6):978–985.

Mokdad, A., Marks, J., Stroup, D., et al. 2004. Actual causes of death in the United States, 2000. *JAMA* 29(10):1238–1245.

Monteon, F., Laidlaw, S., Shaib, J., et al. 1986. Energy expenditure in patients with chronic renal failure. *Kidney Int.* 30(5):741–747.

Navaneethan, S., Yehnert, H., Moustarah, F., et al. 2009. Weight loss interventions in chronic kidney disease: A systematic review and meta-analysis. *Clin J Am Soc Nephrol.* 4:1565–1574.

NHLBI obesity guidelines. 2010. Online. http://www.nhlbi.nih.gov/guidelines/obesity/bmi_tbl.htm (accessed July 2011).

Nikolas, T., Gershon, F., Opotowsky, A., et al. 2004. Awareness of kidney disease in the US population: Findings from the National Health and Nutrition Examination Survey (NHANES) 1999 to 2000. *Am J Kidney Dis.* 44(2):185–197.

Noori, N., Hosseinpanah, F., Nasiri, A., et al. 2009. Comparison of overall obesity and abdominal adiposity in predicting chronic kidney disease incidence among adults. *J Ren Nutr.* 19(3):228–237. Epub March 3, 2009.

Nowicki, M., Murlikiewicz, K., Jagodzinka, M. 2010. Pedometers as a means to increase spontaneous physical activity in chronic hemodialysis patients. *J Nephrol.* 23(3):297–305.

Obermayr, R., Temml, C., Gutjahr, G., et al. 2009. Body mass index modifies the risk of cardiovascular death in proteinuric chronic kidney disease. *Nephrol Dial Transplant.* 24(8):2421–2428. Epub 2009 February 24.

Ouzoni, S., Kouidi, E., Sioulis, A., et al. 2009. Effects of intradialytic exercise training on health-related quality of life indices in haemodialysis patients. *Clin Rehabil.* 23:53–63.

Painter, P. 2009. Implementing exercise: What do we know? Where do we go? *Adv Chronic Kidney Dis.* 16(6):536–544.

Persinger, R., Foster, C., Gibson, M., et al. 2004. Consistency of the talk test for exercise prescription. *Med Sci Sports Exerc.* 36(9):1632–1636.

Sjostrom, L., Narbo, K., Sjostrom, C., et al. 2007. Effects of bariatric surgery on mortality in Swedish obese subjects. *N Engl J Med.* 357(8):741–752.

Soni, R., Weisbord, S., Unruh, M. 2010. Health-related quality of life outcomes in chronic kidney disease. *Curr Opin Nephrol Hypertens.* 19(2):153–159.

Stack, A. and Murthy, B. 2008. Exercise and limitations in physical activity levels among new dialysis in the United States: An epidemiologic study. *Ann Epidemiol.* 18(12):880–888.

Stenvinkel, P. 2010. Chronic kidney disease: A public priority and harbinger of premature cardiovascular disease. *J Intern Med.* 268(5):456–467.

Stolic, R. 2010. Obesity in renal failure: Health or disease? *Med Hypotheses.* 75(6):497–500. Epub 2010 July 24.

Tackling Obesity: The evidence and the uncertainty. The UK Foresight Project. 2007. Online: www.bis.gov.uk/assets/bispartners/docs/obesity/obesity_final_part2.pdf (accessed December 2010).

Teta, D. 2010. Weight loss in obese patients with chronic kidney disease: Who and how? *J Ren Care.* 36(Suppl1):163–171.

Ting, S., Nair, H., Ching, I., et al. 2009. Overweight, obesity and chronic kidney disease. *Nephron Clin Pract.* 112c:c121–c127.

U.S. Department of Health and Human Services (USDHHS). 2008. Physical activity guidelines for Americans [electronic resource]: Be active your way: A fact sheet for adults, Washington, D.C. Online: www.health.gov/PAGuidelines (accessed December 2010).

U.S. Renal Data System (USRDS). 2003. *2003 Annual Data Report: Atlas of End Stage Renal Disease in the United States.* Bethesda, MD: National Institutes of Health, National Institute of Diabetes and Digestive and Kidney Diseases.

Wang, Y., Chen, X., Song, Y., et al. 2008. Association between obesity and kidney disease: A systematic review and meta-analysis. *Kidney Int.* 73(1):19–33. Epub 2007 October 10.

Wassink, A., Van Der Graaf, Y., Soedamah-Muthu, S., et al. 2008. Smart Study Group. Metabolic syndrome and incidence of type 2 diabetes in patients with manifest vascular disease. *Diab Vasc Kid Res.* 5(2):114–122.

Zamojska, S., Szklarek, M., Niewodniczy, M., et al. 2006. Correlates of habitual physical activity in chronic hemodialysis patients. *Nephrol Dial Transplant.* 21:1323–1327.

14 Chronic Kidney Disease and Mineral and Bone Disorder Management

C.J. Parris
Columbia Nephrology

Beth Parris
Blue Cross Blue Shield of South Carolina

CONTENTS

14.1 INTRODUCTION

This chapter discusses chronic kidney disease and mineral bone disorder (CKD–MBD) and the role it plays in the increased incidence of cardiovascular morbidity and mortality in CKD. Just how great is the risk? After adjusting for age, race, and gender, cardiovascular disease (CVD) mortality rates in patients with CKD Stage 5 are 10–20 times those of the general population (Foley et al., 1998). Most patients with advanced CKD present with vitamin D deficiency, secondary hyperparathyroidism (SHPT), hypertension, insulin resistance, vascular calcifications, and dyslipidemia. These comorbidities may start early in Stage 3 CKD and, though they seem dissimilar, have more in common than is apparent at first review (Andress, 2005; Becker et al., 2005; Elder, 2002; Kramer et al., 2005).

As renal function declines, the body tries to maintain calcium homeostasis through adaptive and compensatory mechanisms. These work well up to a point, but as CKD progresses, the compensatory mechanisms begin to fail. There is a decline in urinary phosphorus excretion leading to increased serum phosphorus, which stimulates increased fibroblast growth factor 23 (FGF-23), causing a reduction in active vitamin D, subsequent elevation of parathyroid hormone (PTH), and reduced urinary calcium excretion leading to calcium imbalance. This maladaptive dysregulation leads to elevated phosphorus, worsening SHPT and, if untreated, calcium overload, which contributes to vascular calcifications and increased cardiovascular (CV) morbidity and mortality (Gutierrez et al., 2005; Kalantar-Zadeh et al., 2010; Seiler et al., 2009; Figure 14.1).

Since 1989, the National Kidney Foundation Dialysis Outcomes Quality Initiative (K/DOQI) guidelines have guided the treatment of metabolic bone disorder in dialysis patients. In 2003, the scope of the NKF guidelines was expanded by the K/DOQI. The more recent guidelines

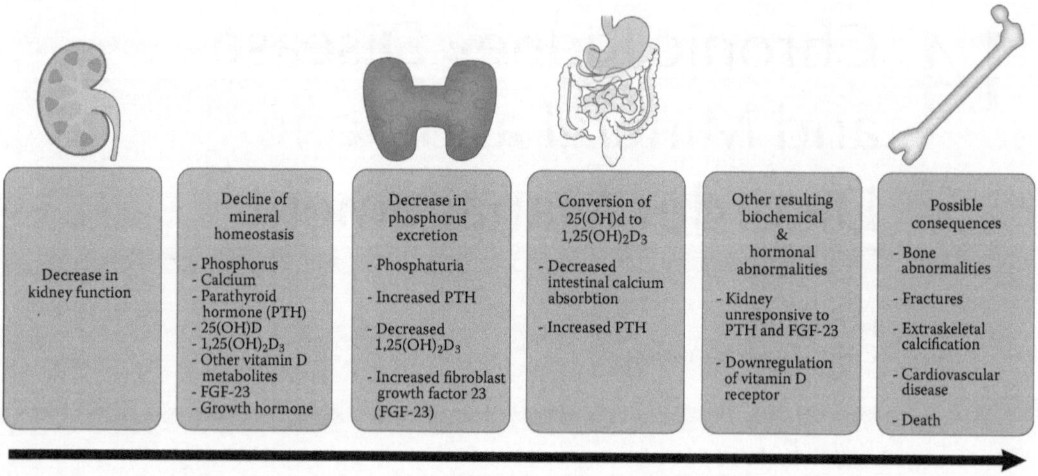

FIGURE 14.1 Progression of bone disease. (Courtesy of Shaun Riffle, University of South Carolina School of Medicine, Columbia, SC.)

revolutionized the care of CKD patients because they not only included recommendations for the dialysis population, but for the first time also made recommendations for all patients with CKD. The guidelines stressed prevention and early diagnosis and continued to focus on treatment. The new guidelines also defined the five stages of CKD and started to shed more light on the comorbidities of CKD. The bone and mineral section of the guidelines included specific recommendations for the prevention and treatment of SHPT (NKF, 2002).

In 2009, the Kidney Disease Improving Global Outcome (KDIGO™) CKD-MBD Guidelines recommended changes to the KDOQI (2003) bone guidelines placing more emphasis on trending mineral and PTH values; attempting to control PTH, phosphorus, and calcium more tightly within the normal range for CKD Stages 3–5; and expanding the recommended PTH range for dialysis patients to 2–9 times normal (KDIGO, 2009). With the release of KDOQI Commentary on KDIGO in February 2010, the guidelines became the accepted standard of care in the United States (Kasiske et al., 2010; Uhlig et al., 2010).

A new system of bundling charges became effective in 2011 with the Centers for Medicare and Medicaid Services (CMS) prospective payment system for the dialysis population. Dialysis companies will no longer be able to charge separately for the IV drugs or for oral drugs with IV equivalents that are used to treat CKD–MBD. Oral medications without IV equivalents, such as phosphorus binders and calcimimetics, will come into the bundle in 2014. Exactly what effect this will have on quality outcomes remains to be seen (CMS, 2008).

14.2 PHOSPHORUS

Phosphorus is one of the most abundant minerals in the human body, second only to calcium. It is stored in bones, teeth, DNA, and cell membranes throughout the body. Inorganic phosphorus is critical for skeletal development and the conversion of food to energy. Phosphorus helps with muscle contraction, nerve conduction, and kidney function. Phosphorus deficiency does not normally occur except with the use of certain products, such as calcium, sevelemer, and antacids that contain aluminum or magnesium, which prevent phosphorus absorption by binding it in the gut. Most phosphorus is intracellular, but a change in pH and serum glucose can cause it to shift in and out of cells, changing the level that is measured without changing the total body phosphorus (KDIGO, 2009). Approximately 700 mg of phosphorus is present in the average adult, of which 85% is contained in bone in the form of hydroxyapatite. Fifteen percent of the extracellular phosphorus is circulating and is measured when a serum phosphorus level is obtained. The Recommended Daily Allowance (RDA) for phosphorus is about 1000 mg for adults, although the average dietary intake is between 800 and 1500 mg/day. Approximately 65% of ingested phosphorus is absorbed in the small intestine, and approximately 200 mg is exchanged between the extracellular pool and bone. The kidneys excrete about 900 mg of excess phosphorus a day. Kidney excretion of phosphorus is the primary method of maintaining phosphorus homeostasis (Brenner, 2008). Foods high in phosphorus are the protein-rich foods like meat, dairy products, and legumes. Approximately 70% of the phosphorus in meat and dairy products is absorbed. Beef and chicken contain about 8 mg phosphorus per gram of protein, much less than low-fat milk, which has 28 mg phosphorus per gram of protein. Balancing a diet containing high biologic value protein, while adhering to a low-phosphorus diet, is difficult at best. Processed meats and cheeses often contain phosphorus additives, which are noted on the list of ingredients but not on the nutrition label. Educating patients to read the list of ingredients will help them to learn which foods to avoid and to make better dietary choices (USDA, 2001).

Recent studies used in the formulation of the KDIGO CKD-MBD guidelines suggest that dialysis patients have higher mortality rates with even a modest elevation in phosphorus. One study looked at the association between higher phosphorus levels and mortality. Of the patients who had phosphorus levels maintained within the KDOQI guidelines, 72% had an increased risk of mortality. A linear relationship was observed between serum phosphorus and mortality, such that with each 0.5 mg/dL increase in phosphorus, there was a corresponding increase in mortality. When phosphorus levels reached 3.5 mg/dL or above, a statistically significant increase in mortality was observed. A 1 mg/dL increase in serum phosphorus was associated with a significant 35% increased risk for acute myocardial infarction (MI) and a 28% increased risk for death or nonfatal MI. This study clearly demonstrated that for dialysis patients, increased phosphorus is associated with an increased risk of cardiovascular morbidity and mortality (Kestenbaum et al., 2005).

It appears that even in the non-CKD population, the risks associated with elevated phosphorus are higher as well. To evaluate this effect, the Framingham Offspring Study evaluated the relationship of serum phosphorus and calcium to the incidence of CVD. Participants were excluded from the analysis if they had CVD or CKD. The primary outcomes were MI, angina, cerebrovascular events, peripheral vascular disease, and congestive heart failure. The analysis revealed that participants with high serum phosphorus levels were associated with an increased risk of CVD (Dhingra et al., 2007). In a second study of non-CKD patients with a recent MI, higher baseline serum phosphorus was associated with a significantly greater risk of MI and death (Tonelli et al., 2005).

To prevent the CKD comorbidities associated with high phosphorus, it is recommended that patients follow a low-phosphorus diet. Though controversial, a low-protein diet of 0.6–0.8 g/kg/day may also slow the progression of kidney disease, reduce proteinuria, and keep serum phosphorus within normal limits (Mitch, 2005). Once the patient has progressed to dialysis, a higher-protein diet is recommended. It is difficult to increase protein intake and at the same time keep phosphorus intake low.

KDIGO and KDOQI Commentary on KDIGO suggest more emphasis should be placed on maintaining phosphorus toward the normal or reference range. The 2003 KDOQI Guidelines suggested that a phosphorus range of 3.5–5.5 mg/dL was optimal, but there is ample evidence, even in the non-CKD population, to suggest that tighter phosphorus control would be beneficial. Data from several large dialysis populations that compared patients with serum phosphorus ≤ 6.5 mg/dL to patients with serum phosphorus > 6.5 mg/dL showed that the higher phosphorus group were at a significantly increased risk of mortality from coronary artery disease (CAD) and sudden death compared to the group with lower phosphorus levels (Ganesh et al., 2001). Another analysis of 40,538 hemodialysis patients found that serum phosphorus levels less than 3 mg/dL and more than 5 mg/dL were associated with increased relative risk of death (Block et al., 2004). Another analysis of 58,000 hemodialysis patients confirmed the increased risk for death associated with high serum phosphorus, but it did not find the same association with low phosphorus after controlling for malnutrition, inflammation, and cachexia syndrome. Therefore, the KDIGO Guidelines do not suggest keeping phosphorus above 3.5 mg/dL as the 2003 KDOQI Guidelines recommended (Kalantar-Zadeh et al., 2006).

The relationship between elevated phosphorus and increased risk of death in the dialysis population is well established. What other modifiable risk factors contribute to vascular calcifications, increased CV events, and death? Actually, an increase in mortality is associated with all mineral and bone parameters, including phosphorus, calcium, and PTH, although the highest mortality is associated with phosphorus (Block et al., 2004). It is important to recognize that diet is not the only source of phosphorus: an elevated PTH can cause resorption of phosphorus and calcium from bone. As CKD progresses, bones increase the production of FGF-23 to try to keep serum phosphorus in the normal range, causing phosphaturia. FGF-23 also suppresses activation of vitamin D by the kidney and contributes to the development of SHPT. Another ominous sign is that dialysis patients with the highest FGF-23 have the highest mortality independent of PTH, calcium, and phosphorus (KDIGO, 2009).

14.3 CALCIUM

The measured serum calcium is a poor reflection of total body calcium. Only 1% of total body calcium is measurable in the serum; the rest is stored in bone. Only ionized calcium, generally 40%–50% of total serum calcium, is physiologically active. Nonionized calcium is bound to albumin and is not physiologically active. In the presence of low serum albumin, there is an increase in ionized calcium relative to total calcium; thus, total serum calcium may underestimate the active serum calcium. A formula for estimating corrected calcium is to add 0.8 mg/dL to the serum calcium for every 1 g decrease in serum albumin below 4 g/dL (KDIGO, 2009).

Serum calcium effectively determines the rate of PTH secretion, since with a slight reduction in serum calcium there is a prompt increase in PTH secretion occurring within a matter of seconds. The rise occurs as a result of preformed PTH being released from stored puvules in the parathyroid glands. If PTH secretion is not effective at maintaining the blood calcium level, increased PTH synthesis occurs over several hours to days. The increased PTH synthesis is mediated through the parathyroid calcium and vitamin D receptors. As CKD progresses, active vitamin D levels fall and further stimulate PTH secretion. PTH causes calcium and phosphorus resorption from bone and reduces calcium excretion by the kidney. PTH then causes increased activation of vitamin D, which increases absorption of calcium and phosphorus in the gut. The net result of increased PTH secretion is an increase in serum calcium (Andress, 2006; Brown et al., 1999; Rodriguez et al., 2006).

In CKD 4 and 5, serum calcium levels decline as active vitamin D levels fall. This results in decreased intestinal absorption of calcium in the gut (Hsu, 2007). By the time most patients reach dialysis, they lack adequate kidney function to excrete calcium and subsequently end up in a positive calcium balance and hypercalcemia (Friis et al., 1968; Popovtzer et al., 1969). Hypercalcemia, more so than hypocalcemia, is associated with increased mortality in the dialysis population. Using a multivariant analysis of a large dialysis population, it was found that the association between serum calcium and relative risk of death was linear with lower risk at lower calcium concentrations. The risk of death with higher calcium was independent of PTH or phosphorus (Kalantar-Zadeh et al., 2006).

The 2003 KDOQI Guidelines called for maintaining the serum calcium in the range of 8.4–9.5 mg/dL, but with the newer 2009 KDIGO and 2010 KDOQI Commentary on KDIGO the stringent control of calcium at the lower end of the normal range has been relaxed and it is now recommended to maintain calcium within the normal or reference range for the lab. Calcium levels that are higher than normal are associated with an increased risk of vascular calcification and result in increased morbidity and mortality. When calcification occurs or when hypercalcemia recurs, care should be exercised to maintain the calcium in the reference range, and the use of calcium-containing phosphorus binders should be avoided (Kasiske et al., 2010).

14.4 PARATHYROID HORMONE

PTH is the primary regulator of calcium as a reduction in calcium leads to a decrease in activation of the calcium-sensing receptor and an increase in secretion of PTH (Potts, 2005). Increased PTH causes resorption of calcium and phosphorus from bone and has an effect on the kidney leading to calcium resorption and phosphorus excretion as well as enhanced production of active vitamin D (Skorecki et al., 2005). The parathyroid gland responds to decreased serum calcium by increasing secretion of preformed PTH within minutes and, with continued stimulation, increased production within hours to days (Silver and Levi, 2005). Overproduction of PTH and subsequent hyperplasia occur over a period of weeks to years, and as this progresses, the PTH-producing cells of the gland increase in number and size. Initially, the hyperplasia is diffuse, but later the glands become nodular and the cells become monoclonal (Rodriguez et al., 2005). Studies show that with diffuse nodular hyperplasia, there is a decrease in the calcium and vitamin D receptors (Tokumoto et al., 2002). This results in the parathyroid gland becoming less responsive to correction of calcium and vitamin D levels, so high PTH output persists (Rodriguez et al., 2005). High levels of PTH cause skeletal and extraskeletal toxicity. The skeletal effects of PTH include high-turnover bone disease (osteitisfibrosa), Brown tumors, bone pain, osteopenia, fractures, hypercalcemia, and hyperphosphatemia and can result in calciphylaxis. The extraskeletal effects of PTH include neuropathy, hypertension caused by changes in the renin-angiotensin system, left ventricular hypertrophy (LVH), myocardial and valvular calcification, glucose intolerance, hyperlipidemia, and anemia. Many of these comorbidities often occur in Stage 3–5 CKD and undoubtedly play a role in the increased morbidity and mortality of CKD (Cunningham, 2000).

Though the 2003 KDOQI Guidelines recommended a fairly narrow range for PTH between 150–300 pg/mL. The KDIGO Guidelines and subsequent KDOQI Commentary have suggested a broader range of 2–9 times the reference range or approximately 130–600 pg/mL. A multivariable analysis suggested that elevations of PTH $\geq$ 600 pg/mL were associated with significantly increased relative risk of death. This result was largely driven by patients with an PTH $\geq$ 900 pg/mL (Block et al., 2004). Excess PTH causes resorption of calcium, magnesium, and phosphorus from the bone leading to their deposition in soft tissues (Moe, 2001). Though calcium and active vitamin D are important regulators of PTH, we also use calcimimetics to target the calcium receptor, suppressing PTH without increasing calcium or phosphorus. When the calcimimetic binds to the PTH calcium receptor it becomes more sensitive to calcium, and PTH secretion is decreased at lower calcium concentrations (Nemeth et al., 2004).

14.5 VITAMIN D

Vitamin D parent compound is derived from dietary sources or produced in the skin from exposure to heat and sunlight. The compound is converted in the liver to 25-hydroxyvitamin D, ergocalciferol. The last step in activating vitamin D to 1, 25 dihydroxyvitamin D occurs in the kidney (Drueke et al., 2006). Active vitamin D then travels throughout the body where it binds to the vitamin D receptors on target organs (Dusso et al., 2005). In 1984, Dr. Slatopolsky demonstrated the ability of the first-generation active vitamin D to suppress PTH in uremic patients; unfortunately, his study also demonstrated that the vitamin D caused a significant increase in serum calcium. The rise in calcium prompted researchers to work to develop new vitamin D analogs that suppress PTH without raising serum calcium (Slatopolsky et al., 1984). Since then, active vitamin D has been used as the mainstay of therapy to try to prevent SHPT. Active vitamin D prevents parathyroid gland hyperplasia, suppresses PTH synthesis and secretion, upregulates vitamin D receptors and calcium-sensing receptors in parathyroid gland, promotes mineral homeostasis by increased absorption of calcium and phosphorus, and helps to maintain normal bone formation (Andress, 2005).

The kidney is not alone in producing active vitamin D; other organs such as lung, colon, prostate, and breast have the 1-α hydroxylase enzyme to convert ergocalciferol to active vitamin D for local use within the organ. It is important to realize that this locally produced active vitamin D does not replace the loss of kidney-activated vitamin D to prevent SHPT as CKD progresses (Drueke et al., 2006). Conversely, giving active vitamin D to treat SHPT does not replace all of the vitamin D needs of the body because the level of active vitamin D obtained in treating SHPT is too low to meet the needs of all the tissues that require it. An ergocalciferol level of at least 30 ng/mL is needed to accomplish this (Goodman and Quarles, 2006).

It is now understood that in many cases, treatment with ergocalciferol does not prevent SHPT in the CKD population. To assess the effect of treatment, a prospective, nonrandomized observational study was performed in vitamin D-deficient patients with stage 3 and 4 CKD. Fifty-two patients with CKD Stage 3 or 4 with vitamin D deficiency and elevated PTH received ergocalciferol. The results revealed that ergocalciferol normalized 25 vitamin D levels in all patients and the median decline in PTH was 13.1% in Stage 3 but only 2.0% in Stage 4. This suggests that ergocalciferol may be a reasonable initial therapy for vitamin D deficiency with elevated PTH levels in Stage 3 CKD; however, it does not appear to have significant benefits in CKD Stage 4 (Zisman et al., 2007). The decline in active vitamin D occurs much earlier than we previously thought. The decline begins in Stage 2 CKD and is near the low end of the normal range by the time patients reach Stage 3. This helps to explain why it is common to see early signs of SHPT in CKD Stage 3. Throughout the early stages of CKD, calcium and phosphorus remain normal or near normal, and do not serve as good markers for developing SHPT. In late Stage 3 CKD, phosphorus and calcium start to become abnormal and SHPT rates are much higher. By CKD Stage 4–5, the majority of the patients have SHPT along with abnormal calcium and phosphorus levels (Levin et al., 2007).

CVD may be improved with active vitamin D supplementation, which inhibits inflammatory markers, modulates immune responses, downregulates renin, stimulates cardiomyocyte remodeling, regulates markers of cardiomyocyte hypertrophy, and may improve LVH in patients undergoing dialysis. Based on these observations, it has been hypothesized that vitamin D may improve CV outcomes including reduced incidence of heart failure, atherosclerosis, and myocardial hypertrophy and, possibly, decreased overall morbidity and mortality (Li et al., 2002; Mathieu and Adornin, 2002; Park et al., 1999; Timms et al., 2002).

A study of 50 dialysis patients, half of whom received active vitamin D after hemodialysis, revealed that the patients treated with active vitamin D had regression of myocardial hypertrophy and a reduction in risk factors for sudden cardiac death. Active vitamin D may be a promising treatment for reducing the rate of sudden cardiac death in the dialysis population (Kim et al., 2006). The fact that vitamin D receptors are ubiquitous throughout the body may explain why so many tissues

TABLE 14.1
Target Ranges for Treatment of CKD–MBD

	Stage 3, 4, and 5 Predialysis	Stage 5 Dialysis
Calcium	Maintain within normal (KDIGO & KDOQI)	Maintain within normal (KDIGO). 8.4–9.5 mg/dL or 2.1–2.375 mmol/L (KDOQI)
Phosphorus	Maintain within normal (KDIGO) 2.7–4.6 mg/dL or 0.87–1.49 mmol/L (KDOQI)	Maintain toward normal (KDIGO) 3.5–5.5 mg/dL or 1.13–1.78 mmol/L (KDOQI)

TABLE 14.2
Target Ranges for Initiating Treatment for intact parathyroid hormone (iPTH)

Stage 3	> Upper limit of normal (KDIGO)35–70 pg/mL (KDOQI)
Stage 4	> Upper limit of normal (KDIGO)70–110 pg/mL (KDOQI)
Stage 5	> Upper limit of normal (KDIGO)150–300 pg/mL (KDOQI)
Stage 5D	2–9 times upper limit of normal (KDIGO)150–300 pg/mL (KDOQI)

TABLE 14.3
Phosphorus-Binding Compounds

Binder Source	Rx	Forms	Content (Mineral/Metal/Element)	Potential Advantages	Potential Disadvantages
Aluminum hydroxide	No	Liquid, tablet, and capsule	Aluminum content varies from 100 to >200 mg/tablet	Very effective phosphate-binding capacity; variety of forms	Potential for aluminum toxicity; altered bone mineralization, dementia; GI side effects
Calcium acetate	Yes/No	Capsule and tablet	Contains 25% elemental Ca^{2+} (169 mg elemental Ca^{2+} per 667 mg capsule)	Effective phosphate binding; potential for enhanced phosphate-binding capability over $CaCO_3$; potentially less calcium absorption	Potential for hypercalcemia-associated risks, including extraskeletal calcification and PTH suppression; more costly than $CaCO_3$; GI side effects
Calcium carbonate	No	Liquid, tablet, chewable, capsule, and gum	Contains 40% elemental Ca^{2+} (200 mg elemental Ca^{2+} per 500 mg $CaCO_3$)	Effective, inexpensive, and readily available	Potential for hypercalcemia-associated risks, including extraskeletal calcification and PTH suppression; GI side effects
Calcium citrate	No	Tablet, liquid, and capsule	Contains 22% elemental Ca^{2+}	Not recommended in CKD	Enhancement of aluminum absorption; GI side effects
Calcium ketoglutarate	—	—	—	—	Similar to other calcium salts; costly; GI side effects; potentially less hypercalcemic than calcium carbonate or acetate; not well studied
Calcium gluconate	—	Tablet and powder	—	—	Similar to other calcium salts; not well studied
Ferric citrate	—	—	—	—	GI side effects; not well studied
Magnesium/calcium carbonate	No	Tablet	~28% elemental Mg^{2+} (85 mg) per total $MgCO_3$ and 25% elemental Ca^{2+} (100 mg) per total $CaCO_3$	Effective; potential for lower calcium load than pure calcium-based binders	GI side effects; potential for hypermagnesemia; not well studied
Magnesium carbonate/calcium acetate	Yes	Tablet	—	—	Lack of availability worldwide; assumed to have similar effects of its components

(Continued)

TABLE 14.3 (Continued)
Phosphorus-Binding Compounds

Binder Source	Rx	Forms	Content (Mineral/Metal/Element)	Potential Advantages	Potential Disadvantages
Sevelamer-HCl	Yes	Caplet	None	Effective; no calcium/metal; not absorbed; potential for reduced coronary/aortic calcification compared with calcium-based binders in some studies; reduces plasma concentration of LDL-C	Costly; potential for decreased bicarbonate levels; may require calcium supplement in presence of hypocalcemia; GI side effects
Sevelamer carbonate	Yes	Caplet and powder	None	Effective; no calcium/metal; not absorbed; assumed to have similar advantages as sevelamer-HCl; potentially improved acid–base balance	Costly; may require calcium supplement in presence of hypocalcemia; GI side effects
Lanthanum carbonate	Yes	Wafer and chewable	Contains 250, 500, or 1000 mg elemental lanthanum per wafer	Effective; no calcium; chewable	Costly; potential for accumulation of lanthanum due to GI absorption, although long-term clinical consequences unknown; GI side effects

Abbreviations: $CaCO_3$, calcium carbonate; CKD, chronic kidney disease; CKD–MBD, chronic kidney disease–mineral and bone disease; GI, gastrointestinal; KDIGO, Kidney Disease: Improving Global Outcomes; LDL-C, low-density lipoprotein cholesterol; PTH, parathyroid hormone; Rx, prescription.

Source: KDIGO, *Kidney Int.*, 76 (suppl 113), S1–S130, 2009. With permission.

are subject to the actions of vitamin D. In addition to the parathyroid gland, vitamin D receptors can be found in the myocytes, smooth muscle, endothelial cells of the CV system, in the liver parenchyma cells, in the thymus, bone marrow, B cells, and T cells, as well as in the gastrointestinal, reproductive, exocrine, respiratory, musculoskeletal, renal, epidermis, central nervous systems, hair follicles, fibroblasts, and stroma of connective tissues. The effect vitamin D deficiency has on these organs and tissues remains a matter of intense research (Andress, 2006).

14.6 SUMMARY

CKD–MBD is a debilitating preventable disease that has effects far beyond bone. Proper evaluation and treatment starting in CKD Stage 3 is imperative to improving outcomes. Recent advances in research have improved the understanding of the comorbidities of CKD, including CKD–MBD, but there is still much work to do. Table 14.1 contains a summary of suggested KDIGO and KDOQI calcium and phosphorus target ranges. Table 14.2 shows initiation ranges for the treatment of the elevated iPTH associated with CKD–MBD. Table 14.3 shows phosphorus-binding compounds.

REFERENCES

Andress, D. 2005. Vitamin D treatment in chronic kidney disease. *Semin Dial.* 18:315–321.

Andress, D. 2006. Vitamin D in chronic kidney disease: A systemic role for selection vitamin D receptor activation. *Kidney Int.* 69:33–43.

Becker, B., Kronenberg, F., Kleistein, J., et al. 2005. Renal insulin resistance syndrome, adiponectin and cardiovascular events in patients with kidney disease: The mild and moderate kidney disease study. *J Am Soc Nephrol.* 16:1091–1098.

Block, G., Klassen, P., Lazarus, J., et al. 2004. Mineral metabolism, mortality, and morbidity in maintenance hemodialysis. *J Am Soc Nephrol.* 15:2208–2218.

Brenner, B.M., ed. 2008. *Brenner and Rector's the Kidney.* 8thed. Philadelphia, PA: Saunders, 156–213.

Brown, A. Dusso, A, Statopolsky, E.1999. Vitamin D. *Am J Physiol.* 277:F157–F175.

Centers for Medicare & Medicaid Services (CMS), HHS. 2008. Medicare and Medicaid Programs; Conditions for coverage for end stage renal disease facilities; Final rule. Available at: http://www.cms.gov/CFCsAndCoPs/downloads/ESRDfinalrule0415.pdf (accessed July 17, 2011).

Cunningham, J. 2000. Are parathyroidectomies still appropriate in chronic dialysis patients? *Semin Dial.* 13:275–278.

Dhingra, R., Sullivan, L., Fox, C., et al. 2007. Relations of serum phosphorus and calcium levels to the incidence of cardiovascular disease in the community. *Arch Intern Med.* 167:879–885.

Drueke, T., Moe, S., Langman, C. 2006. Treatment approaches in CKD. In: Olgaard K, ed. *Clinical Guide to Bone and Mineral Metabolism in CKD.* New York: National Kidney Foundation, 119–127.

Dusso, A., Brown, A., Slatopolsky, E. 2005. Vitamin D. *Am J Physiol Renal Physiol.* 289: F8–28.

Elder, G. 2002. Pathophysiology and recent advances in the management of renal osteodystrophy. *J Bone Miner Res.* 17:2094–2105.

Foley, R., Parfry, P., Sarnak, M. 1998. Clinical epidemiology of cardiovascular disease in chronic renal disease. *Am J Kidney Dis.* 32:S112–S119.

Friis, Hahnemann, S., Weeke, E. 1968. Serum calcium and serum phosphorus in uraemia during administration of sodium phytate and aluminum hydroxide. *Acta Med Scand.* 183:497–505.

Ganesh, S., Stack, A., Levin, N., et al. 2001. Association of elevated serum PO4, CA x PO4 product, and parathyroid hormone with cardiac mortality risk in chronic hemodialysis patients. *J Am Soc Nephrol.* 12:2131–2138.

Goodman, W. and Quarles, L. 2006. Mineral homeostasis and bone physiology. In Olgaard K, ed. *Clinical Guide to Bone and Mineral Metabolism in CKD.* New York: National Kidney Foundation, 2–28.

Gutierrez, O., Isakova, T., Rhee, E., et al. 2005. Fibroblast growth factor-23 mitigates hyperphophatemia but accentuates calcitriol deficiency in chronic kidney disease. *J. Am. Soc. Nephrol.* 16(7):2205–2215.

Hsu C.H. 2007. We have mismanaged calcium and phosphate in renal failure? Available at: http://www.uninet.edu/cin2000/conferences/ChenHsu/ChenHsu.html

Kalantar-Zadeh, K., Kuwae, N., Regidor, D., et al. 2006. Survival predictability of time-varying indicators of bone disease in maintenance hemodialysis patients. *Kidney Int.* 70:771–780.

Kalantar-Zadeh, K., Shah, A., Duong, U., et al. 2010. Kidney bone disease and mortality in CKD: Revisiting the role of vitamin D, calcimimetics, alkaline phosphatase, and minerals. *Kidney Int.* 78:S10–S21.

Kasiske, B., Zeier, M., Chapman, J., et al. 2010. KDIGO clinical practice guideline for the care of kidney transplant recipients: A summary. *Kidney Int.* 77(4):299–311.

KDIGO. 2009. Clinical practice guideline for the diagnosis, evaluation, prevention, and treatment of chronic kidney disease–mineral and bone disorder (CKD–MBD). *Kidney Int.* 76 (suppl 113):S1–S130.

K/DOQI. 2003. Clinical practice guideline for bone metabolism and disease in chronic kidney disease. *Am J Kidney Dis.* (suppl 3).

Kestenbaum, B., Sampson, J., Rudser, K., et al. 2005. Serum phosphate levels and mortality risk among people with chronic kidney disease. *J Am Soc Nephrol.* 16:520–528.

Kim, H., Park, C., Shin, Y., et al. 2006. Calcitriol regresses cardiac hypertrophy and QT dispersion in secondary hyperparathyroidism on hemodialysis. *Nephron Clin Pract.* 102:c21–c29.

Kramer, H., Toto, R., Peshock, R., et al. 2005. Association between CKD and coronary artery calcification: The Dallas Heart Study. *J Am Soc Nephrol.* 16:507–513.

Levin, A., Bakris, G., Molitch, M., et al. 2007. Prevalence of abnormal serum vitamin D, PTH, calcium, and phosphorus in patients with chronic kidney disease: Results of the study to evaluate early kidney disease. *Kidney Int.* 71:31–38.

Li, Y., Kong, J., Wei, M., et al. 2002. 1,25-dihydroxyvitamin D(3) is a negative endocrine regulator of the renin–angiotensin system. *J Clin Invest.* 110:229–238

Mathieu, C. and Adornin, L. 2002. The coming of age of 1,25-dihydroxyvitamin D(3) analogs as immunomodulatory agents. *Trends Mol Med.* 8:174–179.

Moe, S. 2001. *Calcium and Phosphorus Balance in ESRD: Implications and Management.* Cambridge, MA: Genzyme Corporation.

Mitch, W. 2005. Beneficial responses to modified diets in treating patients with chronic kidney disease. *Kidney Int.* 67:S133–S135.

National Kidney Foundation (NKF). 2002. K/DOQI clinical practice guidelines for chronic kidney disease: Evaluation, classification, and stratification. *Am J Kidney Dis.* 39(2 Suppl 1):S1–266.

Nemeth, E., Heaton, W., Miller, M., et al. 2004. Pharmacodynamics of the type II calcimimetic compound cincacalcet HCL. *J Pharmacol Exp Ther.* 308:627–635.

Park, C., Oh, Y., Shin, Y., et al. 1999. Intravenous calcitriol regresses myocardial hypertrophy in hemodialysis patients with secondary hyperparathyroidism. *Am J Kidney Dis.* 33:73–81.

Popovtzer, M., Massry, S., Coburn, J., et al. 1969. The interrelationship between sodium, calcium, and magnesium, excretion in advanced renal failure. *J Lab Clin Med.* 73(5):763–771. Available at: http://www.ncbi.nlm.nih.gov/pubmed?term=Popovtzer%201969%20%20J%20Lab%20Clin%20Med

Potts, J., Jr. 2005. Diseases of the parathyroid gland and other hyper- and hypocalcemic disorders. In: Kasper, D., Braunwald, E., Fauci, A., et al, eds. *Harrison's Principles of Internal Medicine*, 16th edition, New York: McGraw Hill, 2249–2268.

Rodriguez, M., Cañadillas, S., Lopez, I., et al. 2006. Regulation of parathyroid function in chronic renal failure. *J Bone Miner Metab.* 24:164–168.

Rodriguez, M., Nemeth, E., Martin, D. 2005. The calcium-sensing receptor: A key factor in the pathogenesis of secondary hyperparathyroidism. *Am J Physiol Renal Physiol.* 288:F253–F264.

Seiler, S., Heine, G., Fliser, D. 2009. Clinical relevance of FGF-23 in chronic kidney disease. *Kidney Int.* 76:S34–S42.

Silver, J. and Levi, R. 2005. Regulation of PTH synthesis and secretion relevant to the management of secondary hyperparathyroidism in chronic kidney disease. *Kidney Int.* 67 (suppl 95):S8–S12.

Skorecki, K., Green, J., Brenner, B. 2005. Chronic renal failure. In: Kasper, D., Braunwald, E., Fauci, A. eds. *Harrison's Principles of Internal Medicine*, 16th edition, New York: McGraw Hill, 1653–1663.

Slatopolsky, E., Weerts, C., Thielan, J., et al. 1984. Marked suppression of secondary hyperparathyroidism by intravenous administration of 1,25-dihydroxy-cholecalciferol in uremic patients. *J Clin Invest.* 74:2136–2143.

Timms, P., Mannan, N., Hitman, G., et al. 2002. Circulating MMP9, vitamin D and variation in the TIMP-1 response with VDR genotype: Mechanisms for inflammatory damage in chronic disorders? *QJM.* 95:787–796.

Tokumoto, M., Tsuruya, K., Fukuda, K., et al. 2002. Reduced p21, p27 and vitamin D receptor in the nodular hyperplasia in patients with advanced secondary hyperparathyroidism. *Kidney Int.* 62:1196–1207.

Tonelli, M., Sacks, F., Pfeffer, M., et al. 2005. For cholesterol and recurrent events (CARE). *Circulation* 112:2627–2633.

Uhlig, K., Berns, J., Kesterbaum, B., et al. 2010. KDOQI U.S. commentary on the 2009 KDIGO clinical practice guideline for the diagnosis, evaluation, and treatment of CKD-mineral and bone disorder (CKD–MBD). *Am J Kidney Dis.* 55:773–799.

U.S. Department of Agriculture, Agricultural Research Service. 2001. *USDA Nutrient Database for Standard Reference, Release 14.* Nutrient Data Laboratory.

Zisman, A., Hristova, M., Ho, L., et al. 2007. Impact of ergocalciferol treatment of vitamin D deficiency on serum parathyroid hormone concentrations in chronic kidney disease. *Am J Nephrol.* 27:36–43.

15 Diabetes Management

Fran Kittell
University of Wisconsin–Madison

CONTENTS

15.1 INTRODUCTION

Diabetes is the leading cause of kidney disease in the United States. According to the Centers for Disease Control, in 2008 nearly 8% of the population in the United States had diabetes (National Diabetes Fact Sheet, 2008; USRDS, 2009). Diabetes incidence is increasing worldwide, and it has been predicted that this incidence will double by the year 2030 (Wild et al., 2004). The Diabetes and Chronic Kidney Disease Work Group of the National Kidney Foundation Kidney Disease Outcomes Quality Initiative (KDOQI™) states that the burden of diabetic kidney disease (DKD) is appearing in Africa, India, Asia, and the Pacific Islands replacing infectious disease, which was previously thought to be the greatest threat (NKF, 2007). World Kidney Day 2010, under the auspices of the International Society of Nephrology and the International Federation of Kidney Foundations and with the International Diabetes Federation, has now established a day recognizing the need to alert governments, health providers, doctors, and patients of the increasing health and socioeconomic problems related to DKD (Atkins and Zimmet, 2010).

15.2 DEFINITIONS

Diabetes is a group of diseases identified by elevated serum glucose levels resulting from defects in insulin production, insulin action, or both. Most cases of diabetes in the United States are type 2, previously called noninsulin-dependent diabetes mellitus or adult-onset diabetes (National Diabetes Fact Sheet, 2008; NKF, 2007). Those with type 2 diabetes can progress to dependence on insulin as beta cell function decreases and as insulin resistance increases. Approximately 5%–10% of diabetes in the United States is type 1, previously called insulin-dependent diabetes mellitus or juvenile-onset diabetes (National Diabetes Fact Sheet, 2008). People with type 1 diabetes are dependent on exogenous insulin for day-to-day survival (NKF, 2007). Pre-diabetes is another condition in which a person's blood sugar is abnormally elevated but not enough for a diagnosis of type 2 diabetes. Without lifestyle interventions, people with pre-diabetes will develop type 2 diabetes within 10 years. Other names for pre-diabetes include impaired glucose tolerance or impaired fasting glucose (National Diabetes Fact Sheet, 2008).

In the recent past, individuals diagnosed with type 1 diabetes would inevitably suffer from kidney disease, that is, if they were able to survive the associated diabetes complication of cardiovascular disease (CVD). Type 2 diabetes, on the other hand, was considered less severe (benign) and not associated with the consequences of kidney disease. Today, there is sufficient evidence to indicate that the risk of nephropathy with progression to end-stage kidney disease is similar between the two types of diabetes (Hasslacher et al., 1989; NKF, 2007; Ritz and Orth, 1999).

There are a number of possible reasons for the dramatic increase in the number of patients with type 2 diabetes with end-stage kidney disease. The K/DOQI Diabetes and Chronic Kidney Disease Work Group attributes it to the growing worldwide obesity problem and the subsequent diagnosis of type 2 diabetes. Other etiologies may be the accepted use of angiotensin-converting (ACE) inhibitors, angiotensin blockers (ARBs), and statins, which have improved the treatment of hypertension (HTN) and coronary heart disease, enabling more people with type 2 diabetes to live long enough for nephropathy and end-stage kidney disease to develop. Regardless, kidney damage will ensue in either type 1 or type 2 diabetes (NKF, 2007; USRDS, 2009).

DKD, formerly known as diabetic nephropathy, is kidney disease specific to diabetes. Microalbuminuria, defined as albumin–creatinine ratio (ACR) of 30–299 mg/24 h, is the harbinger of the diagnosis of DKD. With the development of more sensitive assays specific for albumin, smaller changes in albuminuria can be detected. The course of DKD can be defined by these progressive incremental losses of urinary albumin expressed in ranges, from the initial appearance of microalbuminuria onto macroalbuminuria, defined as ACR > 300 mg in 24 h, followed by the eventual increase in serum creatinine leading to overt DKD.

One pathological pathway describing elevated plasma glucose levels leading to nephropathy is the advanced glycation end product pathway. This pathway is capable of producing tissue changes that can occur in the glomeruli (EDIC, 2003). Other possible pathological changes explaining DKD include increased glomerular basement membrane thickness, microaneurysm formation, and mesangial nodule formation, or Kimmelsteil-Wilson bodies (Fowler, 2008). Urinary protein losses can be correlated to the estimated glomerular filtration rate (eGFR). The K/DOQI Clinical Practice Guidelines for Diabetes delineate steps for diagnosing DKD; these can be found in Table 15.1 (NKF, 2007).

TABLE 15.1
DKD According to Staging by GFR and Level of Albuminuria

		Albuminuria		
GFR (mL/min)	**CKD Stage**	**Normoalbuminuria**	**Microalbuminuria**	**Macroalbuminuria**
>60	1 + 2	At risk	Possible DKD	DKD
30–60	3	Unlikely DKD	Possible DKD	DKD
<30	4 + 5	Unlikely DKD	Unlikely DKD	DKD

Source: National Kidney Foundation, *Am. J. Kidney Dis.* 49, S22–S23, 2007.
Abbreviations: CKD, chronic kidney disease; DKD, diabetic kidney disease; GFR, glomerular filtration rate.

15.3 GLYCEMIC CONTROL

Optimal glycemic control is paramount in preventing and slowing the complications in both type 1 and type 2 diabetes, including DKD (Kawazu et al., 1994; Loon, 2003; Ritz and Orth, 1999). It is becoming clear that the longer the patient's exposure to hyperglycemia, the greater the risk for complications. More evidence is showing that the more euglycemic the patient, the more delayed the complications of DKD (ADA, 2010b; EDIC, 2003). The Diabetes Control and Complications Trial (DCCT) in 1993 paved the way in clarifying the relationship between intensive diabetic management in type 1 diabetes with goal of achieving near-normal blood glucose levels and the progression of diabetes complications (DCCT, 1993; Delahanty, 1998). Near-normal glycemia resulted in a 39% reduction in the occurrence of microalbuminuria and a 54% reduction in the occurrence of albuminuria (DCCT, 1993). The United Kingdom Prospective Diabetes Study (UKPDS) in 1998 uncovered that in type 2 diabetes every percentage point drop in the hemoglobin A1c blood test can decrease the risk of microvascular complications, including kidney, by 35% (Loon, 2003; National Diabetes Fact Sheet, 2008; UKPDS, 1998). Caught early enough, the Diabetes Prevention Program, a large prevention study of people with prediabetes showed lifestyle intervention including weight loss of at least 7% of initial body weight and increased physical activity of moderate intensity for at least 150 min/week, reduced the development of diabetes altogether by 58%. Lifestyle interventions, in fact, have been found to be more cost-effective than medications (Diabetes Prevention Program Research Group, 2002; National Diabetes Fact Sheet, 2008). This study proved that early lifestyle intervention can reduce the risk of developing type 2 diabetes. This finding becomes more impressive given that clinical trials studying interventions of good glycemic control have excluded those with significant kidney impairment (Williams, 2010).

The KDOQI™ Diabetes and Chronic Kidney Disease Guidelines recommend a target hemoglobin A1c less than 7% for people with diabetes to reduce the development of microalbuminuria, regardless of the stage of kidney disease (NKF, 2007). Risk-to-benefit ratio must be weighed, especially in those with hypoglycemic unawareness and decreased kidney function. Generally, it is known that the risk for hypoglycemia increases for those with chronic kidney disease (CKD) stages 3–5 (Mak and DeFonzo, 1992; Williams, 2009). In fact, end-stage kidney disease without diabetes is the second cause of hypoglycemia in hospitalized patients (Haviv et al., 2000). A number of metabolic abnormalities affect, often in opposition, glycemic control in DKD. One study uncovered that people with type 1 diabetes who received insulin with significant creatinine elevations (mean 2.2 mg/dL) had a fivefold increase in severe hypoglycemic events (Muhlhauser and DeFonzo, 1991; NKF, 2007). Compromised kidney function, particularly when GFR is <20 mL/min, is associated with impaired clearance of insulin and some oral medications (Mak and DeFonzo, 1992; NKF, 2007; Shrishrimal et al., 2009). Normally, the kidney degrades about a third of insulin. With decreased kidney function, the half-life of insulin is prolonged (Wisconsin Diabetes Advisory Group, 2008; NKF, 2007). Also, kidney gluconeogenesis can be diminished with impaired kidney function due to the reduced kidney mass (Gerich et al., 2001; NKF, 2007). On the other hand, peripheral insulin resistance is almost universal in kidney disease, with or without diabetes. This is one possible contributing etiology for the muscle protein catabolism often observed with kidney dysfunction (Cusi et al., 2000). Pancreatic beta cell insulin secretion has been found to be inhibited in the presence of excessive parathyroid hormone (Hajjar et al., 1992; Mak and DeFonzo, 1992). Once dialysis is initiated insulin resistance actually improves, as if the presence of uremic toxins inhibits insulin degradation (Mak and DeFonzo, 1992). One study, in fact, has found that glucose levels are lower on dialysis days, and the risk of hypoglycemia is greater within 24 h of dialysis (Kazempour-Ardebil et al., 2009; Williams, 2010). Another study revealed that glucose tolerance does improve after intravenous administration of 1,25(OH)2D3 for those on dialysis (Mak, 1991). Little data are available for determining the ideal A1c level associated with the better survival for those with diabetes on dialysis, and, given the number of metabolic abnormalities affecting glycemic control, close monitoring of glucose levels is essential to avoid hypoglycemia with subsequent dose reductions of oral medications and insulin likely. In fact, more specifically, when GFR is <50 mL/min, the insulin dose should be reduced by 25%, and by 50% if GFR is <10 mL/min (Aronoff et al., 1983; Bennett et al., 1994). Lastly, individualization, including possibly liberalization, of glycemic goals needs to be evaluated.

Hemoglobin A1c is the gold standard for assessing and monitoring long-term glycemic control in those with diabetes. Percentages of A1c values correlate to average blood glucose over the preceding 60–90 days. In the general population, a strong relationship exists between A1c and mean plasma glucose levels. For every percentage increase in A1c, there is approximately a 35 mg/dL change in mean plasma glucose (Williams, 2010). The K/DOQI Diabetes and CKD work group defers to the American Diabetes Association (ADA) Guidelines for the recommended frequency in measuring A1c twice annually for stable people with diabetes and four times a year in those who are not reaching their glycemic goals or whose therapy has changed (ADA, 2010b; NKF, 2007). Unfortunately, progressive kidney disease can falsely lower the A1c measurement. Low levels of A1c can be attributed to reduced red blood cell mass, reduced red blood cell lifespan, hemolysis, iron deficiency, and hemodilution caused by blood transfusions. On the other hand, a number of variables can falsely elevate levels of A1c, and they include carbamylated hemoglobin interfering with the assay, uremic acidosis, hypertriglyceridemia, hyperbilirubinemia, and alcohol addiction (Joy et al., 2002; NKF, 2007). Initial data regarding glycated albumin as a more sensitive indicator of glycemic control for those with DKD appears promising, but their validity has yet to be determined (Inaba et al., 2007;

TABLE 15.2
Comparison of A1c and Estimated Average Glucose (eAG)

A1c (%)	eAG (mg/dL)
5	97
5.5	111
6	126
6.5	140
7	154
7.5	169
8	183
8.5	197
9	212
9.5	226
10	240
10.5	255
11	269
11.5	283
12	298

Source: American Diabetes Association, Living with diabetes: Estimated average glucose (eAG). http://www.diabetes.org (accessed September 10, 2010). Copyright 2010, American Diabetes Association.

Williams, 2009). Despite A1c's limitations, those with DKD are, still, encouraged to strive for an "as close to normal" (<6%) as possible goal of reaching glycemic levels in the nondiabetic range without significant hypoglycemia to prevent or slow the progression of retinopathy, neuropathy, and possibly macrovascular disease. Once the patient is on dialysis, survival improves with better glycemic control (Nathan et al., 2006; NKF, 2007). It is becoming more apparent that low A1c values may actually be associated with higher mortality rates in patients with diabetes on chronic hemodialysis (HD) (Morioka et al., 2001; Williams, 2009). In fact, extreme high or extreme low A1c is being found to decrease survivability for those with diabetes on dialysis (Joachim, 2010; Williams, 2009; Williams et al., 2010). Recognizing these variables that ultimately affect and make consistent glucose control more difficult as DKD progresses is essential. Consequently, individualizing A1c targets using clinical judgment is essential. Standardized A1c levels are available and can assist the professional in determining estimated average glucose (eAG). The formula describing the relationship between A1c and eAG is: (28.7 × A1c) – 46.7 = eAG (ADA, 2010b; Nathan et al., 2008). See Table 15.2 for comparison chart between A1c and eAG.

15.4 HYPERTENSION

HTN is the second leading cause of kidney disease in the United States (USRDS, 2009). Most of those with DKD have HTN. K/DOQI recommends the target blood pressure for those with DKD, stages 1–4 to be <130/80 mm Hg based upon the Joint National Committee on Prevention, Detection, Evaluation, and Treatment of High Blood Pressure, JNC 7 (Chobanian et al., 2003; Inaba et al., 2007; NKF, 2004, 2007). For those with proteinuria, >1 g protein, target blood pressure is <120/80 mm Hg. The first-line treatment for achieving this goal includes ACE inhibitors or ARBs often in combination with a diuretic. The kidney-protective effects of ACE inhibitors and ARBs include decreasing urinary albumin excretion, slowing the increase in albumin excretion, and delaying the progression from microalbuminuria to macroalbuminuria (Chobanian et al., 2003; NKF, 2004, 2007). A possible explanation for their kidney-protective effects can be their capability of decreasing efferent arteriolar resistance in the kidney thereby decreasing intraglomerular pressure in the kidney. In addition, these agents may affect the permselective characteristics of the glomeruli, which may explain their antiproteinuric qualities (Fowler, 2008; Morelli et al., 1990). Care must be taken for potential hyperkalemia, a side effect of ACE inhibitors and ARBs; although this could be canceled out with the potassium-wasting diuretic. Regardless, even though limiting dietary potassium is typically not necessary until urine output dips to 1000 mL/day, it may be prudent to educate patients with DKD about high potassium-containing foods such as chocolate, nuts, dried fruit, citrus fruit/citrus fruit juice, potatoes, and potassium-containing salt substitutes that they should limit as a precaution. Since most people with DKD have HTN associated with sodium retention, limiting dietary sodium intake to 2.3 g/day is recommended based on the Dietary Approaches to Stop Hypertension (DASH) and the DASH-sodium diets, with modifications for possible potassium and phosphorus limitations. Modifications include a 0.8–1.0 g/day phosphorus limitation and a 2–4 g/day potassium limitation. The DASH diet encourages consumption of fruit, vegetables, and low-fat dairy products, along with whole grains, poultry, fish, and nuts. Only small amounts of red meat, sweets, and sugar-containing beverages are encouraged. The diet also has decreased amounts of total and saturated fat and cholesterol and a slight increase in protein. The DASH diet includes 8–10 servings of fruit and/or vegetables and 2–3 servings low-fat dairy products daily. It leads to an average 11.6/3.5 mm Hg blood pressure reduction. The DASH-Sodium diet recommends a sodium limitation of 1500–2400 mg daily, which can achieve an additional 3.5/2.2 mm Hg blood pressure reduction. This is equal to or greater than what could be achieved with single-drug therapy (Sacks et al., 2001; Wisconsin Diabetes Advisory Group, 2008). A summary of the DASH diet with modifications can be found in Table 15.3 (NKF, 2004). Without lifestyle changes, such as limiting dietary salt, the effects of ACE inhibitors and ARBs will be blunted (NKF, 2007).

TABLE 15.3
Macronutrient Composition and Mineral Content of the Dietary Approaches to Stop Hypertension (DASH) Diet Recommended by JNC 7, with Modifications for Stages 3–4 of CKD

Nutrient	Stage of CKD	
	Stages 1–4	
Sodium (g/day)	<2.4	
Total fat (% of calories)	<30	
Saturated fat (% of calories)	<10	
Cholesterol (mg/day)	<200	
Carbohydrate (% of calories)	50–60	
	Stages 1–2	Stages 3–4
Protein (g/kg/day, % of calories)	1.4 (~18)	0.6–0.8 (~10)
Phosphorus (g/day)	1.7	0.8–1.0
Potassium (g/day)	>4	2–4

Abbreviations: CKD, chronic kidney disease; JNC, Joint National Committee on Prevention, Detection, Evaluation, and Treatment of High Blood Pressure.
Source: National Kidney Foundation, *K/DOQI™ Clinical Practice Guidelines on Hypertension and Antihypertensive Agents in Chronic Kidney Disease*, 2004.

15.5 CVD AND DKD

Hyperglycemia is a primary cause of vascular diabetes complications. Elevated A1c is an independent risk factor for diabetic CVD. When diabetes is complicated by CKD, cardiovascular complications risk increases significantly. Most people with diabetes and CKD have low levels of high-density lipoprotein cholesterol (HDL-C) and high triglyceride levels. Low-density lipoprotein cholesterol (LDL-C) particles in diabetes tend to be smaller and denser (NKF, 2007). Diabetic patients who reach CKD stage 3 are more likely to die of CVD than progress to kidney failure (NKF, 2007; Williams, 2010). The latest studies looking at intensive glycemic control decreasing cardiovascular complications in established type 2 diabetes have proved disappointing. In fact, the Action to Control Cardiovascular Risk in Diabetes Study Group (ACCORD) study was halted due to a 20% increase in mortality from severe hypoglycemic events (ACCORD, 2008; Advance Collaborative Group, 2008; DCCT/EDIC, 2005; Dluhy and McMahon, 2008; Duckworth et al., 2009; Holman et al., 2008; Tkac, 2009). Yet, the ADA continues to recommend target goal of 7% A1c. In those with more established type 2 diabetes, who are at risk for severe hypoglycemia, a less stringent A1c goal of less than 7% needs to be considered using clinical judgment (Skyler et al., 2009). Primary strategies for decreasing cardiovascular risk place greater emphasis on the importance of nonglycemic risk factors, such as blood pressure control, lipid lowering with statin therapy, and lifestyle modifications. Fasting lipid panel is recommended once yearly for all those with diabetes. Therapeutic lifestyle modifications are recommended for those with diabetes and CKD Stages 1–4, no different than for nondiabetic kidney disease. Target goal for LDL-C is <100 mg/dL with less than 70 mg/mL as a therapeutic option. This recommendation does not extend to patients with type 2 diabetes on maintenance HD and no history of CVD, given the weak evidence from the Deutsche Diabetes Dialyse Studie (4D). Study suggesting that for these patients it is too late to improve cardiovascular outcomes (DCCT, 1993; NKF, 2007; Wanner et al., 2005).

15.6 DIABETIC GASTROPATHY

Gastroparesis, according to Parrish (2007), needs to be moved to the top of the list as a possible explanation for unintentional weight loss in one with diabetes on HD (Blair, 2009). Although scant evidence is available to support delayed gastric emptying exclusively in kidney disease, its existence has been documented (Freeman et al., 1985; Ravelli et al., 1992). Delayed gastric emptying is common in diabetes, and prevalence is about equal between both types of long-standing diabetes. It is likely to be more prevalent in those with DKD, particularly given that hyperglycemia diminishes proximal gastric tone, delays frequency and propagation of antral pressure waves, and increases pyloric motility, all of which contribute to delayed gastric emptying (Hebbard et al., 1996; Ma et al., 2009). Consequently, with the growing population of DKD, prevalence of delayed gastric emptying also increases. Generally, diabetic gastropathy refers to a variety of neuromuscular abnormalities of the stomach, including gastric dysrhythmias to antral dilation, antral hypomotility, and gastroparesis. More specifically, the American Gastroenterology Association defines gastroparesis as delayed gastric emptying in the absence of mechanical obstruction (Kock, 1999; Parkman et al., 2004). Symptoms of gastroparesis can include heartburn, early satiety, nausea, vomiting, bloating and halitosis, as well as potentially debilitating deteriorating glycemic control, nutritional status, and quality of life.

Management of diabetic gastroparesis includes tight glycemic control and the use of prokinetic agents. But because domperidone is not available in the United States and cisapride has been withdrawn because of potentially fatal cardiac arrhythmias, only metoclopramide and erythromycin are available, with modest efficacy. To be most effective, metoclopramide has to be taken 20–30 min prior to meals (Beard, 2002). Yet, unfortunately, up to 40% of people cannot tolerate metoclopramide because of central nervous system side effects, such as tremors (Alibibi and McCallum, 1983). Tolerance development decreases erthromycin's effects of accelerated antral contractions and accelerated stomach emptying, further limiting its use as an intervention (Abrahamsson, 2007). A possible nonpharmacologic method of managing gastroparesis is gastric electrical stimulation (GES). With its associated improved gastric emptying, hemoglobin A1c's along with decreased need for nutritional support, and subsequent drop in hospitalization stays, GES is promising but can be costly and is still in its infancy regarding supportive evidence, particularly in determining its true mechanism of action relative to symptom relief (Patrick and Epstein, 2008).

Evidence to support any dietary manipulation for symptom relief is sorely lacking. Yet diet modification, although limited in relieving symptoms, is essential given that few pharmacological treatment options are available for gastroparesis. Large volumes of solid food delay gastric emptying, aggravating symptoms. As a result, small, frequent meals or snacks are suggested. Solid food meals are often better tolerated earlier in the day, with meals becoming more liquid later in the day. Chewing food well and either sitting up 1–2 h after the meal or walking after meal consumption aids in gastric motility. Avoiding excessive fat is often recommended; however, no data exist to support this. In fact, the solid food accompanying the fat may be the contributing aggravator. Because liquid gastric emptying remains unimpaired, fat-containing liquids may not need to be restricted. If the patient is at risk for bezoars, limiting high-fiber foods may be necessary. Lists of foods to avoid can be found in Table 15.4 along with a summary of dietary recommendations (Parrish, 2007). Jejunal tube feedings using any standard polymeric formula, as opposed to a fiber-containing formula associated with bloating and gas, may be necessary if gastroparetic symptoms persist.

15.7 DIETARY CARBOHYDRATE

Optimizing glycemic control through the diabetic exchanges, CHO counting, or glycemic index (GI) is paramount. Although consuming low-GI foods in place of high-GI foods has been found to have some benefit in controlling blood sugars, the total amount of CHO in meals and snacks has been deemed more important than the source (starches or sugars) or type (GI) (ADA, 2008, 2010b; Brand-Miller et al., 2003). Mixed fuel, identified with meals, negates the individual glycemic effect

TABLE 15.4
Diabetic Gastropathy Dietary Recommendations

Mealtime Strategies	Foods to Avoid with Bezoars	
Chew well	Oranges	Green beans
Small meals	Apples	Coconut
Frequent meals	Berries	Figs
Low-fat	Persimmons	Brussel sprouts
Low in insoluble fiber	Sauerkraut	Dried beans and peas
Sit up 1 h after eating/walk after eating	Potato skins	

TABLE 15.5
Kidney Friendly 15 g Glucose Sources

10 jelly beans
8 lifesavers
2 restaurant packets of regular jelly
1 tube frosting
1 tube glucose gel
3 glucose tablets

of the food. This does not mean high-sugar foods are to be encouraged. In fact, as with those without diabetes, discouraging foods containing high amounts of sugar is recommended as they are energy NOT nutrient dense. Prioritizing nutrition messages, including liberalizing CHO's, may be necessary to facilitate compliance. Recommended CHO food sources include whole grains, fruits, vegetables, and nonfat dairy products, with modifications for potassium and phosphorus, which can include but are not limited to whole grain white bread; oat-, wheat-, or corn-based cereals; brown rice; apples with skins, pears, grapes; green beans, carrots, green peppers, broccoli, corn, green peas, and chick pea–based humus.

Adequate fiber intake is also encouraged for a number of reasons: (1) it assists in glycemic control by slowing CHO absorption; (2) its cholesterol lowering effect has possible cardiovascular benefits; and (3) it helps to prevent constipation, particularly for those on peritoneal dialysis, to assist in adequate clearances. One study demonstrated the positive effects of 50 g fiber consumed daily in type 2 diabetes in lowering postprandial hyperglycemia, decreasing hyperinsulinemia, and reducing both cholesterolemia and triglyceridemia (Chandalia et al., 2000).

Because of the potential for widely fluctuating blood sugars, self-monitoring of blood glucose (SMBG) is encouraged three or more times daily, before meals and at bedtime. In the case of hypoglycemia (less than 70 mg/dL plasma glucose), a kidney-friendly 15 g CHO source, preferably pure glucose, is recommended. Fruit and fruit juice are less preferred because they contain fructose and galactose, which must be converted to glucose in the liver before they can effectively raise blood glucose levels (*Diabetes Mellitus*, 2007; McDougall et al., 2001). A list of kidney-friendly 15-g glucose sources can be found in Table 15.5. Be aware of the metabolic repercussions of hyperglycemia, such as hyperkalemia, due to cell shifts and possibly increased thirst and subsequent fluid overload, particularly with lack of polyuria.

15.8 DIETARY PROTEIN

Intake of dietary protein in all stages of CKD appears to have an important impact in those with diabetes (NKF, 2007). Excessive protein consumption leads to hyperemia and renal hyperfiltration (King and Levey, 1993). Renal hyperfiltration, in turn, results in increased intraglomerular pressure, mesangial stretch, solute load, toxins, and overall nephron activity, eventually sclerosing the kidneys (Brenner et al., 1982; Wolk et al., 2007). More specifically, in persons with both diabetes and HTN, a higher protein intake leads to an increase in microalbuminuria (Wrone et al., 2003).

The debate continues over the level of protein restriction that is most effective in decreasing symptoms of uremia, such as nausea and vomiting, while slowing the progression of kidney disease without prompting malnutrition. The Modified Diet in Renal Disease Study looked at this very question with mixed results, although it excluded participants with diabetes. Evidence is limited and often not significant, yet a few studies have suggested that limiting dietary protein intake in those with type 1 diabetes slowed the progression of pathological changes in the DKD kidney. One meta-analysis in particular found that decreasing protein intake to 0.73 ± 0.15 g protein/kg had a greater affect on the rate of GFR decline in diabetic patients than in nondiabetic patients. Fewer studies of type 2 diabetes and dietary protein intake relative to kidney progression are available (Hansen et al., 2002; Kasiske et al., 1998; Pedrini et al., 1996; Walker et al., 1989; Zeller et al., 1991) Even so, the KDOQI™ Diabetes and CKD Guidelines and the ADA recommend a dietary protein intake for people with diabetes and CKD stages 1–4 of 0.8 g/kg/day (Chandalia et al., 2000; NKF, 2007). For CKD stage 5D, the recommended dietary protein intake is no different for one with DKD than for the nondiabetic, 1.2 g protein/kg/day and 1.2–1.3 g protein/kg/day for those on HD and PD, respectively (NKF, 2000; 2007).

People in the United States tend to eat too much protein, consuming approximately 1.04 g protein/kg/day (Wright et al., 2003). To educate a person with DKD to limit protein intake, especially in the face of manipulating several other dietary variables, may prove too daunting. And, apparently, not all protein is created equal. It has been found vegetarians have lower GFRs than omnivores (Margett et al., 1986; Wiseman et al., 1987). The type of protein consumed partially mediates renal hemodynamics. The largest change in postprandial renal hemodynamics appears to be induced by beef, followed by poultry, fish, and plant proteins. Small studies have uncovered promising new evidence regarding the intake of vegetable protein, more specifically, soy protein, regardless of the quantity, as being renal protective by lowering GFR, renal plasma flow, and microalbuminemia in humans compared with the ingestion of animal protein in those with early microalbuminemia or more established macroalbuminemia (Azadbakht and Esmaillzadeh, 2009; Bosch et al., 1986; de Mello et al., 2006; Jibani et al., 2009; Kontessis et al., 1990; Williams et al., 1987). Soybeans contain high concentrations of isoflavones, genistein, and daidzein, which exert estrogen-like effects. The modified DASH diet provides a greater portion of these isoflavones with its emphasis on vegetables, nuts, legumes, fish, and poultry (and little red meat). Whether isoflavones can block the inflammatory responses seen in the progression of kidney disease is still to be seen. In the meantime, recommending a compromise alternating between conventionally low protein and a greater proportion of vegetable protein may help in making the diet more palatable and result in greater compliance (Almeida et al., 2008; Anderson et al., 1998; de Mello et al., 2006; Gross et al., 2002; NKF, 2007; Sacks et al., 2001).

15.9 DIETARY FAT

The recommended fat intake is no different than therapeutic lifestyle interventions suggested for the nondiabetic person suffering from CKD, including limiting saturated fat to less than 7% of total calories, minimizing trans fat, and limiting dietary cholesterol to less than 200 mg/day (ADA, 2008; NKF, 2007). Foods containing saturated fat and trans fat are primary sources of plasma LDL-C (Wisconsin Diabetes Advisory Group, 2008). Saturated fat can be found in meats, whole-fat milk and cheese, butter, lard, ice cream, sausage, and coconut. Lean meat, such as skinless chicken and fish, and low- and nonfat dairy products are to be encouraged. Modified for phosphorus low- and nonfat dairy products include low-fat cream cheese, low- and nonfat cottage cheese, and low-fat brie cheese. Trans fat can be found in fried foods from restaurants, stick margarine, and processed food. Hypertriglyceridemia is frequently observed in those with both types of diabetes. This is due to excess production and slow removal of triglyceride (TG)-rich, very LDLs, particularly following a high CHO meals. These TG-rich lipoproteins have been found to interact with HDL-C, ultimately and effectively decreasing clearance of LDL-C. Dietary recommendations for managing hypertriglyceridemia include weight loss (if necessary) along with limiting intake of CHO, sugar, and alcohol (Haffner, 1998; Sheard and Clark, 2000; Steiner, 1999). Dietary suggestions can include reduced consumption of regular soda, fruit juice, desserts, and other sweetened confections. Alcohol should be limited to one drink per day or less for women and two drinks per day or less for men (ADA, 2008). A fasting lipid panel is recommended annually to monitor cholesterol and triglycerides for those with DKD (ADA, 2008; NKF, 2007; Wisconsin Diabetes Advisory Group, 2008). More recently, it has been found that replacing up to 40% of the calories from CHO with monounsaturated fat, such as olive oil or canola oil, decreases triglyceride levels (ADA, 2004; Garg et al., 1994, 1988; Kris-Etherton, 1999).

15.10 VITAMINS AND MINERALS

The recommendations for vitamins and minerals are no different than for nondiabetic kidney disease. Supplementation with water-soluble vitamins containing the minimum daily requirements is encouraged pre-dialysis with uremia associated with anorexia, overly restrictive dietary protein intake, the need to restrict elevated potassium-containing foods, and the potential for defective metabolic pathways in this milieu (Kopple, 2004; Makoff, 1991). In fact, doses greater than the minimum daily requirements of vitamin B are now discouraged because of a recent unexpected and surprising results found specifically in those with established DKD. Daily doses of 2.5 mg folic acid, 25 mg vitamin B6, and 1 mg vitamin B12 resulted in a greater decrease in GFR and increased vascular events (House et al., 2010). Once on dialysis, all patients are recommended special multivitamins, which are designed to replace the water-soluble vitamins typically lost through the dialysis process. In general, this recommendation is no different than for people on dialysis without diabetes.

15.11 OBESITY AND DKD

Obesity, independent of diabetes and HTN, has been found to be an independent risk factor for the early development of glomerulomegaly, hemodynamic changes with a hyperfiltering kidney, and increased albuminuria (Eknoyan, 2007). Obesity is also associated with the development of type 2 diabetes, through the release of nonesterified free fatty acids, hormones, and adipocytokines (Khaodhiar et al., 2009). Because of the predominance of the combination of obesity and DKD in the CKD arena, weight management becomes an essential component of diet therapy. Much evidence has shown that these processes can be reversed with moderate weight loss (5%–10% of body weight), as previously cited (ADA, 2008; Diabetes Prevention Program Research Group, 2002; Khaodhiar et al., 2009). For successful weight loss, lifestyle intervention of a combination of moderate or vigorous physical activity (30 min or more per day at least 5 days a week) and behavioral modification altering eating habits, including small changes in dietary intake, such as reducing portion sizes, incorporating low-calorie foods for high-calorie foods, and limiting intake of desserts, alcohol, and energy-dense foods are advised for people who have a body mass index (BMI) ≥ 25 kg/m^2 (Wisconsin Diabetes Advisory Group, 2008).

15.12 RENAL REPLACEMENT THERAPY

Evidence is limited on the morbidity and mortality of patients with DKD on various dialysis modalities. Special considerations need to be recognized for patients with DKD on either modality. Hyperglycemia can induce hyperkalemia and increased thirst. Increased thirst, in turn, can lead to fluid overload, requiring high-dextrose-containing bags for optimal fluid removal in peritoneal dialysis or more difficult runs on HD. The feeling of fullness often noted by patients on peritoneal dialysis can exacerbate delayed gastric emptying. The retinopathy often seen in DKD may preclude peritoneal dialysis, where visual acuity is vital in performing connections for an exchange easily.

The weight gain that is a common side effect of peritoneal dialysis is another factor to consider if the patient is already overweight. On the other hand, hypoglycemic events are greater within 24 h of HD, as noted previously (Mak, 1991).

15.13 SYNOPSIS

The complexity of the recommended diet for DKD warrants the involvement of an experienced dietitian. Medical nutrition therapy is an integral component of early diabetes education (Brand-Miller et al., 2003). Once DKD develops, it is recommended that an experienced dietitian who is knowledgeable about both CKD and diabetes participate in the individual's dietary education, pre-dialysis and/or on dialysis. Frequent interaction with a dietitian fostering self-management can improve and achieve dietary intake goals and clinical outcomes (ADA, 2008; NKF, 2007). The recommended diet for DKD should be no different from the diet recommended for nondiabetic CKD. Neither should be partaking in sugary sweets such as, cakes, pies, cookies, candies, and regular soda pop, containing little to no nutritional value. Because the total amount of CHO eaten has been found to be more important than type or source of CHO, the recommended CHO should be no different between nondiabetic and diabetic patients. Liberalizing and encouraging high-fiber CHOs that are relatively lower in phosphorus and potassium-containing fruit and vegetables such as broccoli, corn, green beans, green and red peppers, cucumbers, apples, grapes, berries, pineapple along with whole grain white bread, oat-based cereals and breads, tortillas, popcorn, and pretzels is, again, no different for those with or without diabetes, especially if fluid and protein are restricted, for any modest cardiovascular benefits and for constipation prevention. Limiting protein intake to 0.8 g protein/kg/day for CKD stages 1–4 is recommended just as with nondiabetes. This limitation is more important in individuals with type 2 diabetes because ingested protein has been found to increase serum insulin levels and not serum glucose levels, consequently, protein-containing foods exclusive of complex CHOs are not encouraged to prevent hypoglycemia (ADA, 2008; Gannon and Nuttall, 2001). Of the allowed protein, more fish, poultry (preferably fresh with lower phosphorus content) and plant proteins, particularly soy protein, is encouraged.

A reduction of sodium intake down to 1500 mg is being advocated for all those with HTN, which the U.S. Dietary Guidelines indicate is prevalent by 70% (USDA and USDHHS, 2010). The DASH-sodium diet, as previously mentioned, advocates a 1500–2400 mg sodium limitation, by avoiding packaged, prepared, processed foods. Encourage cooking from scratch, time permitting. A summary of all dietary nutrient recommendations for one with DKD can be found in Table 15.6.

Obtaining a dietary recall of typical dietary intake can help reveal any potential barriers that may need to be addressed. Having the patient attempt to identify these barriers may help empower the patient toward self-management. Encourage needed changes by providing information and offering support. Guide the patient to prioritize suggested recommendations, beginning with vigilance in checking blood sugar, SMBG, at least four times daily, especially given the fluctuating blood sugar levels typically seen in DKD. Insulin doses frequently decrease, and SMBG can prevent hypoglycemia. Often, patients stop testing once they are on dialysis. The random blood glucose testing done at the dialysis treatment center cannot substitute for recommended frequent home testing.

Inform patients to expect shifts in serum levels, such as with serum potassium, and reassure them that they are not to blame. These spikes or nadirs are common in CKD and likely not due to food eaten, but potentially a number of variables, including decreased renal clearance or to medications being prescribed. An example includes ACE inhibitors and not dietary intake causing hyperkalemia. Inform the person that his or her insulin dose will more than likely decrease. Prioritize dietary suggestions as dictated by the constantly changing serum potassium and phosphorus values often seen. Educate the person about anticipated need for and timing of phosphorus binder medication. Make it clear that it is not punishment when binder medications are prescribed; they are needed because the kidneys are unable to clear phosphorus adequately. Focus on including cited preferred foods into dietary patterns.

TABLE 15.6
Recommended Nutrient Intake for DKD, Stages 1–4

Nutrient	Recommendation
Protein (g/kg/day)	0.8–1.0 emphasizing more poultry, fish, plant protein (soy), less red meat; discourage high protein
Total fat (% of calories)	<30%
Saturated fat (% of calories)	< 7%
Monounsaturated fat (% of calories)	Up to 40%, such as olive oil or canola oil
Trans fat	Minimal
Cholesterol (mg/day)	<200
Carbohydrate	Discourage sweets, regular soda, sweetened confections
Total fiber (g/day)	30–50 through fresh fruit/vegetables and whole grains
Sodium (g/day)	1.5–2.4
Potassium (g/day)	Unrestricted until serum levels increase, then 2–4; monitor with ACE-Inhibitor use
Phosphorus (mg/day)	800–1000
Calcium (mg/day)	<2, total between medications and oral intake
Vitamins	<2.5 mg folic acid; <25 mg vitamin B6; <1 mg vitamin B12

Abbreviations: DKD, diabetic kidney disease; ACE, angiotensin-converting enzyme.

Assure patients with DKD that splurging is fine; in fact, work splurges into their recommended food pattern. The dietitian can work favorite foods into the individual's daily food patterns, allowing continued enjoyment. For example, chocolate, if necessary, can be consumed *with* a phosphorus binder medication *and* with a meal for decreased phosphorus and glucose absorption with a mixed-fuel meal. The dietitian need not be thought of as the food police but as an assistant. Remember that diet may be the last means of control for the person. Frequent interactions integrating lifestyle modifications through a series of small changes with the patient, more easily enforced particularly if in-center HD, can improve compliance, creating positive reinforcement.

15.14 CONCLUSION

Diabetes is a progressive disease, and DKD is a phase of the progression. Early on, such as in prediabetes, weight loss, if needed, can delay the onset of type 2 diabetes. Continued weight management along with tight glycemic control is suggested to delay microalbuminuria, or early DKD. In more established DKD, macroalbuminuria, a less stringent (due to the difficulty in avoiding hypoglycemia) but careful glycemic control is advocated to delay the need for renal replacement therapy. SMBG is highly encouraged three or more times daily. Diet therapy is pivotal every step of the way of this progression as it is less expensive, associated with fewer risks and side effects and promotes a healthy lifestyle. Optimal diet therapy includes adequate provision of calories to achieve or maintain an ideal BMI, maintain a positive nitrogen balance, achieve optimal lipid levels, and individualize A1c levels to prevent complications while optimizing the patient's overall health and well-being.

REFERENCES

Abrahamsson, H. 2007. Treatment options for patients with severe gastroparesis. *Gut* 56: 877–883.

Action to Control Cardiovascular Risk in Diabetes Study Group (ACCORD). 2008. Effects of intensive glucose lowering in type 2 diabetes. *N Engl J Med.* 358: 2545–2559.

Advance Collaborative Group. 2008. Intensive blood pressure control and vascular outcomes in patients with type 2 diabetes. *N Engl J Med* 358: 2560–2572.

Alibibi, R. and McCallum, R.W. 1983. Metoclopramide: Pharmacology and clinical application. *Ann Intern Med* 98: 86–95.

Almeida, J., Zelmanovitz, T., Vaz, J., et al. 2008. Sources of protein and polyunsaturated fatty acids of the diet and microalbuminemia in type 2 diabetes mellitus. *J Am Coll Nutr* 27: 528–537.

American Diabetes Association (ADA). 2004. Dyslipidemia management in adults with diabetes. *Diabetes Care* 27: S68–S71.

American Diabetes Association (ADA). 2008. Nutrition recommendations and interventions for diabetes. *Diabetes Care* 31: S61–S78.

American Diabetes Association (ADA). 2010a. Living with diabetes: Estimated average glucose (eAG). http://www.diabetes.org (accessed September 10, 2010).

American Diabetes Association (ADA). 2010b. Standards of medical care in diabetes-2010. *Diabetes Care* 33: S11–S61.

Anderson, J., Blake, J, Turner, J., et al. 1998. Effects of soy protein on renal function and proteinuria in patients with type 2 diabetes. *Am J Clin Nutr* 68: 1347S–1353S.

Aronoff, G., Morrison, G., Golper, T., et al. 1983. Drug prescribing in renal failure. *Am J Kidney Dis* 3: 155–193.

Atkins, R. and Zimmet, P. 2010. Diabetic kidney disease: Act now or pay later. *J Nephrol* 23: 1–4.

Azadbakht, L. and Esmaillzadeh, A. 2009. Soy-protein consumption and kidney-related biomarkers among type 2 diabetics: A crossover, randomized clinical trial. *J Renal Nutr* 19: 479–486.

Beard, P. 2002. Methods for treating diabetic gastroparesis. *J Infus Nurs* 25: 105–108.

Bennett, W., Aronoff, G.R., Golper, T., et al. 1994. *Dosing Guidelines for Adults*. Philadelphia: American College of Physicians.

Blair, D. 2009. Nutrition therapy for gastroparesis. *Renal and Urology News*. http://www.renalandurologynews.com/nutrition-therapy-for-gastroparesis/article/135966/ (accessed October 11, 2010).

Bosch, J., Lew, S., Glabman, S., et al. 1986. Renal hemodynamic changes in humans: Response to protein loading in normal and disease kidneys. *Am J Med* 81: 809–815.

Brand-Miller, J., Petocz, P., Hayne, S., et al. 2003. Low glycemic index diets in the management of diabetes. *Diabetes Care* 26: 2261–2267.

Brenner, B., Meyer, T., Hostetter, T. 1982. Dietary protein intake and the progressive nature of kidney disease. *N Engl J Med* 307: 652–660.

Chandalia, M., Gar, A., Lutjohann, D., et al. 2000. Beneficial effects of high dietary fiber intake in patients with type 2 diabetes mellitus. *N Engl J Med* 342: 1392–1398.

Chobanian, A., Bakris, G., Black, H., et al. 2003. Seventh report of the joint national committee on prevention, detection, evaluation, treatment of high blood pressure. *Hypertension* 42: 1206–1252.

Cusi, K., Maezono, K., Osman, A., et al. 2000. Insulin resistance differentially affects the PI 3-kinase and MAP kinase-mediated signaling in human muscle. *J Clin Invest* 105: 311–320.

Delahanty, L. 1998. Implications of the diabetes control and complications trial for renal outcomes and medical nutrition therapy. *J Renal Nutr* 8: 59–63.

de Mello, V., Zelmanovitz, T., Perassolo, M., et al. 2006. Withdrawal of red meat from the usual diet reduces albuminuria and improves serum fatty acid profile in type 2 diabetes patients with macroalbuminuria. *Am J Clin Nutr* 83: 1032–1038.

Diabetes Control and Complications Trial Research Group. 1993. The effect of intensive treatment of diabetes on the development and progression of long-term complications in insulin-dependent diabetes mellitus. *N Engl J Med* 329: 977–986.

Diabetes Control and Complications Trial/Epidemiology of Diabetes Interventions and Complications (DCCT/EDIC) Study Research Group. 2005. Intensive diabetes treatment and cardiovascular disease in patients with type I diabetes. *N Engl J Med* 353: 2643–2653.

Diabetes Prevention Program Research Group (DCCT). 2002. Reduction in the incidence of type 2 diabetes with lifestyle intervention or metformin. *N Engl J Med* 346: 393–403.

Dluhy, R. and McMahon, G. 2008. Intensive glycemic control in the ACCORD and ADVANCE trials. *N Engl J Med* 358: 2630–2633.

Duckworth, W., Abraira, C., Moritz, T., et al. 2009. Glucose control and vascular complications in veterans with type 2 diabetes. *N Engl J Med* 360: 129–139.

Eknoyan, G. 2007. Obesity, diabetes, and chronic kidney disease. *Curr Diab Rep* 7: 449–453.

Epidemiology of Diabetes Interventions and Complications (EDIC) Study. 2003. Sustained effect of intensive treatment of type I diabetes mellitus on development and progression of diabetic nephropathy. *JAMA* 290: 2159–2167.

Fowler, M. 2008. Microvascular and macrovascular complications of diabetes. *Clinical Diab* 26: 77–82.

Freeman, J., Cobden, I., Heaton, A., et al. 1985. Gastric emptying in chronic renal failure. *Br Med J* 291: 1048.

Gannon, M. and Nuttall, F. 2001. Effect of a high protein, low carbohydrate diet on blood glucose control in people with type 2 diabetes. *J Clin Endocrinol Metab* 86: 1040–1047.

Garg, A., Bantle, J., Henry, R., et al. 1994. Effects of varying carbohydrate content of diet in patients with non-insulin-dependent diabetes mellitus. *JAMA* 271: 1421–1428.

Garg, A., Bonanome, A., Grundy, S., et al. 1988. Comparison of a high-carbohydrate diet with a high-monounsaturated-fat diet in patients with non-insulin-dependent diabetes mellitus. *N Engl J Med* 319: 829–834.

Gerich, J., Meyer, C., Woerle, H. 2001. Renal gluconeogenesis. *Diabetes Care* 24: 382–391.

Gross, J., Zelmanovitz, T., Moulin, C., et al. 2002. Effect of a chicken-based diet on renal function and lipid profile in patients with type 2 diabetes: A randomized crossover trial. *Diabetes Care* 25: 645–651.

Haffner, S. 1998. Management of dislipidemia in adults with diabetes. *Diabetes Care* 21: 160–178.

Hajjar, S., Fadda, G., Thanakitcharu, P., et al. 1992. Reduced activity of Na+-K+ ATPase of pancreatic islets in chronic renal failure: Role of secondary hyperparathyroidism. *J Am Soc Nephrol* 2: 1355–1359.

Hansen, H., Tauber-Lassen, E., Jensen, B., et al. 2002. Effect of dietary protein restriction on prognosis in patients with diabetic nephropathy. *Kidney Int* 62: 220–228.

Hasslacher, C., Ritz, E., Wahl, P., et al. 1989. Similar risks of nephropathy in patients with type I or type II diabetes mellitus. *Nephrol Dial Transplant* 4: 859–863.

Haviv, Y., Sharkia, M., Safadi, R. 2000. Hypoglycemia in patients with renal failure. *Renal Fail* 22: 219–222.

Hebbard, G., Wei, M., Dent, J., et al. 1996. Hyperglycaemia effects proximal gastric motor and sensory function in normal subjects. *Eur J Gastroenterol Hepatol* 8: 211–217.

Holman, R., Paul, S., Bethel, M., et al. 2008. Ten year follow-up of intensive glucose control in type 2 diabetes. *N Engl J Med* 359: 1577–1589.

House, A., Eliasziw, M., Cattran, D., et al. 2010. Effect of B-vitamin therapy on progression of diabetic nephropathy. *JAMA* 303: 1603–1609.

Inaba, M., Okuno, S., Kumeda, Y., et al. 2007. Glycated albumin is a better glycemic indicator than glycated hemoglobin values in hemodialysis patients with diabetes: Effects of anemia and erythropoietin injection. *J Am Soc Nephrol* 18: 896–903.

Jibani, M., Bloodworth, L., Foden, E., et al. 2009. Predominantly vegetarian diet in patients with incipient and early clinical diabetic nephropathy: Effects on albumin excretion rate and nutritional status. *Diabet Med* 8: 949–953.

Joachim, H. 2010. Hemoglobin A1c in hemodialysis patients: Should one size fit all? *Clin J Am Soc Nephrol* 5: 1539–1541.

Joy, M., Cefahe, W., Hogan, S., et al. 2002. Long-term glycemic control measurements in diabetic patients receiving hemodialysis. *Am J Kidney Dis* 39: 297–307.

Kasiske, B., Lakatua, J., Ma, J., et al. 1998. A meta-analysis of the effects of dietary protein restriction on the rate of decline in renal function. *Am J Kidney Dis* 31: 954–961.

Kawazu, S., Tomono, S., Shimizu, M., et al. 1994. The relationship between early diabetic nephropathy and control of plasma glucose in non-insulin dependent diabetes mellitus. The effect of glycemic control on the development and progression of diabetic nephropathy in an eight year follow-up study. *J Diabetes Complicat* 8: 13–17.

Kazempour-Ardebil, S., Tam, F., Lecamwasam, V., et al. 2009. Assessing glycemic control in maintenance hemodialysis patients with type 2 diabetes. *Diabetes Care* 32: 1137–1142.

Khaodhiar, L., Cummings, S., Apovian, C. 2009. Treating diabetes and prediabetes by focusing on obesity management. *Curr Diab Rep* 9: 348–354.

King, A. and Levey, A. 1993. Dietary protein and renal function. *J Am Soc Nephrol* 3: 1723–1737.

Kock, K.1999. Diabetic gastropathy: Gastric neuromuscular dysfunction in diabetes mellitus: A review of symptoms, pathophysiology and treatment. *Dig Dis Sci* 44: 1061–1075.

Kontessis, P., Jones, S., Dodds, R., et al. 1990. Renal, metabolic and hormonal responses to ingestion of animal and vegetable proteins. *Kidney Int* 38: 136–144.

Kopple, J. 2004. Nutritional management of nondialyzed patients with chronic renal failure. In Kopple, J.D. and Massry, S.G. (Eds.), *Nutritional Management of Renal Disease*, 389–404. Philadelphia, PA: Lippincott Williams & Wilkins.

Kris-Etherton, P. 1999. Monounsaturated fatty acids and risk of cardiovascular disease. *Circulation* 100: 1253–1258.

Loon, N. 2003. Diabetic kidney disease: Preventing dialysis and transplantation. *Clinical Diabetes* 21: 55–62.

Ma, J., Rayner, C., Jones, K., et al. 2009. Diabetic gastroparesis: Diagnosis and management. *Drugs* 69: 971–986.

Mak, R. 1991. Intravenous 1,25dihyroxycholecalciferol corrects glucose intolerance in hemodialysis patients. *Kidney Int* 41: 1049–1054.

Mak, R. and DeFonzo, R. 1992. Glucose and insulin metabolism in uremia. *Nephron* 61: 377–382.

Makoff, R. 1991. Water-soluble vitamin status in patients with renal disease treated with hemodialysis or peritoneal dialysis. *J Renal Nutr* 1: 56–73.
Margett, B., Beilin, L., Vandongen, R., et al. 1986. Vegetarian diets in mild hypertension: A randomized controlled trial. *Br Med J* 293: 1468–1471.
McDougall, K., Borman, D., Mitchell, E. 2001. Diabetes care in the dialysis setting. National Kidney Foundation. *Renal Link*. 2: 1–6 (Summer).
Morelli, E., Loon, N., Meyer, T., et al. 1990. Effects of converting enzyme inhibition on the barrier function in diabetic glomerulopathy. *Diabetes* 39: 76–82.
Morioka, T., Tahara, H., Emoto, M., et al. 2001. Glycemic control is a predictor of survival for diabetic patients on hemodialysis. *Diabetes Care* 24: 909–913.
Muhlhauser, I., Toth, G., Sawicki P., et al. 1991. Severe hypoglycemia in type I diabetic patients with impaired kidney function. *Diabetes Care* 14: 344–346.
Munden, J. and Foley, M. (Eds.). 2007. *Diabetes Mellitus: A Guide to Patient Care*. Philadelphia, PA: Lippincott Williams, & Wilkins. pp. 180–222.
Nathan, D., Holman, R., Buse, J., et al. 2006. Management of hyperglycemia in type 2 diabetes: A consensus algorithm for the initiation and adjustment of therapy. *Diabetes Care* 29: 1963–1972.
Nathan, D., Schoenfeld, D., Kuenen, J., et al. 2008. Translating the A1c assay into estimated average glucose values. *Diabetes Care*. 31: 1473–1478.
National Diabetes Fact Sheet. 2008. Department of Health and Human Services, Centers for Disease Control and Prevention.
National Kidney Foundation. 2000. K/DOQI clinical practice guidelines for nutrition in chronic renal failure. *Am J Kidney Dis* 35: S40–S43.
National Kidney Foundation. 2004. National Kidney Foundation: K/DOQI clinical practice guidelines of hypertension and antihypertensive agents in chronic kidney disease. http://www.kidney.org/professionals/KDOQI/guidelines_bp/guide_8.htm (accessed September 11, 2010).
National Kidney Foundation. 2007. KDOQI clinical practice guidelines and clinical practice recommendations for diabetes and chronic kidney disease. *Am J Kidney Dis* 49: S22–S23.
Parkman, H., Hasler, W., Fisher, R. 2004. American Gastroenterological Association technical review on the diagnosis and treatment of gastroparesis. *Gastroenterology* 127:1592–1622.
Parrish, C. 2007. Nutrition concerns for the patient with gastroparesis. *Curr Gastrolenterol Rep* 9: 295–302.
Patrick, A. and Epstein, O. 2008. Review article: Gastroparesis. *Aliment Pharmacol Ther* 27: 724–740.
Pedrini, M., Levey, A., Lau, J., et al. 1996. The effect of dietary protein restriction on the progression of diabetic and nondiabetic renal diseases: A meta-analysis. *Ann Intern Med* 124: 627–632.
Ravelli, A., Ledermann, S., Bissett, W., et al. 1992. Foregut motor function in chronic renal failure. *Arch Dis Child* 67: 1343–1347.
Ritz, E. and Orth, S. 1999. Nephropathy in patients with type 2 diabetes mellitus. *N Engl J Med* 341: 1127–1133.
Sacks, F., Sretkey, L., Vollmier, W., et al. 2001. Effects on blood pressure of reduced dietary sodium and the dietary approaches to stop hypertension (DASH) diet. *N Engl J Med* 344: 3–10.
Sheard, N. and Clark, N. 2000. The role of nutrition therapy in the management of diabetes mellitus. *Nutr Clin Care* 3: 334–348.
Shrishrimal, K., Hart, P., Franklin, M. 2009. Managing diabetes in hemodialysis patient: Observations and recommendations. *Cleve Clin J Med* 76: 649–655.
Skyler, J., Howard, B., Bergenstal, R. 2009. Intensive glycemic control and the prevention of cardiovascular events: Implications of the ACCORD, ADVANCE and VA diabetes trial. A Position Statement of the American Diabetes Association and a Scientific Statement of the American College of Cardiology foundation and the American heart Association. *Diabetes Care* 32: 187–192.
Steiner, G. 1999. Risk factors for macrovascular disease in type 2 diabetes. *Diabetes Care* 22: C6–C9.
Tkac, I. 2009. Effect of intensive glycemic control on cardiovascular outcomes and all-cause mortality in type 2 diabetes: Overview and meta analysis of five trials. *Diabetes Res Clin Pract* 865: S57–S62.
UK Prospective Diabetes Study Group. 1998. Intensive blood glucose control with sulphonylurea or insulin compared with conventional treatment and risk of complications in patients with type 2 diabetes (UKPDS 33). *Lancet* 352: 837–853.
U.S. Department of Agriculture and the U.S. Department of Health and Human Services. 2010. Part A: Executive Summary on the Dietary Guidelines for Americans. http://www.cnpp.usda.gov/Publications/DietaryGuidelines/2010/DGAC/Report/A-ExecSummary.pdf
U.S. Renal Data System, USRDS. 2009. Annual data report: Atlas of chronic kidney disease and end-stage renal disease in the United States. National Institutes of Health, National Institute of Diabetes and Digestive and Kidney Diseases, Bethesda, MD.

Walker, J., Dodds, R., Murrells, T., et al. 1989. Restriction of dietary protein and progression of renal failure in diabetic nephropathy. *Lancet* 334: 1411–1415.

Wanner, C., Krane, V., Marz, W., et al. 2005. Atorvastatin in patients with type 2 diabetes mellitus undergoing hemodialysis. *N Engl J Med* 353: 238–248.

Wild, S., Roglic, G., Green A., et al. 2004. Global prevalence of diabetes: Estimates for the year 2000 and projections for 2030. *Diabetes Care* 27: 1047–1053.

Williams, A., Baker, F., Walls, J. 1987. Effect of varying quantity and quality of dietary protein intake in experimental renal disease in rats. *Nephron* 46: 83–90.

Williams, M. 2010. The role of glycemic control in diabetic ESRD patients. *Renal and Urology News*, March 2010, 227.

Williams, M., Lacson, E., Wang, W., et al. 2010. Glycemic control and extended hemodialysis survival in patients with diabetes mellitus: Comparative results of traditional and time-dependent cox model analysis. *Clin J Am Soc Nephrol* 5: 1595–1601.

Williams, M.E. 2009. Management of diabetes in dialysis patients. *Curr Diab Rep* 9: 466–472.

Wisconsin Diabetes Advisory Group. 2008. Wisconsin diabetes mellitus essential care guidelines. http://dhs.wisconsin.gov/health/diabetes/guidelines.htm (accessed September 7, 2010).

Wiseman, M., Hunt, R., Goodwin, A., et al. 1987. Dietary composition and renal function in healthy subjects. *Nephron* 46: 37–42.

Wolk, R., Moore, E, Foulks, C. 2007. Renal disease. The A.S.P.E.N. Nutrition Support Core Curriculum.

Wright, J., Wang, C., Kennedy-Stephenson, J., et al. 2003. Dietary intake of ten key nutrients for public health, United States: 1999–2000. Advance data from Vital and Health Statistics; no. 334, Hyattsville, Maryland: National Center for Health Statistics.

Wrone, E., Mercedes, C., Palaniappan, L., et al. 2003. Association of dietary protein intake and microalbuminuria in healthy adults: Third national health and nutrition examination survey. *Am J Kidney Dis* 41: 580–587.

Zeller, K., Whittaker, E., Sullivan, L., et al. 1991. Effect of restricting dietary protein on the progression of renal failure in patients with insulin-dependent diabetes mellitus. *N Engl J Med* 324: 78–84.

16 Anemia Management

Emily Dill McDonald
WJB Dorn VA Medical Center

CONTENTS

16.1 INTRODUCTION

Anemia is a common complication of chronic kidney disease (CKD) of any cause. (Besarab and Levin, 2000). A study published in 2004 showed that 28% of Americans with mild CKD (stages 1–3) have anemia, and 87% of those with severe CKD (stages 4 and 5) have anemia (Guralnik et al., 2004). If anemia remains untreated, patients may experience a variety of complications. Published literature reveals that pre-dialysis CKD patients with anemia have an increased risk of morbidity and mortality related to cardiac disease and stroke (Levin, 2003). Because of the long-term effects of untreated anemia, it is important to be able to identify and treat patients appropriately with this potentially serious complication of CKD.

16.1.1 Definition

Anemia is a reduction in one of the red blood cell (RBC) measurements, which include hemoglobin (Hgb), hematocrit (hct), and/or RBC (Beutler and Waalen, 2006). Hgb measures the concentration of oxygen-carrying protein in the blood; the normal range is 13–17 g/dL. Hct is the percent of RBCs in whole blood; the normal range is 36%–50% (Beutler and Waalen, 2006). Finally, RBC is the number of actual RBCs in a specific volume of whole blood; the normal range considered to be 4–6 million cells/mL. Although there are several ways to measure anemia, most guidelines published by healthcare organizations define it using Hgb values.

Patients whose Hgb levels are below the fifth percentile of the normal range as reported by the National Health and Nutrition Examination Surveys (NHANES) database are considered anemic; each set of guidelines varies slightly with its definition (Astor et al., 2002; NKF-K/DOQI, 2006). Because several factors can affect Hgb values, it is important to note that these guidelines pertain to adult patients aged at least 18 years or older and patients of all races. For further discussion of these variables, see Section 16.3.

The World Health Organization (WHO) defines anemia as an Hgb level less than 13 g/dL in males and less than 12 g/dL in females (WHO, 2001). The European Best Practice Guidelines (EBPG) consider males less than 70 years old with a Hgb level less than 13 g/dL or males at least 70 years old or older with a Hgb level of less than 12 g/dL to be anemic. EBPG considers females anemic if the Hgb level is less than 11.5 g/dL (Locatelli et al., 2004). Finally, National Kidney Foundation Kidney Disease Outcomes Quality Initiative (NKF-K/DOQI™) defines anemia as a Hgb level less than 12 g/dL in females and less than 13.5 g/dL in males (K/DOQI 2006). These guidelines are very close in their definitions, but because there are variations, it is important to note which guidelines are used for diagnosing when evaluating patients.

16.2 PATHOPHYSIOLOGY

There are several contributing factors that affect a patient's Hgb level and ultimately cause anemia in patients with CKD. The lifespan of the RBC in a healthy, non-CKD patient is 120 days. The lifespan of the RBC decreases by almost half, to an estimated 60 days, in a stage 5 CKD patient secondary to uremia (Hillman and Finch, 1996).

In addition to uremia, patients with CKD are more likely to have nutrient deficiencies compared to their non-CKD counterparts. These deficiencies are worsened in hemodialysis because nutrients are often removed from the blood during this process. Of note, hemodialysis patients are also at risk for blood loss, exacerbating the anemia initially caused by the inability to produce a sufficient supply of RBC. The most common nutrient deficiencies are B_{12}, folate, and iron deficiencies (NKF-K/DOQI, 2006). These nutrients are important in the production of RBCs, so a deficiency compounds the primary cause of anemia and ultimately worsens the risk and extent of anemia in CKD patients.

Although uremia and nutrient deficiencies can contribute to anemia in a CKD patient, the most common cause of anemia in this population is a decrease in erythropoietin production (McGonigle et al., 1984; NKF-K/DOQI, 2006; Radtke et al., 1979). Erythropoietin is an endogenous hormone produced by the kidneys that is responsible for the division and differentiation of erythroid progenitor cells. In addition, it is responsible for the release of reticulocytes from the bone marrow into the bloodstream (McGonigle et al., 1984; NKF-K/DOQI, 2006; Radtke et al., 1979). Due to the nature of the disease, CKD patients experience a loss of functioning renal mass (McGonigle et al., 1984), which ultimately causes the decrease in erythropoietin hormone production. Published data shows that patients with CKD are unable to produce sufficient erythropoietin to maintain normal Hgb levels. For example, a non-CKD patient responds to low oxygenation by increasing erythropoietin production, but this same compensatory response is not seen in CKD patients (Erslev, 1991).

Literature further explores the correlation between kidney function and anemia, most specifically the severity of anemia to the duration and extent of kidney dysfunction. Typically, patients develop anemia when the estimated glomerular filtration rate (eGFR) falls below 60 mL/min/1.73 m^2 (Astor et al., 2002; McClellan et al., 2004; NKF-K/DOQI, 2006). As CKD progresses, the risk of anemia becomes much greater. The NHANES survey showed the prevalence of anemia increased from 1% in patients with an eGFR of 60 mL/min/1.73 m^2 to 9% at an eGFR of 30 mL/min/1.73 m^2 and, ultimately, to a prevalence of 33%–67% at an eGFR of 15 mL/min/1.73 m^2 (Astor et al., 2002). Anephric patients with the most severe kidney dysfunction correlate with the lowest Hgb levels (Eschbach et al., 1967). KDOQI recommends all patients with an eGFR < 60 mL/min/1.73 m^2 be evaluated for anemia because severity correlates with eGFR.

16.3 SPECIFIC PATIENT POPULATIONS

There are many different factors that can affect Hgb. Diabetic patients are at the highest risk for developing anemia and often develop anemia in earlier stages of CKD when compared to nondiabetic patients. (Bosman et al., 2001). Furthermore, sex and race can play a role in anemia. This complication is more common in males than females and in African Americans compared to Caucasian and Asian patients (Beutler and West, 2005; NKF-KDOQI, 2006; Reed and Diehl, 1991).

Other common factors affecting a patient's Hgb include altitude, gender, age, and smoking (Ruiz-Arguelles, 2006). Patients who live in higher altitudes have shown an increase in erythropoietin production (Richalet et al., 1994). Also, smoking increases carboxyhemoglobin, which in turn increases total Hgb concentrations (NKF-K/DOQI, 2006). In sum, many unique factors can affect a patient's Hgb, all of which should be taken into consideration during a patient evaluation.

16.4 COMPLICATIONS

The signs and symptoms of anemia vary based on severity of the loss of Hgb and also the rate at which the anemia evolved. Patients with CKD typically develop anemia gradually over time; thus, the rate of decline in Hgb does not result in symptoms in this patient population as frequently as with other causes of acute anemia. Ultimately, CKD patients with anemia develop symptoms due to decreased oxygen delivery to tissues.

Most patients with anemia experience fatigue, reduced exercise tolerance, and shortness of breath (Levin, 1999; Locatelli et al., 2004; Ritz and Eisenhardt, 2000). Overall, these symptoms affect patients' quality of life greatly; therefore, this patient population is at an increased risk for developing depression. Furthermore, several published studies indicate an increase in hospitalizations, cardiovascular disease, hospital length of stay, and increase in mortality in pre-dialysis CKD patients (Collins et al., 2001; Dharmarajan et al., 2008; Levin, 1999; Locatelli et al., 2004; Ritz and Eisenhardt, 2000).

As previously mentioned, severe cardiac complications are also associated with anemia. Research shows that anemia both directly and indirectly worsens cardiac function and the symptoms of heart failure in these patients (Levin et al., 1996; USRDS, 2008). The ANCHOR trial found an association with an increase in mortality associated with Hgb levels less than 13–14 mg/dL as compared to Hgb levels of greater than 16–17 mg/dL (Go et al., 2006). These potentially life-altering and even fatal outcomes must be identified early and managed aggressively to prevent these severe complications.

16.5 EVALUATION

Since anemia is a known complication from CKD with potentially fatal consequences, the NKF-K/DOQI guidelines recommend monitoring a patient's Hgb at least annually. Furthermore, the guidelines recommend that a patient with worsening or unstable CKD or who have a history of a previous decline in Hgb levels should be monitored more frequently (NKF-K/DOQI, 2006, 2007).

Patients who are identified as anemic based on the aforementioned guidelines should undergo a thorough workup. Anemia in CKD is most commonly diagnosed by excluding other potential, nonrenal causes of anemia and evaluating the progression and severity of a patient's CKD (NKF-K/DOQI, 2006). This should include the identification or ruling out of other possible causes of anemia, such as bleeding, especially of the gastrointestinal (GI) tract as shown by a stool guaiac test (Goddard et al., 2000; NKF-K/DOQI, 2006). Nutrition deficiencies, malignancies, human immunodeficiency virus (HIV), or other deficiencies may result in anemia as well. It is especially important to investigate additional causes of anemia when the severity of the anemia is disproportionate to the renal dysfunction and/or when a patient experiences leukopenia or thrombocytopenia (NKF-K/DOQI, 2006, 2007).

To evaluate the other potential causes of anemia, several lab tests should be evaluated. A complete blood count shows a patient's Hgb, hct, and RBC and, in addition, shows the white blood cell count (WBC), platelets, reticulocytes, mean corpuscular Hgb (MCH), and mean corpuscular volume (MCV) (Goddard et al., 2000; Morris and Davey, 1996). WBCs and platelets should be reviewed to determine whether other blood disorders are contributing to the anemia. A normal reticulocyte value indicates that the bone marrow is functioning adequately (Morris and Davey, 1996; NKF-K/DOQI, 2006; Wish, 2006).

MCH shows the average amount of oxygen-carrying Hgb in a RBC. RBCs that are larger (macrocytic) are most likely to have a higher MCH; whereas, RBCs that are smaller (microcytic) are most likely to have a lower MCH (hypochromic) (Goddard et al., 2000).

MCV indicates the average volume of the RBC; normal MCV is 80–100 fL (Morris and Davey, 1996). RBCs that are within this range are termed *normocytic*. Microcytic indicates an MCV value less than 80 fL, while macrocytic is defined by a value greater than 100 fL. Iron deficiency or genetic Hgb, formation disorders result in anemias that are microcytic. Macrocytic anemia is usually associated with B_{12}/folate deficiency (Goddard et al., 2000; Morris and Davey, 1996).

Most patients with an anemia due to chronic disease, including CKD, are normochromic and normocytic (NKF-K/DOQI, 2006). Although erythropoietin deficiency is the primary cause of anemia in CKD, the literature does not support evaluating erythropoietin levels. These levels do not help distinguish between the causes of anemia (McGonigle et al., 1984; Radtke et al., 1979).

By evaluating these lab results, the cause and severity of the anemia most likely can be identified. The Hgb, instead of hct, is the best indicator for the severity of the anemia (K/DOQI, 2006). Hgb is more stable and can be measured directly. Conversely, hct is unstable and is usually affected by extended storage and changes in temperature (Morris and Davey, 1996). Also, the measure of hct is not standardized. Some literature indicates that hct can be affected by increase in serum glucose, which further affects its instability (Van Duijnhoven and Treskes, 1996).

Although Hgb is a stable measure, there can be a dilutional affect (NKF-K/DOQI, 2006; WHO, 2001). This is not a major concern for nonhemodialysis patients or for peritoneal dialysis patients, but it should be taken into consideration with patients on hemodialysis.

Iron deficiency is the most common cause of treatment failure in anemic patients, and it should be considered when evaluating a patient's lab work. The lab work for iron deficiency includes: ferritin, transferrin, iron levels, and transferrin saturation (TSAT) (NKF-K/DOQI, 2006; Wish, 2006). TSAT and ferritin are used to evaluate the availability of iron for erythropoiesis. TSAT is an estimate of the amount of iron immediately available for delivery to the bone marrow. It is calculated by finding the ratio of iron to total iron binding capacity and is reported as a percentage. Ferritin is an indirect measure of iron storage (Wish, 2006). It is important to note that ferritin can be affected by liver disease, infection, and inflammation, which can cause a false elevation and mask a possible depletion. Finally, transferrin is the carrier of iron from storage to the bone marrow for incorporation into RBC; it can be affected by a person's poor nutrition (Wish, 2006).

16.6 TREATMENT OF ANEMIA

16.6.1 Goals of Therapy

Overall, the target Hgb value for CKD patients should be individualized to optimize their quality of life and management of comorbidities. The literature supports that aiming for a Hgb of 11 g/dL will improve a patient's quality of life without increasing their risk of adverse reactions (NKF-K/DOQI,

2006). This published data encompasses dialysis (peritoneal and hemodialysis) and nondialysis patients.

Along with this data, further evidence shows little benefit and possibly even harm with regard to morbidity and mortality if the targeted Hgb is 13 g/dL or higher (Clement et al., 2009; K/DOQI, 2006; Palmer et al., 2010; Phrommintikul et al., 2007). It was because of this data that NKF-K/DOQI guidelines were revised in 2007 to reflect a change in the recommended Hgb target range. Those recommendations were to treat to a goal Hgb range of 11–12 g/dL but not to exceed 13 g/dL (Collins et al., 2001). More recent recommendations based on an Food and Drug Administration (FDA) Safety Alert are to treat to a goal Hgb of 10–11 g/dL (FDA Drug Safety Communication: Modified dosing recommendations to improve the safe use of erythropoiesis-stimulating agents [ESAs] in chronic kidney disease, June 24, 2011).

Although the Hgb range of 10–11 g/dL is recommended by the guidelines, it is relatively difficult to maintain patients within this narrow window because of variables related to the laboratory and the individual treatment response of patients. The FDA previously recommended aiming for a Hgb range of 10–12 g/dL (USFDA, 2007b). They joined KDOQI in the recommendation to not exceed a Hgb of 13 g/dL. The FDA has placed alerts with regard to Hgb range in product labeling for ESAs.

Treatment of anemia has both short-term and long-term effects. Increasing oxygen-carrying capacity by increasing Hgb ultimately decreases shortness of breath and fatigue, increases energy, and improves the patient's quality of life (Foley et al., 2009; Hampl et al., 2002; Silverberg, 2003). Published literature shows that patients who reach an Hgb of at least 11 g/dL have improvement in all-cause mortality, stabilization of left ventricular hypertrophy (LVH), fewer hospitalizations, and improving quality of life (Hampl et al., 2002; Silverberg, 2003).

16.6.2 Iron Therapy

Iron stores must be adequate to ensure that a patient will have maximum benefit and response to erythropoietic agents (Besarab et al., 2000; Fishbane, 2007; Lexi-Comp, 2011; NKF-K/DOQI, 2006). In addition to ensuring appropriate response to ESAs, other goals of iron therapy include avoiding storage depletion, preventing iron deficiency, and achieving and maintaining target Hgb levels (NKF-K/DOQI, 2006). Before starting iron therapy, lab work must be evaluated to assess the extent of the iron deficiency.

Iron therapy should be initiated when TSAT is less than or equal to 20% and ferritin is less than 100–500 ng/mL for nondialysis and peritoneal dialysis patients, and less than 200–500 ng/mL for hemodialysis patients (NKF-K/DOQI, 2006). Iron should not be used when ferritin levels are greater than 500 ng/mL.

Both oral and intravenous administrations are effective in repleting iron (Eschbach et al., 1989; Fick et al., 2003; Stoves et al., 2001). No matter the choice of iron formulation or route of administration for replacement, iron therapy should be started prior to initiation of ESAs. ESAs will increase the need for iron; thus, iron stores need to be sufficient to cover the demand (Charytan et al., 2005; Lexi-Comp, 2011). Data on safety endpoints and efficacy comparing oral iron versus intravenous (IV) iron have shown conflicting results (Fishbane, 2007). At this time, K/DOQI guidelines recommend that either IV or oral therapy can be given to nondialysis CKD and peritoneal dialysis Stage 5 CKD patients.

Increasing a patient's dietary iron intake may be an effective supplement to oral or IV iron. Iron is primarily absorbed in the duodenum with only about 1–2 mg absorbed out of every 20 mg of iron consumed (NKF-K/DOQI, 2006). Patients who are considered healthy respond to iron deficiency by increasing the absorption of dietary iron by 25%–30%. It is speculated that CKD patients do not have this same response. Because of these factors, replacing iron by increasing dietary intake most likely will not replete a patient to the desired goals.

Increasing dietary intake of iron may be an option as adjunctive therapy for certain patients. Foods containing heme iron have increased bioavailability of iron because it is absorbed better than other sources of iron (Bothwell, 1995; Halberg, 1981). Heme iron sources include poultry, fish, and ground beef. Nonheme iron sources also provide iron, but the absorption is about 33%–50% less than from heme sources. Iron-fortified foods, lentils, beans, and spinach are examples of nonheme iron sources (Bothwell, 1995; Halberg, 1981).

Furthermore, other nutrients may indirectly affect iron absorption from food. Ascorbic acid may increase the absorption of iron (Siegenberg et al., 1994). In contrast, food containing phenols (tea), phytates (bran), polyphenols (berries and bright colored vegetables), and calcium (dairy) may inhibit or decrease iron absorption (Siegenberg et al., 1994; see Table 16.1).

There are several options for oral iron replacement, which vary by formulation and amount of elemental iron. To treat an iron deficiency, the goal iron dose from oral supplements should be 200 mg of elemental iron daily (NKF-K/DOQI, 2006). The formulations include ferrous sulfate, fumarate and gluconate, and polysaccharide iron complex. Depending on the formulation, oral iron must be taken from once daily to up to three times daily in order to reach the elemental iron intake goal (Fishbane, 2007). Ferrous sulfate is the least expensive formulation but requires more frequent dosing at three times daily to achieve this goal of 200 mg of elemental iron per day (Fishbane, 2007; see Table 16.2).

Oral iron may be more convenient for a nonhemodialysis patient because it can be administered at home, thereby preventing extra visits to the medical center for administration. Unfortunately, the side effects typically limit the efficacy and increase the risk of treatment failure with this class of medications. The most common side effects are those of the GI tract, most often constipation (Fishbane, 2007; NKF-K/DOQI, 2006). Other GI side effects include cramping, nausea, and diarrhea (Lexi-Comp, 2011). Patients should be educated that stools may become darker and harder due to the increase in iron (Fishbane, 2007; Lexi-Comp, 2011). It is important to note that the incidence of GI side effects increases as the dose increases. Reducing the dose or changing formulations may reduce the incidence of these side effects (Fishbane, 2007; NKF-K/DOQI, 2006). Furthermore, because the side effects, especially constipation, may be worse in the elderly population, it is advised to limit the dose to ferrous sulfate 325 mg daily in this patient population (Fick et al., 2003).

Ensuring appropriate absorption of the elemental iron is important to achieve maximum effects from this supplementation. An acidic environment is needed to achieve the greatest absorption of iron. Patients should be educated to take their iron supplementation in between meals; bedtime administration may be effective in minimizing the effects from food. Antacids such as histamine-2 (H_2) receptor antagonists and proton pump inhibitors will further inhibit the absorption from this medication (Fishbane, 2007; Lexi-Comp, 2011). Products with calcium will have similar effects in minimizing the acidic environment and affecting iron absorption (Lexi-Comp, 2011). Unfortunately,

TABLE 16.1
Foods and Dietary Intake Affecting Iron Absorption

Effect	Food and/or Nutrient	Mechanism
Increase absorption	Poultry, fish, ground beef	Direct source of heme iron Greater bioavailability versus nonheme iron
	Beans, lentils, spinach	Direct source of nonheme iron
	Ascorbic acid (vitamin C)	Indirectly via improving absorption of iron from food
Decrease absorption	Tea (phenols) Bran (phytates) Berries and bright colored vegetables (polyphenols) Dairy (calcium)	Indirectly inhibits absorption of iron from food

TABLE 16.2
Oral Iron Formulations (Recommended Goal Dose: 200 mg of Elemental Iron)

Iron Formulation	Brand Name	Strength of Tablet (Amount of Elemental Iron)	Elemental Iron (mg/g) of Drug	Percentage Availability of Elemental Iron (%)
Ferrous sulfate	Ferrous sulfate	325 mg (65 mg)	200	20
	Fer-Gen-Sol®	125 mg (25 mg)		
	Fer-In-Sol®	125 mg (25 mg)		
	Feratab®	300 mg (60 mg)		
Ferrous fumarate	Ferrous fumarate	325 mg (107 mg)	330	33
	Hemocyte®	324 mg (106 mg)		
	NephroFer®	350 mg (115 mg)		
	Feostat®	100 mg (33 mg)		
Ferrous gluconate	Ferrous gluconate	325 mg (36 mg)	120	11
	Fergon®	225 mg (27 mg)		
Iron polysaccharide	Niferex-150®	150 mg (150 mg)	1000	100
	Ferrex-150®	150 mg (150 mg)		
	Niferex®	50 mg (50 mg)		

the effects of food on iron absorption may limit its usefulness in preventing or minimizing potential GI side effects.

The newer formulations of iron, such as polysaccharide iron complex and heme iron polypeptide, were developed to decrease the administration frequency, to maximize iron absorption in the GI tract, and to potentially limit the GI side effects. At this time, data shows that patients on these formulations do meet treatment goals, but there is limited information comparing older versus newer formulations with regard to efficacy and adverse events (Fishbane and Besarab, 2007). Ferrous sulfate is less expensive and should be used as initial iron replacement therapy. If a patient is unable to tolerate one formulation, then it is appropriate to try others.

If a patient is unable to take oral iron for any reason, or if he has consistent IV access and makes regular visits to a doctor's office (usually hemodialysis patients), IV iron is an option for replacement therapy. IV iron therapy is also appropriate in patients who do not meet their goal TSAT and ferritin levels after 2 months of oral iron or if the target Hgb range is not met with use of ESAs (NKF-K/DOQI, 2006).

The three IV iron formulations are iron dextrin, ferric gluconate, and iron sucrose. These medications are given infrequently, and the doses are much larger than those of oral iron. Prior to starting IV iron, patients should be evaluated for underlying infection or inflammatory diseases, as these patients are not candidates for this route of administration (Canziani et al., 2001; Parkkinen et al., 2000). Because of safety concerns, ferric gluconate and iron sucrose are preferred over iron dextran (NKF-K/DOQI, 2006).

Iron dextran is the oldest of the three formulations, and it has a significantly higher incidence of anaphylaxis and other side effects compared to the other two formulations. Since there is the risk of serious side effects, iron dextran requires a test dose prior to administering the maintenance dose (Fishbane, 2003). Typical iron dextran doses are 500–1000 mg/dose repeated as needed to replete stores appropriately (Charytan et al., 2001; Michael et al., 2002).

Ferric gluconate and iron sucrose can be dosed anywhere from 100 to 400 mg per dose and repeated as needed to replete stores (Fishbane, 2007; Silverberg, 2003). Although these formulations do not have as high a risk of anaphylaxis as iron dextran and do not require a test dose, precautions should be taken and there should be close monitoring for potential adverse events (Fishbane, 2003; NKF-K/DOQI, 2006).

The most common side effect of all IV-iron formulations is hypotension, which can be minimized by administering a lower dose or slowing the rate of administration (Fishbane, 2003). Other side effects include nausea and vomiting, which also can be minimized by slowing the rate (Michael et al., 2002). Unfortunately, the more serious side effects such as anaphylaxis and iron overload cannot be avoided by changing the rate of administration. Should a patient experience these events, intervention must be made to prevent serious harm to the patient. Iron overload is a serious risk typically seen when iron is administered when a patient's ferritin is greater than 800 ng/mL (NKF-K/DOQI, 2006; Morris and Davey, 1996). It is especially noted with IV iron because of the high iron load given at one time. Ultimately, deposits form and cause dysfunction of the liver, pancreas, and heart (NKF-K/DOQI, 2006; Parkkinen et al., 2000). Should a patient experience iron overload, deferoxamine or phlebotomy should be used. Although the actual risk of iron overload is not well studied, there have not been data to show added benefit when ferritin levels are greater than 500 ng/mL (NKF-K/DOQI, 2006).

Precautions against infection and inflammation should be taken when considering treatment with IV iron (Canziani et al., 2001; Parkkinen et al., 2000). These symptoms can be a sign of infection or chronic oxidative stress. Although somewhat controversial, there are data stating that exposure to iron increases a patient's risk of bacterial infections (Canziani et al., 2001; Parkkinen et al., 2000). The data proposes that because bacteria uses iron for cellular functioning, administration of IV iron in high doses will worsen the acute state. Guidelines recommend withholding iron supplements for a patient during an infectious state (NKF-K/DOQI, 2006).

Another controversial debate surrounding iron therapy is the increase in oxidative stress created by the replacement. Authors propose that this increase in oxidative stress can worsen cardiovascular disease (Agarwal et al., 2004; Kletzmayr and Horl, 2002). At this time, there is no evidence to show that iron replacement increases a patient's risk of morbidity or mortality. Further research is needed prior to making recommendations on this concern.

Monitoring iron therapy should include iron labs (ferritin, iron levels, transferring, and TSAT) monthly during initial treatment. Once the patient is stable, monitoring can be extended to 3-month intervals. As stated earlier, KDOQI states that the goal of hemodialysis patients is ferritin of >200 ng/mL and a TSAT of >20% (NKF-K/DOQI, 2006; Silverberg, 2003). Nonhemodialysis patients and peritoneal dialysis patients should aim for a ferritin of >100 ng/mL and also a TSAT of >20% (NKF-K/DOQI, 2006).

These goals should be closely monitored to ensure there is sufficient iron for RBC production and to decrease the patient's risk for iron overload. Again, there are no data to show added benefit with a ferritin level greater than 500 ng/mL (NKF-K/DOQI, 2006). It is also important to note that once a patient's iron has been repleted, iron replacement must be continued, especially with concomitant use of ESA therapy. ESA therapy will stimulate an increase in RBC production, thus increasing iron consumption.

16.6.3 ESA Therapy

All agents that augment erythropoiesis through direct or indirect action on erythropoietin receptors are considered ESAs. The actions of these proteins stimulate erythroid progenitor cells to divide and differentiate; ultimately, the release of reticulocytes from the bone marrow to the bloodstream is induced (Clement et al., 2009; USFDA, 2007b). Because the rates of making and releasing blood cells are increased, the consumption of the nutrients needed for making these cells, such as iron, B_{12}, and folate, also increases. This reiterates the importance of ensuring that iron is repleted prior to initiating ESA therapy.

There are many benefits to ESA therapy. Overall, ESA therapy has been proven to significantly reduce the need for blood transfusions in anemic patients, thus often decreasing need for hospitalization (Revicki et al., 1995). Furthermore, treatment with ESAs have reduced or even alleviated the symptoms most often associated with anemia, and this treatment has (not yet proven) potential to improve patients' cardiac health (Fink et al., 2001; Revicki et al., 1995). Most recent reports have shown an improvement in cardiovascular outcomes when patients' anemia is treated with ESAs.

Because the benefit can be so great, the FDA recommends CKD patients with a Hgb less than 10 mg/dL should be evaluated for the use of ESA therapy (Clement et al., 2009; USFDA, 2007b). If patients have an active malignancy or a history of malignancy, then ESAs should be initiated with caution. Again, ESA therapy should not be initiated until any iron deficiency has been corrected. The lowest possible dose in order to achieve a goal Hgb range of 10–12 mg/dL should be used (Clement et al., 2009; USFDA, 2007b).

Drug options available in the United States, which increase erythropoiesis include epoetin alpha (Procrit® and Epogen®) and darbepoetin (Aranesp®) (USFDA, 2007b). Epoetin beta is not available in the United States. Both medications have the same site of action, and both are proteins created to mimic the endogenous hormones produced by the kidneys. Because of the slight difference in darbepoetin's structure compared to that of epoetin's, darbepoetin has a higher molecular weight. This increased weight extends its duration of action; thus, epoetin is referred to as short-acting, whereas darbepoetin is referred to as long-acting.

Both medications can be administered IV or subcutaneously (Ateshkadi et al., 1993). Subcutaneous dosing is usually chosen based on its convenience for patients, specifically patients not on dialysis who do not visit the clinic regularly. IV epoetin is most commonly used in hemodialysis patients because it can be administered during their hemodialysis sessions, decreasing the need for additional needle sticks. Epoetin is usually administered one to three times weekly. Current literature shows that patients respond to therapy similarly with each dosing interval (McGowan et al., 2008; Provenzano et al., 2005). Darbepoetin can be administered weekly or every other week (Suranyi et al., 2003). Recently, the dosing interval of darbepoetin was extended to monthly dosing, without affecting the response to therapy (Jadoul et al., 2004).

Epogen is usually dosed based on vial size; the typical starting dose is Epogen 10,000 units weekly or 20,000 units every other week. Should a patient's Hgb prior to treatment be greater than 10 mg/dL, a provider should use clinical judgment with regard to possibly starting a lower dose (Table 16.3).

The most common side effects with either of these formulations are hypertension and seizures (Phrommintikul et al., 2007; Vaziri, 1999). These are typically associated with an increased rate of rise of the Hgb. Thus, patients should be monitored closely upon initiating ESA therapy in order to appropriately monitor the effects of the ESA on Hgb.

Hypertension is a potentially serious side effect of ESA medications, and patients should be monitored closely for changes in blood pressure (NKF-K/DOQI, 2006). Hypertension is more commonly seen in dialysis patients than nondialysis patients, but owing to potential complications, all patients with uncontrolled hypertension should be cautiously started on ESAs. It is not a contraindication, but measures should be taken to better monitor and control the blood pressure. KDOQI

TABLE 16.3
Comparison of Epoetin Alpha to Darbepoetin

	Epoetin alpha	Darbepoetin
Brand Name	Procrit or Epogen	Aranesp
Route of Administration	Subcutaneous (SQ) or IV	SQ or IV
Half-life (IV administration)	4–13 h	21 h (IV) 49 h (SQ)
Time to Onset of Full Effect	2–3 weeks	2–6 weeks
Dosing Frequency	Three times weekly to weekly	Every other week to monthly
Side Effects	Injection site reaction, nausea/vomiting, hypertension, stroke, seizures	Injection site reaction, nausea/vomiting, hypertension, stroke, seizures

guidelines recommend withholding ESA therapy based on blood pressure only when the hypertension does not respond to antihypertensive therapy.

Another serious side effect with ESA therapy is the risk of thromboembolism and/or stroke (Phrommintikul et al., 2007). This side effect is more often associated with ESA use when a patient's Hgb is above the range of 10–12 g/dL (Clement et al., 2009; USFDA, 2007b). ESAs should not be administered in patients with a Hgb greater than 13 g/dL (Clement et al., 2009; Fishbane, 2007; Ofsthun et al., 2003; USFDA, 2007b; Wish, 2006). This was the reason for the FDA's Black Box Warning, issued in 2007. The warning reads, "In clinical studies, patients experienced greater risks for death, serious cardiovascular events, and stroke when administered erythropoiesis-stimulating agents (ESAs) to target hemoglobin levels of 13 g/dL and above. Individualize dosing to achieve and maintain hemoglobin levels within the range of 10–11 g/dL. Again, patients should be monitored closely to minimize this adverse event" (Clement et al., 2009; USFDA, 2007b).

This warning is located in the package insert of all ESA medications. Along with close monitoring of actual Hgb levels, the package inserts provide guidance on the rate of rise of the Hgb. The manufacturers recommend a maximum rate of 1 g/dL rise in Hgb over a 2-week period. Should the rate exceed this recommendation, then the ESA dose should be reduced by 25%. On the contrary, if the rate of rise is not at least 1 g/dL over 4 weeks, then the dose should be increased by 25% (Clement et al., 2009; USFDA, 2007b). These recommendations and guidelines reiterate the importance of checking an Hgb every 2 weeks until stable.

As stated above, monitoring of ESAs focuses primarily on the Hgb values. Initially, a patient's Hgb should be checked every 2 weeks. Once the Hgb is stable, the time period for checking the Hgb is extended to every 4 weeks. The importance of checking the Hgb so often centers on prevention of potentially serious side effects and ensuring an appropriate response to therapy.

Although recommendations have been made to check the Hgb at least every 2 weeks initially, it is important to note that in order to see the maximum effects from a certain dose, the appropriate time must be given for the increase in erythropoiesis and RBC production rate. This can take as few as 4 weeks or up to 16 weeks. Therefore, adjustments for doses of ESA medications should not occur more often than every 2–4 weeks (Clement et al., 2009; Collins, 2002; USFDA, 2007b).

Along with Hgb monitoring, other routine labs should be drawn, such as iron labs, B_{12}/folate, and thyroid function studies. These do not need to be drawn monthly once stable but, again, should be monitored on a periodic basis.

Some patients may have resistance to ESA therapy despite constant monitoring and dose adjustments. These patients should have a thorough workup to review the possibilities for infection, inflammation, blood loss, aluminum toxicity, elevated parathyroid hormone, hypothyroidism, and malnutrition specifically related to B_{12} and folate (NKF-K/DOQI, 2006). The most common reason for ESA resistance is iron deficiency. Thus, iron should be replete prior to initiating ESA therapy (Fernandez-Rodriguez et al., 1999; NKF-K/DOQI, 2006).

Unfortunately, despite proper monitoring and dose adjustments, some patients fail therapy. Prior to determining that a patient has failed ESA therapy, the provider must ensure that the patient's iron is replete. Furthermore, the patient should have received adequate dosing of ESA therapy for at least 4–6 months. Adequate dosing is defined as 450 units/kg/week with IV administration or 300 units/kg/week with subcutaneous administration. Even after reaching the therapeutic range for the Hgb, a patient is at risk of failing ESA treatment should the Hgb not remain in the desired range (NKF-K/DOQI, 2006).

16.7 NONPHARMACOLOGICAL TREATMENT

16.7.1 L-Carnitine

The mechanism in which L-carnitine contributes to anemia is unknown. Several reports postulate that carnitine is necessary for increased formation of colony-forming-unit erythroid in the bone marrow; this has been reported in mice (Kitamura et al., 2005). Another speculation is that carnitine is necessary for the RBC phospholipid membrane. When this component is reduced or absent, the RBC becomes deformed and is very fragile, which ultimately reduces the half-life of the cell (Eknoyan et al., 2003).

Hemodialysis patients are thought to be especially at risk of a deficient carnitine state. There is also speculation that CKD patients, nondialysis, and dialysis patients, have a reduction in activity in the pathway required to convert acyl coA to acyl carnitine, ultimately creating a deficiency (Evans, 2003). This deficiency may contribute to anemia in CKD patients via the pathways previously discussed. In order to correct this deficiency, L-carnitine has been used in dialysis patients to treat anemia, with or without concomitant ESA therapy (Eknoyan et al., 2003; Evans, 2003).

The adverse events associated with L-carnitine are minimal, but some patients have reported seizures with IV L-carnitine (Kitamura et al., 2005). Researchers are concerned with potential accumulation of harmful products of L-carnitine metabolism (Bain et al., 2006; Evans, 2003). Small studies using oral L-carnitine doses ranging from 0.5 to 2 g daily for up to 3 years have not shown harm to the patients; these doses were well tolerated (Golper et al., 2003). There is not current evidence comparing IV versus oral L-carnitine.

It is important to note that D-carnitine and DL-carnitine should not be used. D-carnitine is not used for fatty acid metabolism; thus, it will not affect the RBC membrane. DL-carnitine has been associated with neuromuscular dysfunction(McGowan et al., 2008).

A study published by Kooistra showed an association with anemic dialysis patients requiring higher doses of epoetin therapy when the serum free carnitine levels were low (Kooistra et al., 1991). Other small studies, randomized and nonrandomized, show that patients have an improvement in hct or Hgb with L-carnitine administration, and at times a decrease in ESA doses is required to maintain a therapeutic Hgb (Hurot et al., 2002; Kooistra et al., 1991). On the other hand, data from randomized, placebo-controlled trials show no significant difference in Hgb for anemic dialysis patients.

Should a dialysis patient not respond to conventional therapy, it is reasonable to try L-carnitine (McGowan et al., 2008). KDOQI guidelines for nutrition in adult anemia patients recommend oral or IV L-carnitine 1 g after dialysis (NKF-K/DOQI, 2000). Patients should be assessed every 3 months for response to therapy; L-carnitine should be discontinued at 9–12 months if no response (Evans, 2003). The NKF Carnitine Consensus Conference noted concern over the use of oral carnitine due to unknown risks associated with its breakdown in the GI tract (Evans, 2003). Overall, KDOQI guidelines for anemia state that there is insufficient evidence to support use of L-carnitine in anemia due to CKD (NKF-K/DOQI, 2000, 2006). Again, the hesitation pertains to the small size and poor study designs of the trials supporting use of L-carnitine.

16.7.2 Ascorbic Acid (Vitamin C)

It has been proposed that ascorbic acid improves a patient's anemia through several possible mechanisms. Iron needs an acidic environment for absorption, so vitamin C may help with iron absorption if it is administered 30 min prior to the iron supplement (Bridges and Hoffman, 1986). Also, vitamin C may increase the release of iron from ferritin providing more iron to be transported to the bone marrow for incorporation into RBC production (Bridges and Hoffman, 1986; Lipschitz et al., 1971). Lastly, ascorbic acid may have antioxidant properties.

Ascorbic acid is available in both oral and IV formulations, but most studies have researched the use of IV ascorbic acid in hemodialysis patients only. Some literature has reported the use of ascorbic acid in doses of 150–200 mg daily in order to normalize vitamin C levels in dialysis patients (Descombes et al., 1993).

A meta-analysis of trials in anemic hemodialysis patients comparing ascorbic acid with standard of care was published in 2009 (Deved et al., 2009). It found that the populations with ascorbic acid had significantly increased Hgb levels, decreased epoetin doses, and improved transferrin saturation. Despite the significant findings, there was no report on specific patient outcomes and few reports of adverse events. In addition, the studies were small, which limits the power of the outcomes (Deved et al., 2009). There have been some randomized controlled trials with ascorbic acid in dialysis patients. Most of the data are conflicting and, again, side effects were commonly not reported (Attallah et al., 2006; Keven et al., 2003).

Because adverse events are rarely reported in the studies, the safety and long-term efficacy with oral or IV ascorbic acid is unknown. The primary concern about the use of ascorbic acid is the potentially harmful pro-oxidant effects (Chen et al., 2003). Ascorbic acid may increase oxalate in the body, which can create crystals with different cations, such as calcium and iron (Canavese et al., 2005). These crystals could potentially affect organs should they accumulate. This effect may be seen with either IV or oral administration. Because of this concern, some authors of trials recommend using IV ascorbic acid only in patients unable to achieve target Hgb levels with adequate iron stores and sufficient epoetin doses (Ballal et al., 1991; Sezer et al., 2002; Tarng and Huang, 1998).

Furthermore, these trials were with dialysis patients and used IV ascorbic acid with doses ranging from 100 to 500 mg. These trials usually assessed patients for response after 8 weeks, and then therapy was discontinued (Ballal et al., 1991; Sezer et al., 2002; Tarng and Huang, 1998). Based on the trial designs, if a patient receives ascorbic acid for treatment of anemia, then it should be administered intravenously and for a short duration.

The K/DOQI guidelines state there is insufficient evidence to support use of ascorbic acid. The EBPGs state that use of ascorbic acid to correct ascorbic acid levels may reduce the hyporesponsiveness to epoetin and/or treatment with iron for iron deficiency.

16.7.3 Androgens

Before the development of ESAs, androgens were used regularly in the treatment of anemia. Androgens were thought to possibly increase endogenous erythropoietin production, sensitivity of erythroid progenitor cells to erythropoietin, and possibly increase RBC survival (Sheashaa et al., 2005). Currently, there is very limited data to support the use of androgens in conjunction with ESAs or instead of ESAs. Potential side effects of androgens include acne, priapism, liver dysfunction, and hepatocellular carcinoma (Eussen et al., 2005; Gaughan et al., 1997). The risk of androgen use outweighs the benefits, especially in women (NKF-K/DOQI, 2006).

Current guidelines, including K/DOQI and the European Best Practices Guidelines, state that the risks with androgens outweigh the potential, limited benefit. K/DOQI states that androgens should not be used in treatment of anemia in CKD.

16.7.4 B_{12}/Folate

As mentioned previously, a deficiency in B_{12} and folate may cause anemia and potentially worsen anemia due to CKD. The treatment of macrocytic anemia due to folate and/or B_{12} deficiency can be treated through several different avenues (see "Evaluation" for more information on diagnosis.).

B_{12} (cyanocobalamin) can be replaced both orally and parenterally. Replacement doses are much higher than the recommended dietary intake of B_{12} (Kuzminski et al., 1998). Literature shows that patients respond equally to both oral and intramuscular administration (Bolaman et al., 2003; Butler et al., 2006). Parenteral B_{12} injections are given in doses of 1000 mcg (Kuzminski et al., 1998). During initial treatment, the doses are administered daily and are titrated downward over time. After this phase, doses are administered monthly until the deficit is corrected (Delpre et al., 1999). Injections are a good option for patients with compliance concerns.

The use of oral formulations is limited by compliance and absorption. To ensure appropriate absorption, high doses of oral B_{12} should be used at doses of 1000–2000 mcg daily (Bolaman et al.,

2003). Other options for B_{12} replacement are sublingual and nasal spray, although data are limited (Cunningham et al., 1981; Slot et al., 1997). With either route of administration, B_{12} treatment has few adverse events and is inexpensive (Butler et al., 2006).

Once B_{12} treatment has been initiated, then folic acid should also be replaced if patient is considered deficient (USFDA, 2007a). Although the recommended daily intake of folic acid is 200 mcg/day, the recommended dose for replacement therapy is 1–5 mg daily; the most common dose is 1 mg daily. Folic acid replacement is administered orally for at least 1 month up to 4 months. Some reports have associated folic acid treatment with malignancies, so treatment should be limited to appropriate use in a deficiency (USDA, 2009). Because the replacement doses of B_{12} and folate are much higher than the recommended dietary intake, these doses are rarely found in over-the-counter multivitamins (Table 16.4).

16.7.5 Multivitamins

Malnutrition does contribute to anemias, especially in CKD patients. Unfortunately, several factors can contribute to malnutrition in CKD patients. These factors include a decrease in oral intake due to a change in taste, anorexia, depression, or dislike for the restricted diets required due to their renal disease (NKF-K/DOQI, 2000, 2006). Many CKD patients must restrict their intake of protein, which is a major source of dietary iron (NKF-K/DOQI, 2000). Furthermore, dialysis patients are at risk of malnutrition for the reasons stated above, which is worsened by the affects of dialysis itself. Dialysis removes nutrients, especially water-soluble vitamins, and also causes blood loss. Dialysis patients are also in a higher catabolic state, which increases the use of nutrients (NKF-K/DOQI, 2000).

Because they are at risk for loss of water-soluble vitamins, dialysis patients should be monitored closely for deficiencies. There are special formulations of vitamin supplements that take into consideration CKD patients. These formulations contain vitamin B, vitamin C, and folic acid. It is important to note that there are currently no data supporting regular vitamin therapy other than supplementation to correct deficiencies.

16.7.6 Other

Patients who are symptomatic and anemic, especially those with blood loss, should be considered for blood transfusions. The risk of transfusions, such as infections and fluid overload, should be discussed at length with patients. The risks should also be weighed versus the benefits; thus, the recommendation is to use transfusion only in symptomatic patients (NKF-K/DOQI, 2006).

TABLE 16.4
Comparison of Treatment for Common Nutritional Deficiencies

Nutrient Deficiency	Therapy	Adjunctive Therapy
Iron	Hemodialysis IV iron with dialysis sessions CKD (nondialysis) or peritoneal dialysis Oral iron[a]	Consider increasing dietary iron intake but use caution with other dietary restrictions, especially in patients with kidney disease. See Table 16.1
B12	Dose = 1000– 2000 mcg Route: IM, oral, sublingual, or intranasal	Fish, poultry, eggs
Folate	1 mg daily by mouth	Leafy green vegetables, whole grains

[a] If unable to tolerate or unable to reach treatment goals, then switch to IV iron.

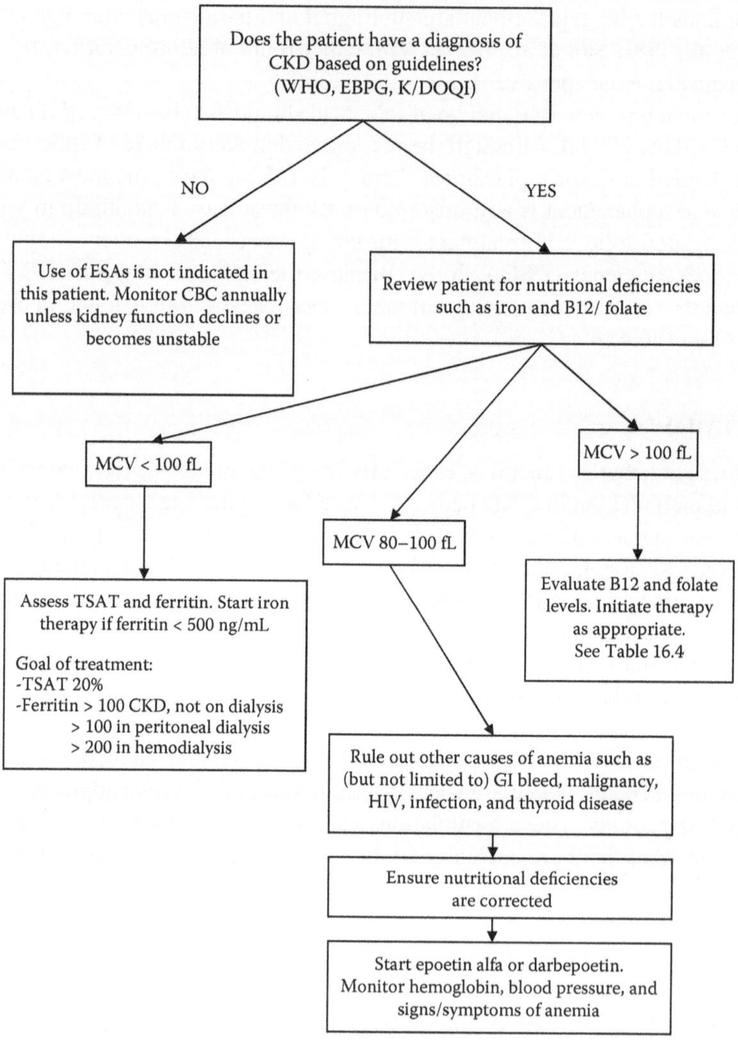

FIGURE 16.1 Work-up of anemia. *Abbreviations*: CBC, complete blood count; CKD, chronic kidney disease; ESA, erythropoietin-stimulating agents; GI, gastrointestinal; HIV, human immunodeficiency virus; MCV, mean corpuscular volume; TSAT, transferrin saturation.

16.8 SUMMARY

Patients with CKD should be monitored closely for anemia (Figure 16.1). Should their Hgb values fall below the desired range, a thorough workup to determine the underlying cause should be undertaken. There are many treatment options to correct deficiencies of both hormones and nutrients. No matter the course of treatment, all patients should be followed closely in order to prevent potentially harmful and even fatal outcomes due to poorly controlled anemia.

REFERENCES

Agarwal, R., Vasavada, N., Sachs, N., et al. 2004. Oxidative stress and renal injury with intravenous iron in patients with chronic kidney disease. *Kidney Int.* 65(6):2279–2289.

Astor, B., Muntner, P., Levin, A., et al. 2002. Association of kidney function with anemia: The Third National Health and Nutrition Examination Survey (1988–1994). *Arch Intern Med.* 162(12):1401–1408.

Ateshkadi, A., Johnson, C., Oxton, et al. 1993. Pharmacokinetics of intraperitoneal, intravenous and subcutaneous recombinant human erythropoietin in patients on continuous ambulatory peritoneal dialysis. *Am J Kidney Dis*. 21(6):635–642.

Attallah, N., Osman-Malik, Y., Frinak, S., et al. 2006. Effect of intravenous ascorbic acid in hemodialysis patients with EPO-hyporesponsive anemia and hyperferritinemia. *Am J Kidney Dis*. 47(4):644–654.

Bain, M., Faull, R., Milne, R., et al. 2006. Oral L-carnitine: Metabolite formation and hemodialysis. *Curr Drug Metab*. 7(7):811–816.

Ballal, S., Domoto, D., Polack, D., et al. 1991. Androgens potentiate the effects of erythropoietin in the treatment of anemia of end-stage renal disease. *Am J Kidney Dis*. 17(1):29–33.

Besarab, A., Amin, N., Ahsan, M., et al. 2000. Optimization of epoetin therapy with intravenous iron therapy in hemodialysis patients. *J Am Soc Nephrol*. 11(3):530–538.

Besarab, A. and Levin, A. 2000. Defining a renal anemia management period. *Am J Kidney Dis*. 36(6 Suppl 3):S13–S23.

Beutler, E. and Waalen, J. 2006. The definition of anemia: What is the lower limit of normal of the blood hemoglobin concentration? *Blood* 107(5):1747–1750.

Beutler, E. and West, C. 2005. Hematologic differences between African-Americans and whites: The roles of iron deficiency and alpha-thalassemia on hemoglobin levels and mean corpuscular volume. *Blood* 106(2):740–745.

Bolaman, Z., Kadikoylu, G., Yukselen, V., et al. 2003. Oral versus intramuscular cobalamin treatment in megaloblastic anemia: A single-center, prospective, randomized, open-label study. *Clin Ther*. 25(12): 3124–3134.

Bosman, D., Winkler, A., Marsden, J., et al. 2001. Anemia with erythropoietin deficiency occurs early in diabetic nephropathy. *Diabetes Care* 24(3):495–499.

Bothwell, T. 1995. Overview and mechanisms of iron regulation. *Nutr Rev*. 53(9):237–245.

Bridges, K. and Hoffman, K. 1986. The effects of ascorbic acid on the intracellular metabolism of iron and ferritin. *J Biol Chem*. 261(30):14273–14277.

Butler, C., Vidal-Alaball, J., Cannings-John, R., et al. 2006. Oral vitamin B12 versus intramuscular vitamin B12 for vitamin B12 deficiency: A systematic review of randomized controlled trials. *Fam Pract*. 23(3):279–285.

Canavese, C., Petrarulo, M., Massarenti, P., et al. 2005. Long-term, low-dose intravenous vitamin C leads to plasma calcium oxalate supersaturation in hemodialysis patients. *Am J Kidney Dis*. 45(3):540–549.

Canziani, M., Yumiya, S., Rangel, E., et al. 2001. Risk of bacterial infection in patients under intravenous iron therapy: Dose versus length of treatment. *Artif Organs*. 25(11):866–869.

Charytan, C., Levin, N., Al-Saloum, M., et al. 2001. Efficacy and safety of iron sucrose for iron deficiency in patients with dialysis-associated anemia: North American clinical trial. *Am J Kidney Dis*. 37(2):300–307.

Charytan, C., Qunibi, W., and Bailie, G. 2005. Venofer Clinical Studies Group. Comparison of intravenous iron sucrose to oral iron in the treatment of anemic patients with chronic kidney disease not on dialysis. *Nephron Clin Pract*. 100(3):c55–c62.

Chen, W., Lin, Y., Yu, F., et al. 2003. Effect of ascorbic acid administration in hemodialysis patients on in vitro oxidative stress parameters: Influence of serum ferritin levels. *Am J Kidney Dis*. 42(3):158–166.

Clement, F., Klarenbach, S., Tonelli, M., et al. 2009. The impact of selecting a high hemoglobin level on health-related quality of life for patients with chronic kidney disease: A systematic review and meta-analysis. *Arch Intern Med*. 169(12):1104–1112.

Collins, A. 2002. Influence of target hemoglobin in dialysis patients on morbidity and mortality. *Kidney Int Suppl*. 80:44–48.

Collins, A., Li, S., St. Peter, W., et al. 2001. Death, hospitalization and economic associations among incident hemodialysis patients with hematocrit values of 36 to 39%. *J Am Soc Nephrol*. 12(11):2465–2473.

Cunningham, J., Sharman, V., Goodwin, F., et al. 1981. Do patients receiving haemodialysis need folic acid supplements? *Br Med J* (Clin Res Ed). 282(6276):1582.

Delpre, G., Stark, P., and Niv, Y. 1999. Sublingual therapy for cobalamin deficiency as an alternative to oral and parenteral cobalamin supplementation. *Lancet* 354(9180):740–741.

Descombes, E., Hanck, A., and Fellay, G. 1993. Water soluble vitamins in chronic hemodialysis patients and need for supplementation. *Kidney Int*. 43(6):1319–1328.

Deved, V., Poyah, P., James, M., et al. 2009. Ascorbic acid for anemia management in hemodialysis patients: a systematic review and meta-analysis. *Am J Kidney Dis*. 54(5):1089–1097.

Dharmarajan, T., Pankratov, A., and Morris, E. 2008. Anemia: Its impact on hospitalizations and length of hospital stay in nursing home and community older adults. *J Am Med Dir Assoc*. 9(5):354–359.

Eknoyan, G., Latos, D., and Lindberg, J.2003. National Kidney Formation Carnitine Consensus Conference. Practice recommendations for the use of L-carnitine in dialysis-related carnitine disorder. National Kidney Foundation Carnitine Consensus Conference. *Am J Kidney Dis.* 41(4):868–876.

Erslev, A. 1991. Erythropoietin. *N Engl J Med.* 324(19):1339–1344.

Eschbach, J., Downing, M., Egrie, J., et al. 1989. USA multicenter clinical trial with recombinant human erythropoietin (Amgen) results in hemodialysis patients. *Contrib Nephrol.* 76:160–165.

Eschbach Jr., K., Funk, D., Adamson, J., et al. 1967. Erythropoiesis in patients with renal failure undergoing chronic dialysis. *N Engl J Med.* 276(12):653–658.

Eussen, S., de Groot, L., Clarke, R., et al. 2005. Oral cyanocobalamin supplementation in older people with vitamin B12 deficiency: A dose-finding trial. *Arch Inter Med.* 165(10):1167–1172.

Evans, A. 2003. Dialysis-related carnitine disorder and levocarnitine pharmacology. *Am J Kidney Dis.* 41(4 Suppl 4):S13–S26.

Fernandez-Rodriguez, A., Guindeo-Casasus, M., Molero-Labarta, T., et al. 1999. Diagnosis of iron deficiency in chronic renal failure. *Am J Kidney Dis.* 34(3):508–513.

Fick, D., Cooper, J., Wade, W., et al. 2003. Updating the Beers criteria for potentially inappropriate medication use in older adults: results of a US consensus panel of experts. *Arch Intern Med.* 163(22): 2716–2724.

Fink, J., Blahut, S., Reddy, M., et al. 2001. Use of erythropoietin before the initiation of dialysis and its impact on mortality. *Am J Kidney Dis.* 37(2):348–355.

Fishbane, S. 2003. Safety in iron management. *Am J Kidney Dis.* 41(Suppl 5):18–26.

Fishbane, S. 2007. Iron management in nondialysis-dependent CKD. *Am J Kidney Dis.* 49(6):736–743.

Fishbane, S. and Besarab A. 2007. Mechanism of increased mortality risk with erythropoietin treatment to higher hemoglobin targets. *Clin J Am Soc Nephrol.* 2(6):1274–1282.

Foley, R., Curtis, B., and Parfrey, P. 2009. Erythropoietin therapy, hemoglobin targets and quality of life in healthy hemodialysis patients: A randomized trial. *Clin J Am Soc Nephrol.* 4(4):726–733.

Gaughan, W., Liss, K., Dunn, S., et al. 1997.A 6-month study of low-dose recombinant human erythropoietin alone and in combination with androgens for the treatment of anemia in chronic hemodialysis patients. *Am J Kidney Dis.* 30(4):495–500.

Go, A., Yang, J., Ackerson, L., et al. 2006. Hemoglobin level, chronic kidney disease, and the risks of death and hospitalizations in adults with chronic heart failure: The Anemia in Chronic Heart Failure: Outcomes and Resource Utilization (ANCHOR) study. *Circulation* 113(23):2713–2723.

Goddard, A., McIntyre, A., and Scott, B. 2000. Guidelines for the management of iron deficiency anaemia. British Society of Gastroenterology. *Gut* 46(Suppl 3–4):IV1–IV5.

Golper, T., Goral, S., Becker, B., et al. 2003. L-carnitine treatment of anemia. *Am J Kidney Dis.* 41(4 Suppl 4):S27–S34.

Guralnik, J., Eisenstaedt, R., Ferrucci, L., et al. 2004. Prevalence of anemia in persons 65 years and older in the United States: Evidence for a high rate of unexplained anemia. *Blood* 104(8):2263–2268.

Halberg, L. 1981. Bioavailability of dietary iron in man. *Annu Rev Nutr.* 1:123–147.

Hampl, H., Stenberg, C., Berweck, S., et al. 2002. Regression of left ventricular hypertrophy in hemodialysis patients is possible. *Clin Nephrol.* 58(Suppl 1):S73–S96.

Hillman, R. and Finch, C. 1996. *Red Cell Manual.* 7th edition. Philadelphia, PA: Davis.

Hurot, J., Cucherat, M., Haugh, M., et al. 2002. Effects of L-carnitine supplementation in maintenance hemodialysis patients: A systematic review. *J Am Soc Nephrol.* 13(3):708–714.

Jadoul, M., Vanrenterghem, Y., Foret, M., et al. 2004. Darbepoetinalfa administered once monthly maintains haemoglobin levels in stable dialysis patients. *Nephrol Dial Transplant.* 19(4):898–903.

Keven, K., Kutlay, S., Nergizoglu, G., et al. 2003. Randomized, crossover study of the effect of vitamin C on EPO response in hemodialysis patients. *Am J Kidney Dis.* 41(6):1233–1239.

Kitamura, Y., Satoh, K., Satoh, T., et al. 2005. Effect of L-carnitine on erythroid colony formation in mouse bone marrow cells. *Nephrol Dial Transplant.* 20(5):981–984.

Kletzmayr, J. and Horl, W. 2002. Iron overload and cardiovascular complications in dialysis patients. *Nephrol Dial Transplant.* 17(Suppl 2):25–29.

Kooistra, M., Struyvenberg, A., and van Es, A. 1991. The response of recombinant human erythropoietin in patients with the anemia of end-stage renal disease is correlated with serum carnitine levels. *Nephron* 57(1):127–128.

Kuzminski, A., Del Giacco, E., Allen, R., et al. 1998. Effective treatment of cobalamin deficiency with oral cobalamin. *Blood* 92(4):1191–1198.

Levin, A. 1999. How should anaemia be managed in pre-dialysis patients? *Nephrol Dial Transplant.* 14(Suppl 2):66–74.

Levin, A. 2003. Clinical epidemiology of cardiovascular disease in chronic kidney disease prior to dialysis. *Semin Dial.* 16(2):101–105.

Levin, A., Singer, J., Thompson, C., et al. 1996. Prevalent left ventricular hypertrophy in the predialysis population identifying opportunities for intervention. *Am J Kidney Dis.* 27(3):347–354.

Lexi-Comp Online. February 2011. *Pediatric Lexi-Drugs Online.* Hudson, OH: Lexi-Comp, Inc.

Lipschitz, D., Bothwell, T., Seftel, H., et al. 1971. The role of ascorbic acid in the metabolism of storage iron. *Br J Haematol.* 20(2):155–163.

Locatelli, F., Aljama, P., Barany, P., et al. 2004. Revised European best practice guidelines for the management of anaemia in patients with chronic renal failure. *Nephrol Dial Transplant.* 19(Suppl2):ii, 1–47.

McClellan, W., Aronoff, S., Bolton, W., et al. 2004. The prevalence of anemia in patients with chronic kidney disease. *Curr Med Res Opin.* 20(9):1501–1510.

McGonigle, R., Wallin, J., Shadduck, R., et al. 1984. Erythropoietin deficiency and inhibition of erythropoiesis in renal insufficiency. *Kidney Int.* 25(2):437–444.

McGowan, T., Vaccaro, N., Beaver, J., et al. 2008. Pharmacokinetic and pharmacodynamic profiles of extended dosing of epoetinalfa in anemic patients who have chronic kidney disease and are not on dialysis. *Clin J Am Soc Nephrol.* 3(4):1006–1014.

Michael, B., Coyne, D., Fishbane, S., et al. 2002. Sodium ferric gluconate complex in hemodialysis patients: Adverse reactions compared to placebo and iron dextran. *Kidney Int.* 61(5):1830–1839.

Morris, M. and Davey, F. 1996. Basic examination of blood. In Henry, J.B., ed. *Clinical Diagnosis and Management by Laboratory Methods.* Philadelphia, PA: WB Saunders, 549–593.

National Kidney Foundation (NKF) K/DOQI. 2000. Clinical Practice Guidelines for nutrition in chronic renal failure. *Am J Kidney Dis.* 35(6 Suppl 2):S1–S140.

National Kidney Foundation (NKF) K/DOQI. 2006. Clinical Practice Guidelines for anemia in chronic kidney disease. *Am J Kidney Dis.* 47(5 Suppl 3):S11–S145.

National Kidney Foundation (NKF) K/DOQI. 2007. Clinical Practice Guidelines and Clinical Practice Recommendations for anemia in chronic kidney disease: 2007 Update of Hemoglobin Target. *Am J Kidney Dis.* 50(3):471–530.

Ofsthun, N., Labrecque, J., Lacson, E., et al. 2003. The effects of higher hemoglobin levels on mortality and hospitalization in hemodialysis patients. *Kidney Int.* 63(5):1908–1914.

Palmer, S., Navaneethan, S., Craig, J., et al. 2010. Meta-analysis: Erythropoiesis-stimulating agents in patients with chronic kidney disease. *Ann Intern Med.* 153(1):23–33.

Parkkinen, J., von Bonsdorff, L., Peltonen, S., et al. 2000. Catalytically active iron and bacterial growth in serum hemodialysis patients after intravenous iron-saccharate administration. *Nephrol Dial Transplant.* 15(11):1827–1834.

Phrommintikul, A., Haas, S., Elsik, M., et al. 2007. Mortality and target haemoglobin concentrations in anaemic patients with chronic kidney disease treated with erythropoietin: A meta-analysis. *Lancet* 369(9559):381–388.

Provenzano, R., Bhaduri, S., and Singh, A. 2005. PROMPT Study Group. Extended epoetinalfa dosing as maintenance treatment for the anemia of chronic kidney disease: The PROMPT study. *Clin Nephrol.* 64(2):113–123.

Radtke, H., Claussner, A., Erbes, P., et al. 1979. Serum erythropoietin concentration in chronic renal failure: Relationship to degree of anemia and excretory renal function. *Blood* 54(4):877–884.

Reed, W. and Diehl, L. 1991. Leukopenia, neutropenia and reduced hemoglobin levels in healthy American blacks. *Arch Intern Med.* 151(3):501–505.

Revicki, D., Brown, R., Feeny, D., et al. 1995. Health-related quality of life associated with recombinant human erythropoietin therapy for predialysis chronic renal disease patients. *Am J Kidney Dis.* 25(4):548–554.

Richalet, J., Soububielle, J., Atenzana, A., et al. 1994. Control of erythopoiesis in humans during prolonged exposure to the altitude of 6,542m. *Am J Physiol.* 266(3 Pt 2):R756–R764.

Ritz, E. and Eisenhardt, A. 2000. Early epoetin treatment in patients with renal insufficiency. *Nephrol Dial Transplant.* 15(Suppl3):40–44.

Ruiz-Arguelles, G. 2006. Altitude above sea level as a variable for definition of anemia. *Blood.* 108(6):2131; author reply.

Sezer, S., Ozdemir, F., Yakupoglu, U., et al. 2002. Intravenous ascorbic acid administration for erythropoietin-hyporesponsive anemia in iron loaded hemodialysis patients. *Artif Organs.* 26(4):366–370.

Sheashaa, H., Abdel-Razek, W., El-Husseini, A., et al. 2005. Use of nandrolonedecanoate as an adjuvant for erythropoietin dose reduction in treating anemia in patients on hemodialysis. *Nephron Clin Pract.* 99(40):c102–c106.

Siegenberg, D., Baynes, R., Bothwell, T., et al. 1994. Ascorbic acid prevents the dose-dependent inhibitory effects of polyphenols and phytates on nonheme-iron absorption. *Am J Clin Nutr.* 53(2):537–541.

Silverberg, D. 2003. Outcomes of anaemia management in renal insufficiency and cardiac disease. *Nephrol Dial Transplant.* 18(Suppl 2):ii, 7–12.

Slot, W., Merkus, F., Van Deventer, S., et al. 1997. Normalization of plasma vitamin B_{12} concentration by intranasal hydroxocobalamin in vitamin B_{12}-deficient patients. *Gastroenterology* 113(2):430–433.

Stoves, J., Inglis, H., and Newstead, C. 2001. A randomized study of oral vs. intravenous iron supplementation in patients with progressive renal insufficiency treated with erythropoietin. *Nephrol Dial Transplant.* 16(5):967–974.

Suranyi, M., Lindberg, J., Navarro, J., et al. 2003. Treatment of anemia with darbepoetinalfa administered de novo once every other week in chronic kidney disease. *Am J Nephrol.* 23(2):106–111.

Tarng, D. and Huang, T. 1998. A parallel, comparative study of intravenous iron versus intravenous ascorbic acid for erythropoietin-hyporesponsive anaemia in haemodialysis patients with iron overload. *Nephrol Dial Transplant.* 13(11):2867–2872.

U.S. Department of Agriculture (USDA), Agricultural Research Service. 2009. USDA National Nutrient Database for Standard Reference, Release 22. Nutrient Data Laboratory Home Page. Available at: http://www.ars.usda.gov/ba/bhnrc/ndl

U.S. Food and Drug Administration (USFDA). February 2007a. Folic acid: Prescribing information. Silver Spring, MD: U.S. Food and Drug Administration.

U.S. Food and Drug Administration (USFDA). March, 2007b. Epogen (epoetinalfa), procrit (epoetinalfa), aranesp (darbepoetinalfa) for injection: Prescribing information. Silver Spring, MD: U.S. Food and Drug Administration (USFDA).

U.S. Renal Data System (USRDS). 2008. Annual data report: Atlas of chronic kidney disease and end-stage renal disease in the United States. Bethesda, MD: National Institutes of Health, National Institute of Diabetes and Digestive and Kidney Diseases.

Van Duijnhoven, H. and Treskes, M. 1996. Marked interference of hyperglycemia in measurements of mean (red) cell volume by Technicon H analyzers. *Clin Chem.* 42(1):76–80.

Vaziri, N. 1999. Mechanism of erythropoietin-induced hypertension. *Am J Kidney Dis.* 33(5):821–828.

Wish, J. 2006. Assessing iron status: beyond serum ferritin and transferrin saturation. *Clin J Am Soc Nephrol.* 1(Suppl 1):S4–S8.

World Health Organization (WHO). 2001. *Iron Deficiency Anemia: Assessment, Prevention and Control. A Guide for Program Managers.* Geneva, Switzerland: World Health Organization.

17 Enteral and Parenteral Nutritional Support

Kyle Thompson
Appalachian State University

Lynn K. Thomas
University of South Carolina School of Medicine

CONTENTS

17.1 INTRODUCTION

When renal dysfunction is present in a critically ill patient, intensive nutritional management is required. Critically ill patients with renal disease tend to present as complicated cases, are often malnourished, and may exhibit numerous nutrition-related metabolic aberrations. This chapter discusses the practice of enteral and parenteral nutritional support in critically ill patients with renal disease.

17.2 DEFINITION AND PURPOSE OF ENTERAL NUTRITION

Enteral nutrition (EN) is the process of providing nutrients through a tube that delivers food directly into the stomach or small bowel. Alternatively called tube feeding, EN may be administered through a nasal tube into the stomach or small bowel, or via a tube placed in the stomach or small bowel through the abdominal wall.

The purpose of EN is to meet nutritional requirements when the patient's gastrointestinal tract is functional but he or she is unable to meet nutrient needs through oral intake. Compared with parenteral nutrition, enteral feeding is associated with improved maintenance of gastrointestinal mucosal function and fewer infectious complications. Enteral feeding is also much less expensive than parenteral nutrition. Therefore, it should be used preferentially to parenteral nutrition or in combination with parenteral nutrition if nutrient needs cannot be met by the enteral route alone (Druml, 2010). Parenteral nutrition should be reserved for patients who are unable to utilize nutrients taken in via the gastrointestinal route.

17.2.1 Goals of EN Therapy

Goals of EN therapy include improving or maintaining nutritional parameters, including lab values, weight, and quality of life. EN is also used to prevent the development of nutrient deficiencies that may negatively impact patient outcomes.

Evidence indicates that EN substantially increases total dietary intake; however, data to associate improved intake with better clinical outcomes are lacking. EN has been associated with improved serum albumin, which is an important indicator of prognosis in renal disease (Stratton et al., 2005).

17.2.2 Indications for EN

For all patients with renal disease, whether acute or chronic, EN should be considered if oral intake from meals, snacks, and oral supplements is inadequate to meet estimated or measured needs for a period ranging from several days to 2 weeks (National Kidney Foundation/KDOQI, 2000).

The feeding route should be considered. Nasogastric or percutaneous endoscopic gastrostomy (PEG) tube placements are preferred for patients on fluid restriction. Feeding into the stomach allows for the use of hypertonic 1.5–2 cal/mL formulas. Placement of a PEG tube is usually contraindicated in patients receiving peritoneal dialysis because of a significantly heightened risk of infection. The presence of pancreatitis or gastroparesis may require placement of the feeding tube tip into the small bowel rather than the stomach (Krenitsky, 2004). These feedings will require more volume in order to reach recommended calorie and protein levels.

A thorough nutrition assessment should be performed prior to initiating EN to determine whether the patient may benefit from enteral feedings. Assessment should include all relevant anthropometric, clinical, biochemical, and dietary parameters. Particular considerations in nutrition assessment for critically ill patients with renal disease include an evaluation of treatable problems that may be causing nutrition difficulties, paying attention to medications with nutrition-related side effects, and assessing the patient's current level of renal function. For patients receiving hemodialysis, the dialysis regimen and the possible presence of uremia should be considered as a source of eating problems (Krenitsky, 2004).

If possible and prudent per patient's condition, oral diet and oral supplementation should be attempted prior to initiation of enteral feeding. If no trial of oral feeding is possible, in most cases the patient should receive EN within 24–48 h of entering the intensive care unit (ICU) (McClave et al., 2009).

17.2.3 Delivery of EN Therapy

Nutrient needs for critically ill renal patients vary with the type of illness. Table 17.1 provides suggested macronutrient recommendations for various categories of renal disease. Clinical judgment is important in individualizing the nutrition prescription to the patient, taking into account age, body size, therapeutic goals, and overall medical condition. The nutrition prescription should be adjusted as needed based on careful monitoring of the patient's condition throughout the clinical course.

When estimating calorie needs in the ICU setting, it is important to take into account calorie-providing medications such as the sedative Diprivan® (propofol), delivered in a 10% lipid emulsion providing 1.1 cal/mL. In addition, IV fluids that provide calories, such as solutions containing 5% dextrose (providing 170 cal/L) should be included in the total calorie count to avoid overfeeding (Fuhrman, 2004).

17.2.4 Selection of Formula

Formula selection for critically ill renal patients depends on the patient's nutritional status, including laboratory values, and the patient's degree of renal function.

Many renal patients are able to tolerate standard enteral formulas. Standard formulas are less expensive than disease-specific formulas, and may result in fewer gastrointestinal complications

TABLE 17.1
Daily Nutrient Requirements

	Acute Kidney Injury	CKD	Dialysis
Fluids	Output plus 500 ccs	Restrict as necessary	Output plus 1000 ccs
Energy[a]	30–35 kg	30–35 kg	30–35 kg
Protein[b]	0.6–0.8 g/kg	0.6–0.75 g/kg	1.2–1.4 g/kg
Sodium	1–2 g	1–3 g	2 g
Potassium	Serum within normal limits (WNL)	Unrestricted unless elevated	2g
Calcium	Serum WNL	Serum WNL	<2.0 g
Phosphorus	Serum WNL	10–12 mg/g/protein	12–15 mg/g/protein
Vitamins/minerals	Follow Recommended Daily Allowance (RDA)	B-complex plus C, Individualized vitamin D, iron, and zinc	Ascorbic acid 60–100 mg Pyridoxine 2 mg B123 μg Vitamin E 15 IU Zinc 15 mg No vitamin A or K Individualize vitamin D and iron RDA others

Abbreviation: CKD, chronic kidney disease.

[a] For some critical care situations, energy needs may be reduced temporarily to 20–25 kcal/kg.

[b] Increase amount if renal replacement therapy is used. Usually in the 1.0–1.7 g/kg/day range depending on the type of therapy.

due to osmolalities, which are typically lower than those of disease-specific formulas (Mueller and Bloch, 2008).

If nutrition assessment reveals no electrolyte irregularities which might require a disease-specific formula, the patient may be started on a standard enteral formula and monitored for fluid status and electrolyte changes. If fluid volume is a concern, a 2-cal/mL formula may be selected to deliver adequate nutrients in a smaller amount of formula (Wolk et al., 2007).

Hyperpotassemia, hypermagnesemia, and hyperphosphatemia are the most common issues that prompt selection of a disease-specific formula (Marian and McGinnis, 2007).

Renal-specific enteral formulas are designed to provide lower intakes of magnesium, sodium, phosphorus, and potassium compared to standard formulas (Chen and Peterson, 2009). See Table 17.2 for a comparison of renal-specific formulas to standard formulas.

Little research has been done to date regarding outcomes of standard formulas versus disease-specific formulas (Chen and Peterson, 2009; Malone, 2005; Stratton et al., 2005; Table 17.2).

TABLE 17.2
Standard and Renal-Specific Formulas (Oral Supplement and Tube Feeding)

Product	Calorie (s/mL)	CHO (g/L)	PRO (g/L)	FAT (g/L)	Na	K (mg/L)	PO_4 (mg/L)	Vitamin A (IU)	%H_2O (L)
Boost® (Nestle')	1.0	173	42	17.8	550	1690	1270	5400	85
Boost® Glucose Control (Nestle')	1.1	84	58.2	49	1099	1099	928	5063	85
Boost Plus® (Nestle')	1.5	190	59	58	720	1610	1270	5400	78
Ensure® (Abbott)	1.1	164	36	24	800	1480	1000	5000	83
Ensure Plus® (Abbott)	1.5	200	54.9	53.3	880	2114	840	5000	68
Glucerna® (Abbott)	1.5	133	82.5	75	1380	2520	1000	8660	76
Nepro® (Abbott)	1.8	161	81	96	1060	1060	720	3180	73
Novasource® Renal (Nestle')	2	200	74	100	900–1600	810–1100	650	3300	70
Nutren Renal® (Nestlé)	2	205	70	104	740	1256	700	4996	70
Re/Gen HP/ HC® Shelf Stable (Nutra/ balance)	2	261	67	67	1000	1277	377	n/a	n/a
Suplena® Carb Steady (Abbott)	1.8	196	45	96	802	1137	717	3165	74

17.2.4.1 Acute Kidney Injury

In acute kidney injury (AKI), standard tube feedings are appropriate unless a fluid restriction is indicated, in which case a high-calorie (2 cal/mL) standard formula may be used. Because patients with AKI are often in a catabolic state, protein should not be restricted; a standard high-protein formula may be considered.

Suggested energy ranges are 25–35 cal/kg/day (Cano et al., 2009). The AKI staging system developed by Mehta et al. (2007) recommends estimating daily requirements at the higher end of the range based on advanced disease state and comorbidities (Stages 2 and 3) (Table 17.3). Daily protein requirements can also be based on stage of AKI. Restrictions are not generally advised since inadequate protein intake increases the risk for malnutrition.

In the advanced stages of AKI, patients often require renal replacement therapy (RRT). This can be either intermittent or continuous dialysis. While on RRT, calories, fluids, and protein allowances can be increased as warranted.

17.2.4.2 Chronic Renal Failure

Patients with chronic renal failure should receive either a standard formula or disease-specific formula based on the results of a thorough nutritional assessment. Standard formulas should be used preferentially to disease-specific formulas if the patient's nutritional status permits. Energy and nutrient requirements should be based on stage of chronic kidney disease (CKD) and any comorbidities that necessitate further adjustments. Refer to Table 17.1 for daily nutrient requirements for dialysis patients.

17.2.4.3 Hemodialysis

For hemodialysis patients, prescribe either a standard formula or a renal-specific formula as indicated by the results of the nutritional assessment. If a standard formula is indicated, consider a standard high-protein formula due to the increased protein losses associated with dialysis. All standard formulas are low in sodium, but keep in mind any potassium and phosphorus restrictions when using the high-protein formulas (Malone, 2005).

TABLE 17.3
Classification/Staging System for Acute Kidney Injury[a]

Stage	Serum Creatinine	Urine Output Criteria
1	Increase in serum creatinine of more than or equal to 0.3 mg/dL (≥26.4 μmol/L) or increase to more than or equal to 150%–200% (1.5- to 2-fold) from baseline	Less than 0.5 mL/kg/h for more than 6 h
2[b]	Increase in serum creatinine to more than 200%–300% (>2- to 3-fold) from baseline	Less than 0.5 mL/kg/h for more than 12 h
3[c]	Increase in serum creatinine to more than 300% (>3-fold) from baseline (or serum creatinine of more than or equal to 4.0 mg/dL [≥354 μmol/L] with an acute increase of at least 0.5 mg/dL [44 μmol/L])	Less than 0.3 mL/kg/h for 24 h or anuria for 12 h

[a] Modified from RIFLE (Risk, Injury, Failure, Loss, and End-stage kidney disease) criteria. The staging system proposed is a highly sensitive interim staging system and is based on recent data indicating that a small change in serum creatinine influences outcome. Only one criterion (creatinine or urine output) has to be fulfilled to qualify for a stage.

[b] 200%–300% increase = 2- to 3-fold increase.

[c] Given wide variation in indications and timing of initiation of renal replacement therapy (RRT), individuals who receive RRT are considered to have met the criteria for stage 3 irrespective of the stage they are in at the time of RRT.

Source: Mehta, R., et al., 2007 *Crit. Care.*, 11, R31–R39, 2007.

17.2.5 Administration of Enteral Formula

For most patients, it is prudent to begin feeding at about 50% the desired rate, gradually advancing the rate of feeding by 10 mL/h every 8–12 h until the goal rate is reached. With medically fragile patients such as the frail elderly, the malnourished patient, or the patient with a history of severe gastrointestinal disease, the clinician may wish to initiate and advance feedings at a slower rate. Patients must be closely monitored for metabolic problems during the initiation of EN.

Restriction of potassium and phosphorus during feeding initiation can lead to the development of the medical emergency of hypokalemia and/or hypophosphatemia, especially if the patient is taking phosphate-binding medications (Charney and Charney, 2002). Discontinuation or dose reduction of phosphate binders may be indicated, especially if the patient is receiving a renal formula and is not receiving any oral nutrition. Elderly, malnourished, and patients with a history of alcohol abuse are especially prone to electrolyte abnormalities. In some cases, a phosphorus supplement may be required to maintain adequate levels. Consider the patient's overall plan for the administration of medications, as adjustment of either the medication or the tube feeding schedule may be required to maximize the benefits of medications and nutrition.

17.2.6 Monitoring and Adverse Reactions

Careful monitoring of patients receiving EN in the critical care setting is essential to achieve desired outcomes. The nutritional parameters that should be monitored include fluid status, serum electrolytes, indicators of protein status, glycemic markers, clinical course, and factors involved in the transfer of nutrition care from one setting to another.

In order to assist in the difficult task of monitoring a renal patient's weight, dry weight may be measured or estimated. Once the patient's dry weight is established, subsequent fluid weight gains can be monitored. Intake and outtake records are helpful in assessing fluid weight status. Fluid weight gain should be kept within a desired range. Fluid restriction can be used to manage fluid weight gain, and high-calorie enteral formulas can assist in meeting fluid intake goals. Weight should be monitored daily in the critical care setting (Furhman, 2004).

Electrolyte status should be monitored closely. As previously discussed, it is best not to use a renal formula on a default basis, but to use a standard formula if possible, owing to the possibility of hypokalemia or hypophosphatemia. Electrolytes may be modified by adjusting the type of enteral formula used, and by means of appropriate supplementation and/or medications. Electrolytes should be monitored daily until stability is achieved, and then should be monitored several times per week while the patient is in the critical and acute care settings (Fuhrman, 2004).

Protein indicators for renal patients include albumin and prealbumin. Albumin is associated with prognosis in renal patients, but is a reflection of underlying disease rather than nutritional status. Prealbumin is inversely associated with acute-phase reactants such as C-reactive protein (Krenitsky, 2004). If a patient could benefit from additional protein, a high-protein formula may be provided. Alternatively, a protein powder or liquid protein supplement may be administered through the feeding tube.

The most common metabolic anomaly of critical illness is hyperglycemia. Because nearly two-thirds of persons with renal disease also have type 1 or type 2 diabetes, hyperglycemia is a major issue for renal patients in critical care settings. Hyperglycemia should be closely monitored and carefully managed, since both critical illness and diabetes may increase blood glucose levels by promoting insulin resistance and increased gluconeogenesis (Fuhrman, 2004). In the order of increasingly aggressive management, subcutaneous insulin, sliding scale insulin, or a continuous insulin drip may be used to manage blood glucose levels. If the patient is capable of oral intake, oral hypoglycemic agents may also be used. Blood glucose should be monitored 4–6 times per day in the critical care setting (Fuhrman, 2004).

TABLE 17.4
Suggested Minimal Monitoring

Weigh every other day until stable then weekly for acute care and monthly for long-term care. Daily weights may be required in intensive care settings and for dialysis patients.
Basic electrolytes plus calcium, magnesium, and phosphorous, complete blood count initially then every 10 days. Do more frequently in intensive care situations. Do monthly or at least quarterly in long-term care and in the dialysis clinic.
Albumin initially, then every month. Other more frequent assays and monitoring parameters are used in intensive care.
Monitor glucose readings until feeding or nutrition support is at final rate and blood sugars are stable.
Check inputs and outputs according to unit policies.

The patient's clinical course should be monitored (Table 17.4), including overall medical condition, overall nutrition status, medications, concurrent therapies, and discharge planning (Wolk et al., 2007).

As the patient progresses through the continuum of care, it is important to consider nutritional factors that may affect the patient in subsequent nutrition care settings. Collaboration of nutrition care with future caregivers, including clinicians in acute care facilities, case managers/social workers, long-term care providers, homecare staff, and family members will help to ensure a smoother transition for the patient to other care settings. If the patient receives regular hemodialysis, the renal dietitian who works with the patient at the dialysis center may provide valuable assistance in ensuring optimal nutrition care throughout the nutrition-care process.

17.2.7 Transitional Enteral Feedings

If the patient's clinical condition improves so that he or she can begin taking nutrients by mouth, a transitional feeding plan should be implemented. Diet restrictions should be implemented based on nutritional assessment; no restriction should be imposed without clinical justification because of the risk of promoting poor intake and subsequent malnutrition (Krenitsky, 2004).

Begin oral feedings with small amounts of the appropriate foods. Gradually increase the amount of oral intake and decrease the amount of tube feeding over a period of 2 days to 1 week. Initiate a calorie count when oral intake begins. When the patient is able to consume ≥75% of calories by mouth for 2–3 consecutive days, it is appropriate to discontinue the tube feeding. Continue to monitor the patient's oral intake by calorie count until adequate oral intake is established. Assess nutrition education needs and provide appropriate diet education to the patient and the patient's family (Marion and McGinnis, 2007).

17.3 INDICATIONS FOR PARENTERAL NUTRITION

Indications for parenteral nutrition in renal patients are similar to those for other critically ill patients. Parenteral nutrition is usually reserved for patients who are too ill to maintain adequate oral nutrition and cannot tolerate enteral nutrition because of gastrointestinal complications. Provision of parenteral nutrition to renal patients is similar to that for other critically ill patients.

Parenteral nutrition is associated with increased risk of infections compared to EN, and it is much more costly than enteral feedings. Parenteral nutrition also requires a greater fluid volume to deliver nutrients than EN (Krenitsky, 2004).

Parenteral nutrition may be contraindicated in patients for whom intravenous access cannot be established or who have a poor prognosis (Fuhrman, 2004).

17.3.1 Goals of Parenteral Nutrition

The goals of parenteral nutrition therapy are to meet the patient's nutrient needs, appropriately manage fluids and electrolytes, maintain or improve nutritional status, and prevent development of nutrient deficiencies (Fuhrman, 2004).

17.3.2 Delivery of Parenteral Nutrition

Refer to Table 17.1 for macronutrient recommendations for several renal conditions.

When determining a recommended dextrose concentration for parenteral feedings, note that it may be possible to control fluid load by using a higher-dextrose concentration. Be sure to consider all sources of dextrose being provided to the patient, including those in IV fluids, before writing a nutrition prescription. The glucose utilization rate should not exceed 4–6 mg/kg/min in the critically ill patient.

Standard amino acid formulas such as 4.25%, 8.5%, and 10% Travasol® are typically used to provide protein parenterally to renal patients. Specialty amino acid formulas for renal patients have been used in the past, but these are rarely used today because they do not improve outcomes (Barber et al., 2007).

Lipid emulsion may be used to meet energy needs when controlling fluids. A 10% lipid emulsion contains 1.1 cal/mL, and a 20% lipid emulsion contains 2.0 cal/mL. All sources of lipid calories should be considered, including sedative medications such as propofol (Diprivan), which contains 1.1 cal/mL.

Overall fluid load should be monitored and adjusted based on patient tolerance and needs. Monitor electrolytes carefully and adjust as needed to maintain appropriate serum parameters. Electrolytes may be adjusted by changes in the parenteral infusion, by intravenous supplementation (although this adds to the fluid load), or by medication adjustments (Wolk et al., 2007).

A standard vitamin and trace-mineral infusion should be added to the solution bag. It is thought that vitamin and mineral requirements are changed in renal patients, but there is no parenteral vitamin and mineral preparation designed especially for renal patients. Vitamin A may be elevated in end-stage renal disease patients; however, because renal patients receiving parenteral nutrition are usually not eating, the standard vitamin preparation should not be problematic (Wilkens and Juneja, 2008).

17.3.3 Administration of Parenteral Nutrition

Parenteral nutrition should be initiated slowly at a rate of 20–30 mL/h. Monitor metabolic parameters carefully during initiation. Be especially vigilant for electrolyte irregularities, which may indicate development of refeeding syndrome, especially in malnourished patients. If the patient tolerates the infusion, advance by 10–15 mL/h at intervals of 8–12 h until goal rate is reached (Fuhrman, 2004).

17.3.4 Monitoring Parenteral Nutrition

Monitoring requirements are similar to those for any critically ill patient.

Monitor indicators of fluid status, including daily weights, intake and output records, and renal function indicators. Electrolytes should be monitored daily until stable. Once stable, electrolytes may be monitored several times per week (see Table 17.4).

Hyperglycemia should be closely monitored and carefully managed, since both critical illness and diabetes may increase blood glucose levels by promoting insulin resistance and increased gluconeogenesis (Fuhrman, 2004). In order of increasingly aggressive management, subcutaneous insulin, sliding scale insulin, or a continuous insulin drip may be used to manage blood glucose levels. If the patient is capable of oral intake, oral hypoglycemic agents may also be used. Blood glucose should be monitored 4–6 times per day in the critical care setting (Fuhrman, 2004).

Ensure that a standard vitamin and trace-element infusion is provided.

The patient's clinical course should be monitored, including overall medical condition, overall nutrition status, medications, concurrent therapies, and discharge planning (Wolk et al., 2007). Monitoring the patient for coordination of care issues is similar to that of the patient receiving EN.

If the patient's condition permits, it is to the patient's advantage to transition to enteral/oral feedings as soon as possible. Monitoring of traditional nutrition parameters, such as appetite and diet records (if the patient is consuming oral nutrients), are helpful in determining an appropriate timetable for transitioning to gastrointestinal feedings.

17.3.5 Adverse Reactions

Refeeding syndrome can occur in malnourished patients. Symptoms include generalized fatigue, edema, hemolysis, and cardiac arrhythmias. To avoid the associated adverse reactions of hypophosphatemia, hypomagnesemia, and hypokalemia, initiate parenteral nutrition slowly and monitor closely. Make immediate adjustments for electrolyte aberrations (Kumpf and Gervasio, 2007).

17.3.6 Transitional Feedings

If the patient's clinical condition improves to the point that the patient can begin taking nutrients enterally or by mouth, a transitional feeding plan should be implemented. Transitional feedings may occur in the renal patient in much the same way as with the patient without kidney disease; the difference lies in tailoring the oral diet to the patient's degree of renal function and oral capability. Diet restrictions should be implemented based on the results of nutritional assessment; if restrictions are not clinically indicated they should not be imposed.

Enteral feedings may begin slowly based on patient tolerance. Even small amounts of enteral feeding may promote improved mucosal function and help to promote its important immune functions in decreasing infections (Charney, 2004; Druml and Kierdorf, 2009). Enteral feedings may begin at 20%–30% goal rate, then increase by 10–15 mL/h every 8–12 h until the goal rate is reached. As increasing amounts of enteral feeding are tolerated, decrease the parenteral infusion. When enteral feeds reach 60% of the goal rate, the parenteral infusion may be stopped. Monitor blood glucose levels closely during this process. Monitor the patient's tolerance of EN. If the patient is unable to tolerate the full dose of EN, a combination of EN and parenteral nutrition may be used to meet the patient's nutrient needs, ensuring that the patient receives the important benefits of EN (Marion and McGinnis, 2007).

Begin oral feedings with small amounts of appropriate foods; gradually increase the amount of oral intake and decrease the amount of tube feeding or parenteral nutrition over a period of 2 days to 1 week. Initiate a calorie count, comparing oral intake with estimated needs. When the patient is consuming ≥60% of calories by mouth, it is appropriate to discontinue the tube feeding and/or parenteral feeding.

If the patient remains unable to meet nutrient needs by mouth, consideration may be given to cyclic tube feedings or parental feedings, perhaps at night, to achieve nutrient needs. Collaboration with other members of the health care team is essential in smoothing this transition for the patient (Fuhrman, 2004).

17.4 INTRADIALYTIC PARENTERAL NUTRITION: INTRODUCTION AND GOAL OF THERAPY

The goal of all nutrition therapy is to improve the markers for malnutrition, and when appropriate, facilitate weight gain. Intradialytic parenteral nutrition (IDPN) is one of the strategies that can be employed in the effort to improve severe malnutrition in stage 5 CKD patients receiving dialysis. It is considered an advanced therapy and is tried only after dietary counseling, oral nutrition supplements, and tube feedings have failed.

17.4.1 Definition

IDPN is a solution of carbohydrate, amino acids, lipids, electrolytes, and vitamin/minerals that is infused during a patient's usual dialysis treatments. It is usually administered during the last 90 min of treatment. The delivery schedule is based on the premise that extra parenteral nutrients can be delivered and excess fluids extracted with no change in the dialysis regimen. It is thought that IDPN can be used as an aggressive clinical strategy to reverse malnutrition in the stage 5 CKD patient (Pupim et al., 2002).

Intraperitoneal nutrition (IPN) is similar to IDPN. This type of therapy is used to help improve hypoalbuminemia in patients receiving peritoneal dialysis. Protein and amino acid losses in the dialysate can reach 15 g/day. These losses contribute to chronic malnutrition (Wang et al., 2003). IPN solution replaces a portion of the glucose dialysate for one or two exchanges each day when continuous ambulatory peritoneal dialysis is being used. For patients using continuous cycler-assisted peritoneal dialysis, the IPN can be added to the last fill or given as a manual exchange during the day. Twenty to forty grams of amino acids can be administered to counteract daily losses and provide additional protein to reverse malnutrition (Fuhrman, 2009).

17.4.2 Malnutrition: Causes and Management

Malnutrition is a frequent problem in patients with stage 5 CKD. In adults, protein-energy malnutrition is strong predictor of morbidity and mortality. Causes include inadequate food intake, nutrient losses during dialysis, chronic inflammation, metabolic alterations, and catabolic responses to other chronic diseases (Kopple, 2000; Moore and Lindenfield, 2007).

Every malnourished patient is closely followed by the dietitian assigned to each clinic. A detailed nutrition assessment is completed as soon as a patient is recognized as being malnourished. Comorbid conditions affecting nutritional status should be identified and corrected at this time, if possible. Counseling, including meal planning with the patient and family members or caregivers, is the first strategy employed. Food supplements are suggested if dietary management fails to improve nutrition status. Two kinds of supplements are often recommended: either powdered protein supplements that are mixed with other foods or concentrated liquid supplements that provide both extra calories and protein. At this point in the therapy, appetite stimulants such as megestrol acetate are frequently tried.

If malnutrition cannot be reversed with aggressive oral intake, then enteral tube feedings are prescribed. Tube feedings require precise management of fluid status; delivery methods must be planned around visits to the dialysis clinic. Low-volume intermittent feedings can be used to complement inadequate oral intake or to provide the complete daily nutrient requirements. Unfortunately, tube feedings tend to be underutilized because of patient resistance (Wong et al., 2003).

In some instances, where a tube feeding is not practical, such as in peritoneal dialysis, amino acid solutions are used in place of dextrose exchanges up to twice a day. The amount of protein delivered by this method is limited due to restrictions on osmolarity during exchanges, but improvements in serum albumin have been documented (Kopple, 1999).

Parenteral nutrition, usually given either as a cyclic or a 24/7 infusion, is preferred over IDPN. Barriers to home parenteral nutrition frequently include patient adherence, lack of family support, inadequate home environment, and expense. IDPN has found a niche by virtue of being given at the dialysis clinic under medical supervision. According to a recent study with IDPN patients treated from 3 to 12 months, response to therapy appears to be associated with the severity of hypoalbuminemia. Severe hypoalbuminemia was defined as greater or equal to 3 g/dL (Dezfuli et al., 2009). This finding may help redefine IDPN criteria.

17.4.3 Criteria

To be eligible for IDPN, all previous trials of oral and enteral therapy must have failed. An inadequate nutrition status must be evidenced by persistent, severe protein malnutrition or severe energy

TABLE 17.5
Typical Measures to Determine Nutritional Status

Monthly	Quarterly	Biannual	As needed
Stabilized serum albumin	Percent of standard body weight or normal body mass index (10% weight loss over ≤ 3 months)	Subjective global assessment	Prealbumin
Percent of usual post treatment weight		Dietary interview	Stabilized serum creatinine or urea nitrogen
nPNA (protein equivalent of total nitrogen appearance)			Skin fold thickness or mid-arm muscle area, circumference

malnutrition with significant weight loss. K/DOQI™ Nutrition Guideline 19 outlines indications for nutritional support (Kopple, 2000). The indications include a documented period of inadequate intake, evidence of failed dietary therapy, and the need to combine IDPN with current oral intake to meet daily nutrient needs. Table 17.5 contains the typical biochemical and anthropometric measurement parameters used to justify the use of IDPN.

Inclusion criteria are similar for Medicare and most private insurers. The official Medicare language states: "If the medical record, including the judgment of the attending physician, indicates the impairment will be long and indefinite duration, the test of permanence is met. Unless there are contraindications, there must be a reasonable trial of both oral and enteral nutrition if the gastrointestinal tract is functional." (Medicare Manual, 2010).

IPN can be provided, according to K/DOQI guidelines, for peritoneal dialysis patients who are malnourished and consume inadequate energy and protein. They must be unable to tolerate an adequate oral diet or tube feeding. Inclusion criteria generally follow the standards set by the Centers for Medicare and Medicaid Services.

17.4.4 Formulations

IDPN solutions are typically 500–1000 mL in total volume. They are packaged as a 2-in-1 (dextrose and amino acids) or 3-in-1 (dextrose, amino acids, and lipids) admixtures. These mixtures can also contain vitamins, minerals, and electrolytes if needed. The admixtures are formulated to provide between 500 and 1200 calories and 1.2–1.4 g protein/kg (Wolk et al., 2007). Concentrations vary according to tolerance and considerations of chronic diseases such as diabetes mellitus (Table 17.6). Intravenous lipids are the most challenging of the macronutrients secondary to the potential for free-fatty-acid toxicity. In the serum, free fatty acids are bound to the albumin. Therefore, patients with low albumin levels have increased concentrations of unbound free fatty acids, which can cause cardiac and pulmonary injuries (How and Lau, 2004; Table 17.4).

IPN solutions contain the usual dialysate and amino acids based on the patient's usual peritoneal exchange prescription. For example, an amino acid solution of 1.5% would provide 30 g of protein in a 2 L volume of 2.5% dextrose (Fuhrman, 2009).

17.4.5 Delivery Methods

IDPN delivery is started below goal rate in order to assess patient tolerance. It usually requires at least three dialysis treatments to advance to complete nutrient delivery. The rate of infusion is generally determined by dividing the IDPN volume by the dialysis treatment time. The rate should not exceed 350 mL/h.

TABLE 17.6
Typical IDPN Formulations

Prescription[a]	Total Volume (mL)	Formula Composition = Calories	Total Calories
250 mL D50	500	125 g dextrose = 425	525
250 mL 10% AA		25 g protein = 100	
250 mL D70	800	175g dextrose = 595	815
550 mL 10% AA		55 g protein = 220	
250 mL D50	950	125 g dextrose = 425	1025
500 mL 10% AA		50 g protein = 200	
200 mL 20% lipids		200 mL lipids= 400	
250 mL D30	975	75 g dextrose =255	905
500 mL 10% AA		50 g protein = 200	
225 mL 20% lipids		225 mL lipids = 450	

[a] "D" indicates dextrose and "AA" indicates amino acids.

17.4.6 Advantages and Disadvantages

IDPN is administered during dialysis. Patient compliance is not a problem. It is also very convenient, with no extra dialysis treatments required. No additional access is necessary, and staff is on hand to monitor for intolerances or imbalances. The amount of ultrafiltration can be adjusted to compensate for extra fluid removal.

Evidence supporting the use of IDPN is limited. Most studies have small sample sizes. The majority of the data were compiled in the 70s, 80s, and early 90s before tighter Medicare regulations reduced the number of patients eligible for treatment. These studies did observe improvements in appetite, increases in serum albumin, total protein, and transferrin indices (Chertow et al., 1994; McCann et al., 1999; Pupim et al., 2002, 2004). In 1999, a 9-month study by Mortelmans et al. (1999) showed an increase in body weight and improvement in albumin and transferrin parameters of nutrition status.

IDPN is only delivered three times per week. This may not be sufficient for many severely malnourished patients, especially where gastrointestinal function is marginal. It often takes an extended amount of time to see improvements in nutritional status. The IDPN solution composition varied in the early studies, so no optimal solution has been defined (Wolk et al., 2007). Glucose metabolism changes, lipid intolerance, and refeeding syndrome are concerns with this IDPN therapy. In some cases, hypoglycemia reactions occur at the end of treatment (Burrowes et al., 1993). A recent 2-year multicenter, prospective randomized study showed that the use of IDPN did not improve survival. It reported no definite advantage over oral nutritional supplementation (Cano et al., 2007).

The cost of IDPN therapy is high. Medicare requires that specific criteria be met before reimbursement is allowed. Evidence of effectiveness is based mostly on individual reports or small studies. There is a lack of large prospective studies available to help the clinician decide risk/benefit ratio. However, there are certain circumstances in which the use of IDPN appears to be a reasonable method of nutrient replenishment.

17.4.7 Team Approach to Nutrition Support in Renal Disease

Many members of the health care team must collaborate to successfully care for the critically ill patient with renal disease. A nutrition support team consisting of a physician, a registered dietitian, a registered nurse, a registered pharmacist, a social worker, and appropriate therapists may work together to promote optimal outcomes for the patient. The patient is the beneficiary when members of the health care team cultivate excellent working relationships in order to develop trust and camaraderie, as well as promote a learning environment that supports collaboration and information sharing.

17.5 CONCLUSION

The provision of nutrition support to renal patients is similar to the provision of nutrition support to patients with normal kidney function. Renal patients require additional monitoring to promote maintenance of appropriate metabolic parameters. Skilled intervention by dietetics professionals is essential to achieving excellent outcomes in these complicated patients.

REFERENCES

Barber J., Rollins, C., Sacks, G. 2007. Parenteral nutrition formulations. In *The A.S.P.E.N. Nutrition Support Core Curriculum*. Silver Spring, MD: American Society for Parenteral and Enteral Nutrition, 277–299.

Boost®, Boost Plus, Boost Glucose Control, Novasourse® Renal, and Nutren® Renal. Available at: www.nestle-nutrition.com/products (accessed January 2011).

Burrowes, J., Alto, A., Kaufman, A. 1993. Intradialytic parenteral nutrition: A practical approach. *Am Nephrol Nurses Assoc J*. 20:671–677.

Cano, N., Aparicio, M., Brunori, G., et al. 2009. ESPEN guidelines on parenteral nutrition: Adult renal failure. *Clin Nutr.* 28:401–414.

Cano, N., Fouque, D., Roth, H., et al., and the French Study Group for Nutrition in Dialysis. 2007. Intradialytic parenteral nutrition does not improve survival in malnourished hemodialysis patients: A 2 year multicenter, prospective, randomized study. *Am Soc Nephrol.* 18:2583–2591.

Charney, P. 2004. Parenteral nutrition in kidney disease. In L. Byham-Gray, and K. Wiesen, (Eds.), *A Clinical Guide to Nutrition Care.* Chicago, IL: American Dietetic Association, Renal Practice Group, 151–158.

Charney, P. and Charney, D. 2002. Nutrition support in renal failure. *Nutr Clin Pract.* 17:226–235.

Chen, Y. and Peterson, S. 2009. Enteral Nutrition formulas: Which formula is right for your adult patient? *Nutr Clin Pract.* 24:344.

Chertow, G. Ling, J. Lew, N., et al. 1994. The association of intradialytic parenteral nutrition administration with survival in hemodialysis patients. *Am J Kidney Dis.* 24:912–920.

Dezfuli, A., Scholl, D., Lindenfield, S., et al. 2009. Severity of hypoalbuminemiapredicts response to intradialytic parenteral nutrition in hemodialysis patients. *J Renal Nutr.* 19:291–297.

Druml, W. 2010. Nutrition support in acute renal failure. In *Handbook of Nutrition and the Kidney*, Sixth Edition. Philadelphia, PA: Lippincott Williams & Wilkins, Wolters Kluwer, 84.

Druml, W. and Kierdorf, H. 2009. Parenteral nutrition in patients with renal failure. The German Association for Nutritional Medicine. *German Medical Science* v. 7. doi: 10.3205/000070 (accessed January 12, 2011).

Ensure®, Ensure Plus®, Glucerna®, Nepro®, and Suplena®. Available at: www.abbott.com/products (accessed January 2011).

Fuhrman, M. 2004. Parenteral nutrition in kidney disease. In L. Byham-Gray, and K. Wiesen, (Eds.), *A Clinical Guide to Nutrition Care.* Chicago, IL: American Dietetic Association, Renal Practice Group, 158–174.

Fuhrman, M. 2009. Intradialytic parenteral nutrition and intraperitoneal nutrition. *Nutrit Clin Pract.* 24:470–480.

How, P. and Lau, A. 2004. Intradialytic parenteral nutrition. *Pharmacotherapy* 24:12–18.

Kopple, J. 1999. Therapeutic approaches to malnutrition in chronic dialysis patients: The different modalities of nutritional support. *Am J Kidney Dis.* 33:180–185.

Kopple, J. for the K/DOQI Nutrition Work Group Membership. 2000. National Kidney Foundation. Kidney disease outcomes quality initiative: Clinical practice guidelines for nutrition in chronic renal failure. *Am J Kidney Dis.* 35 (suppl. 2):S17–S104.

Krenitsky, J. 2004. Nutrition in renal failure: Myths and management. *Pract Gastroenterol.* 20:40–59.

Kumpf, V. and Gervasio, J. 2007. Complications of parenteral nutrition. In Gottschlich, M. (Ed.), *The A.S.P.E.N. Nutrition Support Core Curriculum.* Silver Spring, MD: American Society for Parenteral and Enteral Nutrition, 323–339.

Malone, A. 2005. Enteral formula selection: A review of selected product categories. *Pract Gastroenterol.* 28: 45–74.

Marian, M., and McGinnis, C. 2007. Overview of enteral nutrition. In M. Gottschlich (Ed.), *The A.S.P.E.N. Nutrition Support Core Curriculum.* Silver Spring, MD: American Society for Parenteral and Enteral Nutrition, 187–208.

McCann, L., Feldman, C., Hornberger, J. 1999. Effect of intradialytic parenteral nutrition on delivered Kt/V. *Am J Kidney Dis.* 33:1131–1135.

McClave, S., Martindale, R., Vanek, V., et al. 2009. Guidelines for the provision and assessment of nutrition support therapy in the adult critically ill patient. *J Parenter Enteral Nutr*. 33 (3):277–316.

Medicare Manual. 2010. Medicare National Coverage Determinations Manual. Chapter 1, Part 3, Section 180.2. Revision 113, 02–19-10. Available at: www.cms.gov/manuals/downloads/ncd103c1_Part3.pdf

Mehta, R., Kellum, J., Shah, S., et al. 2007. Acute kidney injury network: Report of an initiative to improve outcomes in acute kidney injury. *Crit Care*. 11:R31–R39.

Moore, E., and Lindenfield, S. 2007. Intradialytic parenteral nutrition: A nutrition support intervention for high risk malnutrition in chronic kidney disease. *Support Line*. 29:6–16.

Mortelmans, A., Duym, P., Vanderbroucke, J., et al. 1999. Intradialytic parenteral nutrition in malnourished hemodialysis patients; a prospective long-term study. *J PEN*. 23:90–95.

Mueller, C. and Bloch, A. 2008. Intervention: Enteral and parenteral nutrition support. In L. Mahan and S. Escott Stump (Eds.), *Krause's Food and Nutrition Therapy*. St. Louis, MO: Saunders, 506–528.

National Kidney Foundation/KDOQI. 2000. *Clinical Practice Guidelines for Nutrition in Chronic Renal Failure*. Available at: http://www.kidney.org/professionals/KDOQI/guidelines_updates/doqi_nut.html

Pupim, L., Flakoll, P., Brouillete, J., et al. 2002. Intradialytic parenteral nutrition improves protein and energy homeostasis in chronic hemodialysis patients. *J Clin Invest*. 110:483–492.

Pupim, L., Flakoll, P., Ikizler, T. 2004. Nutritional supplementations acutely increases albumin fractional synthetic rate in chronic hemodialysis patients. *J Am Soc Nephrol*. 15:1920–1926.

Re/Gen Hp/HC® shelf stable. Available at: www.nutra-balance-products.com (accessed January 2011).

Stratton, R.J., Bircher, G., Foque, D., et al. 2005. Multi-nutrient oral supplements and tube feeding in maintenance dialysis: A systematic review and meta-analysis. *Am J Kidney Dis*. 46:387–405.

Wang, A., Sanderson, J., Sea, M., et al. 2003. Important factors other than dialysis adequacy associated with inadequate dietary protein and energy intakes in patients receiving maintenance peritoneal dialysis. *Am J Clin Nutr*. 77:834–841.

Wilkens, K. and Juneja, V. 2008. Medical nutrition therapy for renal disorders. In L. Mahan and S. Escott Stump (Eds.), Krause's *Food & Nutrition Therapy*, 12th edition. St. Louis, MO: Saunders, 921–958.

Wolk, R., Moore, E. and Foulks, C. 2007. Renal disease. In M. Gottschlich (Ed.), *The A.S.P.E.N. Nutrition Support Core Curriculum*. Silver Spring, MD: American Society for Parenteral and Enteral Nutrition, 591–592.

Wong, P., Smith, P. and Rodgers, D. 2003. The use of intradialytic parenteral nutrition to treat malnutrition: A case study. *CANNT J*. 13:31–46.

18 Nutrition in Kidney Transplantation

Nicole Armellino-Nitti
Loyola University Medical Center

Tamara Karosanidze
University of Virginia Health System

CONTENTS

18.1 INTRODUCTION: HISTORY AND STATISTICS

The field of transplantation has progressed dramatically over the past 60 years. The very first attempt at kidney transplantation between humans took place in 1936 when a Russian surgeon, Yuri Voronoy, transplanted a kidney from a deceased donor to a uremic patient. Unfortunately, the graft did not produce any urine and the recipient lived only 2 days. Many other attempts at human kidney transplantation followed. The first successful kidney transplant was performed in 1954 at the Peter Bent Brigham Hospital in Boston, where a surgical team led by Dr. Joseph Murray transplanted a kidney from a healthy male donor into his identical twin brother. The transplant was successful secondary to the genetic matching of donor and recipient without the aid of iatrogenic immune-suppression. However, advances in immune-suppressive therapy would be needed to make transplantation of solid organs between genetically diverse humans a routine and reliable practice (Linden, 2009).

In 2009 more than 16,000 renal transplants were performed in the United States. Presently, more than 86,000 individuals are waiting to receive a kidney (OPTN, 2010).

18.2 LIVING KIDNEY DONATION AND DONOR ASSESSMENT

Given the large number of patients awaiting kidney transplantation and the scarcity of deceased organs, living kidney donation surgery is a lifesaving option for many people with stage 5 chronic kidney disease (CKD). In fact, 6387 lives were changed in 2009 by living kidney donations. This represents 38% of all kidney transplants performed that year (OPTN, 2010).

There are many advantages to living donation: a kidney from a living donor usually starts to work immediately after transplant; the graft has a longer life span; the surgery can be scheduled ahead of time; and a living kidney donation permits other transplant candidates on the waiting list to get their transplants sooner (St. Luke's Episcopal Hospital, Texas Medical Center, 2009).

Living kidney donation surgery is generally accepted as a safe procedure for the donor. Researchers have shown that the remaining kidney is efficient in removing waste and excess fluid from the blood. It grows bigger and assumes the work of both kidneys (St. Luke's Episcopal Hospital, Texas Medical Center, 2009).

Requirements for kidney donation can vary from one transplant center to another nationwide. Generally, donors have to be between the ages of 18 and 65; be nonsmokers; and have no evidence of malignancy, human immunodeficiency virus (HIV), Hepatitis B, diabetes, hypertension (HTN), kidney disease, or an active mental illness. They should preferably have the same blood type as the recipient and a negative cross-match. Donors must be at a healthy weight prior to donation; therefore, many transplant centers decline overweight volunteers until they achieve weight loss (St. Luke's Episcopal Hospital, Texas Medical Center, 2009).

Assessment of nutritional status is one of the many components of the living kidney donor-evaluation process. As mentioned earlier, if a potential donor is overweight or obese, he or she will be required to lose weight in order to be able to donate his or her kidney. A registered dietitian's role is to provide nutrition counseling for successful weight loss. Emphasis is placed on healthy eating and increased physical activity (PA).

18.3 DISEASES LEADING TO STAGE 5 CKD REQUIRING TRANSPLANTATION

It is important to understand the etiology of kidney disease as the renal pathology may influence the likelihood of recurrence of disease and can also lead to the development of comorbidities. In the adult population, the diseases, conditions, and medications that may lead to end-stage kidney disease necessitating transplant include glomerular disorders; diabetes (type 1 or type 2); cystic ailments; hypertensive nephrosclerosis; renovascular conditions; autoimmune diseases; nephrotoxic medications; tubular and interstitial disorders; neoplasms; graft failure; and congenital, familial, or metabolic disorders. Table 18.1 depicts kidney diseases that may lead to kidney transplant (OPTN, 2010). The most common causes of kidney disease leading to transplantation in adults are diabetes (both type 1 and type 2), HTN, glomerulonephritis, polycystic kidney disease, and congenital diseases; however, diabetes, HTN, and glomerulosclerosis account for nearly 80% of all patients with end-stage renal disease (Cupples and Ohler, 2003; Figure 18.1). In the pediatric population, the most common causes of kidney disease leading to transplantation are aplasia/hypoplasia/dysplasia of the kidney; obstructive uropathy; focal

TABLE 18.1
Indications for Renal Transplant

Diagnosis Categories	Kidney Diseases
Glomerular diseases	Anti-glomerular basement membrane antibody disease (GMB), chronic glomerulonephritis or glomerulosclerosis, focal segmental glomerulosclerosis (FSGS), membrane nephropathy, hemolytic uremic syndrome, Alport's syndrome, amyloidosis, Henoch-Schoenlein purpura, sickle cell anemia
Diabetes	Type 1 or type 2
Cystic diseases	Polycystic kidneys, medullary cystic kidneys, acquired cystic disease
Hypertensive nephrosclerosis	Hypertensive nephrosclerosis
Renovascular and other vascular diseases	Chronic nephrosclerosis, malignant hypertension, polyarteritis, progressive systemic sclerosis, renal artery thrombosis, scleroderma
Autoimmune	IgA nephropathy, Goodpasture's disease, Wegener's disease, systemic lupus erythematosis
Nephrotoxic agents	Cyclosporine, gentamicin, nonsteroidal anti-inflammatory agents, analgesics, intravenous contrast dyes, antibiotic, cancer chemotherapy, radiation, heroin
Congenital, rare familial, and metabolic disorders	Congenital obstructive uropathy, cystinosis, Fabry's disease, hypoplasia/dysplasia/aplasia/dysgenesis/agenesis; nephrophthisis; prune belly syndrome
Tubular and interstitial diseases, urinary tract abnormalities	Acquired obstructive or analgesic or pyelonephritis/reflux, oxalate nephropathy, gout, nephritis, nephrolithiasis, acute tubular necrosis, cortical necrosis, sarcoidosis, urolithiasis, posterior ureteral valves, neurogenic bladder, Fanconi's syndrome
Neoplasms	Incidental carcinoma, lymphoma, myeloma, renal cell carcinoma, Wilms' tumor
Re-transplant/Graft failure	Retransplant/graft failure
Other	Rheumatoid arthritis, familial nephropathy, nephrotic syndrome, human immunodeficiency virus (HIV) nephropathy

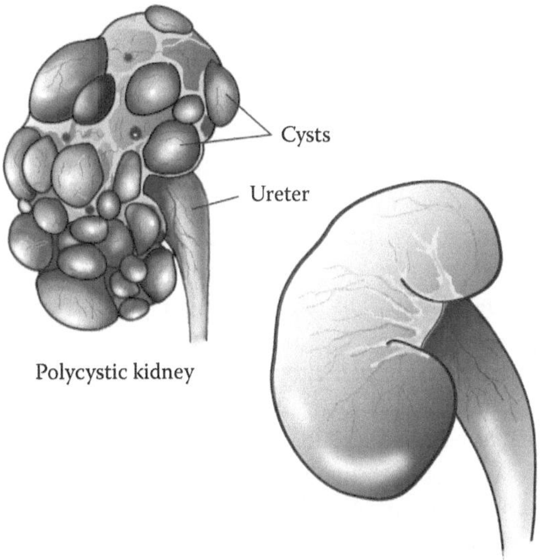

FIGURE 18.1 Polycystic kidney. (Courtesy of the National Institute of Diabetes and Digestive and Kidney Diseases, National Institutes of Health.)

segmental glomerulosclerosis; reflux nephropathy; and chronic glomerulonephritis according to the Annual Report of the North American Pediatric Renal Trials and Collaborative Studies (NAPRTCS), 2007 (USRDS, 2010).

18.4 KIDNEY TRANSPLANT EVALUATION PROCESS

The transplant process begins with a referral from the patient's primary care provider to a transplant center where they determine if the patient has end-stage disease necessitating a transplant. The evaluation for kidney transplant and acceptance criteria vary from program to program. Patients must undergo various tests and procedures and then all the results are brought to a multidisciplinary board to determine if the patient is a suitable candidate for transplantation. If and when the patient is deemed to be an acceptable transplant candidate, the patient is added to the national transplant waiting list or may have a living related or unrelated donor matched for transplantation.

The transplant evaluation process begins with an extensive history and physical examination to determine if the patient can physiologically tolerate the transplant with a low risk of long-term morbidity and mortality. The cause of kidney disease must be determined, and the patient may undergo radiologic and invasive testing to determine the stage of kidney disease. The patient may also need imaging of the kidney via renal or abdominal ultrasound, computed tomography (CT), or magnetic resonance imaging (MRI). Imaging will provide information regarding the size and any structural abnormalities of the kidneys. The patient may also undergo other radiologic or diagnostic tests, including a chest X-ray, electrocardiogram, voiding cystourethrogram, and mammograms in women over 40. The patient may also need pulmonary function tests, cardiac echocardiogram, cardiac stress tests, cardiac catheterization, abdominal CT, MRI, or other noninvasive vascular studies if those are indicated by the exam or other findings.

The patient must undergo various laboratory tests of the blood and urine, including a complete metabolic panel, complete blood count, prothrombin time, partial thromboplastin time, international normalized ratio, liver function, hepatitis B and C, cytomegalovirus, HIV, Epstein–Barr virus (EBV), herpes simplex virus, varicella zoster virus, and a venereal screening test for syphilis. Urine analysis and cultures are tested, and a 24-h urine collection is obtained to evaluate for protein and creatinine. Other laboratory tests include ABO blood typing, tissue typing, cross-match, and panel reactive antibodies.

Other evaluations include a psychosocial assessment completed by a social worker to determine the long-term success of the patient. This involves the review of psychiatric, substance abuse, and social histories, as well as family and other social support systems. Patients may be required to join a support group or attend a rehabilitation program if, for example, they have had a history of substance abuse. They are also questioned about compliance history as medication compliance and regular attendance to posttransplant clinic appointments are of utmost importance to ensure the best opportunity for graft function. A patient's mental status, perceived health, coping style and skills, as well as quality of life are also examined. Finally, a patient's culture and religion may be considered for any hidden concerns such as objections to any blood or blood products from certain religious faiths.

Finally, a nutrition evaluation is completed by a registered dietitian to determine if the patient is at increased nutrition risk before or after the transplant. This involves taking a detailed diet history, including discussing dietary or herbal supplement use and analyzing anthropometric data including height, weight, body mass index (BMI), ideal body weight, percent ideal body weight, and recent weight change. The registered dietitian provides appropriate education pending the progression of kidney disease for both pretransplant and posttransplant phases. Often, patients are required to follow a low-potassium, low-sodium, and low-phosphorus diet pretransplant with moderate intake of protein depending on the need for dialysis. Following the transplant, the patient may only need to follow a heart-healthy/cardiac diet depending on the clinical course and graft function. The nutrition assessment and diets for both the pre- and posttransplant periods are discussed in greater detail later in the chapter.

When a donor (deceased or living) becomes available, the organ and tissue must be matched by tissue typing, cross-matching, and antibody screening. Tissue typing is used to determine tissue compatibility between the donor and candidate. Cross-matching is a blood test to determine how the recipient will react to the donor. A positive cross-match means the organ is incompatible, whereas a negative cross-match means the organ is compatible. Antibody screening is used to determine if the transplant candidate has antibodies that would react to the donor's antigens. When a kidney from a deceased donor becomes available, it is offered to the first person on the transplant list. The transplant, however, cannot take place if the recipient is not healthy enough to undergo an immediate major surgery. Factors affecting the final decision for a transplant include tissue match, blood type, length of time on the waiting list, immune status, and the distance between the donor and the recipient.

It is also important to note contraindications to kidney transplantation. If a patient has reversible kidney disease, active infection or chronic untreated infection, untreatable end-stage diseases of other organs or a limited life expectancy as defined by the transplant center, transplantation may not be appropriate. In terms of age, chronological age itself is not a contraindication as much as physiological age. Medical issues to consider are advanced extra-renal diseases such as peripheral vascular disease or advanced coronary artery disease as well as improving glycemic control in patients with diabetes. Medication compliance, substance abuse, and uncontrolled psychiatric disorders also need to be addressed. If a patient is rejected for transplantation based on medical or psychosocial findings, he or she may be referred to different transplant centers for another evaluation or may even be reevaluated at a later time if there are altered circumstances.

18.5 NUTRITION ASSESSMENT: PRETRANSPLANT

A detailed nutrition assessment prior to transplant is essential to determine those patients at nutrition risk. A nutrition assessment comprises the medical history, including the diagnosis necessitating kidney transplant; previous surgeries, in particular abdominal surgeries; and co-morbid conditions including other medical histories. Additional considerations include any gastrointestinal issues such as nausea, vomiting, diarrhea, constipation, gastrointestinal bleeding, abdominal pain, and difficulties chewing or swallowing. The current diet prescription is also considered to determine its appropriateness.

The dietitian obtains a nutrition history comprising a diet recall or diet history, previous or current enteral or parenteral nutrition support, the use of vitamin and/or mineral supplementation, and any other dietary restrictions. A diet recall or diet history is needed to determine the quality and quantity of intake and evaluate the need for suitable nutrition education. A physical examination is also completed and is essential to assess edema, ascites, dental and oral health, muscle or fat wasting, and mental status. Anthropometric data and the weight history are also considered to determine weight loss or gain. Weight is particularly important in the renal transplant patient because pretransplant obesity correlates with increased operating time, wound complications, and hospitalizations (Singh et al., 2005) in the short term, and can have lasting effects on chronic renal allograft dysfunction (Meier-Krieshe et al., 1999) and cardiac function (Lentine et al., 2008).

Laboratory data, particularly serum sodium, predialysis blood urea nitrogen and creatinine, glucose, potassium, magnesium, calcium, phosphorus, albumin, and the lipid profile are evaluated to determine the need for dietary modifications. It is important to optimize glycemic control, lipids, and electrolytes prior to transplant for ideal transplantation and to ensure proper healing. The dietitian determines the most appropriate diet for the patient based on current renal status and past medical history (e.g., diabetes or cardiovascular disease [CVD]) and aims to correct any electrolyte imbalances.

The dietitian will then determine the most appropriate diet, making recommendations for calories, protein, and fluid. Calorie recommendations depend on a patient's need to maintain, gain, or lose weight. Typically, energy needs for pediatric CKD patients are similar to those of healthy children of the same age and activity level and are adjusted for height and weight. Energy needs remain the same for pediatric patients on hemodialysis but are decreased for children on peritoneal dialysis because of the absorption of dextrose from the dialysate (National Kidney Foundation, 2009). Adult patients require 20–35 cal/kg of body weight but need to be adjusted according to weight status (Brown et al., 2010). The European Society for Clinical Nutrition and Metabolism recommends providing at least 30–35 cal/kg of body weight per day for stable adult CKD patients on hemodialysis (Cano et al., 2009). The reason for an increase in calories is the catabolic state in patients with CKD. Protein needs will vary depending on the patient's need for dialysis. Recommendations for children on hemodialysis are the dietary reference intake (DRI) plus 0.1 g/kg body weight per day and between 0.15 and 0.3 g/kg body weight plus DRI per day for peritoneal dialysis (National Kidney Foundation, 2009). The ultimate goal for children with CKD is normal growth and development, bone development, and metabolic homeostasis. A protein restriction of 0.6–0.8 g protein per kilogram of body weight per day in the adult patient may be warranted if the patient has renal insufficiency or failure but is not on dialysis (Beto and Bansal, 2004). The protein recommendation for stable patients on maintenance hemodialysis is 1.2 g protein per kilogram of body weight per day and 1.3 g of protein per kilogram body weight per day for those on continuous ambulatory peritoneal dialysis (Cano et al., 2006; Kopple, 2001). The increase in protein is needed to replace albumin and amino acids lost during the dialysis treatment. Together the increase in calories and protein protect against the protein-calorie malnutrition that may occur when inadequate calories and/or protein are available to spare protein use as energy. Fluid parameters depend on the severity and treatment of CKD. In the early stages of kidney disease, there is usually no fluid restriction with normal urine output (Beto and Bansal, 2004). Adult patients receiving hemodialysis may consume 1000 mL of fluid plus any additional amount equal to urine output; patients on peritoneal dialysis may consume 1500–2000 mL of fluid daily (Beto and Bansal, 2004). Typically, the patient will need to follow a 2 g sodium, 2 g potassium, and 2 g phosphorus diet, but this may be adjusted depending on serum laboratory values.

The dietitian will also need to assess diet compliance. The patient is expected to follow the appropriate diet as instructed by the dietitian but may have some difficulties along the way. The dietitian will troubleshoot and provide additional resources as needed. It is important for the patient to communicate any questions or concerns to the dietitian regarding the diet (Figure 18.2).

18.6 NUTRITION ASSESSMENT: POSTTRANSPLANT

18.6.1 Short-Term Nutrition Goals

Following transplantation, during the acute phase (for 4–6 weeks after surgery), patients have increased nutrient needs. Adequate calorie and protein provision is necessary to promote healing of surgical anastomosis and to prevent infections. Usually, adult and pediatric patients are started on a clear liquid diet 24–48 h following transplantation and quickly advanced to solid foods. Need for specific dietary restrictions will be driven by patient's graft function, thus nutrition recommendations should be made on an individual basis. Enteral or parenteral nutrition is rarely needed in renal transplant recipients (RTRs) unless postoperative complications prevent adequate nutrient delivery via the oral route. If enteral nutrition is initiated, a standard polymeric, isotonic formula is usually used. Specialized infant formulas such as SimilacPM® 60/40 (Abbot Nutrition) or Good Start®(Nestle Nutrition) are justified when the transplanted kidney is not functioning properly. Similarly, Nepro®, Suplena® (Abbot Nutrition), Magnacal® (Novartis), Novasource Renal® (Nestle Nutrition), or Renal Cal® (Nestle Nutrition) are used in adult patients or older children with suboptimal kidney function (Blue, 2002; Connolly, 2002).

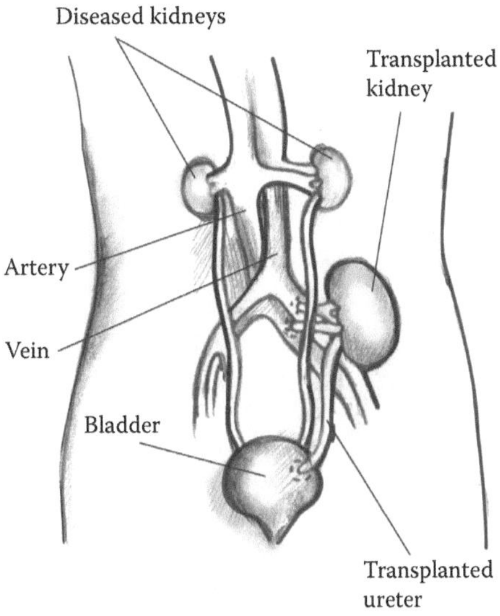

FIGURE 18.2 Transplanted kidney. (Courtesy of the National Institute of Diabetes and Digestive and Kidney Diseases, National Institutes of Health.)

18.6.1.1 Nutrient and Energy Requirements

Protein needs are elevated because of high nitrogen losses, high doses of corticosteroid medications, stress of surgery, catabolism of muscle, and pre-existing malnutrition. The patient's dry body weight or adjusted body weight should be used when estimating protein needs. Usually, 1.3–1.5 g protein are provided, with higher amounts (up to 2 g protein/day) supplied to adult patients requiring peritoneal dialysis and those with other losses from drains and wounds (Blue, 1992; Connolly, 2002; Kent, 2008; Teplan et al., 2009). Pediatric RTRs have elevated protein needs for the first 3 months following surgery. Dry weight or ideal body weight for height/length is used for calculating needs. Two to three grams of protein/kg are provided in children under the age of 10, and 2 g protein/kg body weight in patients over the age of 10 (Connolly, 2002). Without adequate protein, patients are more likely to experience delayed wound healing, are more susceptible to infections, and can develop gastrointestinal and decubital ulcers (Blue, 2002; Martins et al., 2004).

Calorie needs of adult kidney transplant patients can be estimated using the Harris-Benedict equation with a stress factor of 1.3–1.5 or calculated based on calories/kilogram dry body weight or adjusted body weight. Most sources recommend 30–35 cal/kg body weight (Blue, 1992; Teplan et al., 2009), but overweight patients and patients without active infections or fever may only need 20–30 cal/kg (Blue, 2002). The need for more calories in the early phase of kidney transplantation is due to surgical stress and high doses of immunosuppressive medications although research on energy expenditure of postrenal transplant patients is limited. Martins et al. (2004) reported results of a pilot study (unpublished work) where indirect calorimetry was used to measure energy expenditure in seven RTRs during 1 month after surgery and found their energy expenditure to be significantly higher (27 cal/kg) than that of healthy individuals (23 cal/kg). Calorie requirements of pediatric patients are summarized in Table 18.2 (Connolly, 2002).

18.6.1.2 Nutrition-Related Complications

Hyperglycemia is common during the acute posttransplant phase and results from steroids, stress of surgery, and infections. High blood sugars are managed by exogenous insulin and a carbohydrate-controlled diet. Patients are advised to limit intake of simple sugars (Kent, 2008).

TABLE 18.2
Calorie Requirements of Pediatric Renal Transplant Recipients

Age	Calorie Requirements (kg)
Infants (0–1 years)	
0–6 months	≥108
7 months–1 year	≥98
Toddlers (1–3 years)	102
Children (4–10 years)	
4–6	90
7–10	70
Adolescents (11–18 years)	
Girls 11–14	47
Girls 15–18	40
Boys 11–14	55
Boys 15–18	45

Fat restriction is not recommended during the acute posttransplant phase in adult or pediatric patients. However, dyslipidemia resulting from long-term use of antirejection medications does warrant following a "heart-healthy" diet during the chronic posttransplant period (Connolly, 2002; Kent, 2008).

Fluid and electrolyte requirements during the acute posttransplant phase will vary from patient to patient and should be individualized based on patient's clinical condition. Usually, sodium is not restricted in patients during the acute posttransplant phase unless there is evidence of poor allograft function or exacerbation of HTN. In this case, a 2 g sodium diet is recommended (Kent, 2008).

Antirejection medications can cause changes in serum potassium, phosphorus, and/or magnesium levels. Patients are closely monitored and recommendations for supplementation are based on laboratory results.

Mild hyperkalemia is commonly seen in RTRs. Dietary potassium restriction (2 g/day) is often necessary for potassium levels above 5 mmol/L. Hyperkalemia often occurs when high-dose calcineurin inhibitors administered in the acute post-operative phase. Other medications, such as angiotensin-converting enzyme inhibitors, angiotensin receptor blockers, and beta blockers may also exacerbate hyperkalemia when given concurrently. Depending on the severity of hyperkalemia, in addition to dietary restriction, administration of diurctics, potassium exchange resin (sodium polystyrene or kayexalate), and/or insulin with glucose and calcium gluconate may be necessary. Hypokalemia is more common with the administration of sirolimus in kidney transplant patients in which case a potassium supplementation is needed (Pham et al., 2010).

Hypophosphatemia is another common laboratory abnormality following successful kidney transplantation. The causes of low phosphorus levels are many and include considerable initial diuresis (most commonly seen in living-donor kidney transplant recipients), magnesium depletion, glucosuria, corticosteroid use, and a faulty renal phosphate reabsorption caused by allograft injury. Rhabdomyolysis, left ventricular dysfunction, insulin resistance, and osteomalacia are just a few of the negative consequences of severe hypophosphatemia. Mild hypophosphatemia (phosphorus > 2 mg/dL) may be treated with increased dietary phosphorus intake, whereas a more severe hypophosphatemia (phosphorus < 2 mg/dL) may require administration of oral phosphorus tablets or an intravenous supplementation (Pham et al., 2010; Teplan et al., 2009).

Hypomagnesemia following renal transplantation is quite common and is brought on by the loss of magnesium through urine while on cyclosporine or tacrolimus therapy. Patients with diabetes and those on loop diuretics may also be more prone to having low magnesium levels. Since patients may have inadequate dietary intake of magnesium, oral supplementation is usually warranted. Oral magnesium supplements (400–800 mg magnesium oxide three times a day) are provided, but intravenous magnesium supplementation is necessary in severe hypomagnesemia (<1 mg/dL) (Pham et al., 2010).

18.6.2 Long-Term Nutrition Goals, Nutrition-Related Complications and Management

Patients who undergo a kidney transplant are at an increased risk for several complications including weight gain, diabetes, HTN, dyslipidemia, CVD, infection, fractures, and malignancies. These complications contribute to an increase in morbidity and mortality. The long-term objective for the post kidney transplant patient is to optimize overall health for not only the individual but also for the functioning of the graft.

18.6.2.1 Posttransplant Weight Gain

Posttransplant weight gain and obesity have an impact on the kidney transplant recipient. Obesity, as defined by a BMI greater than 35 kg/m^2 is a predictive factor for an increased risk of diabetes, wound complications, metabolic syndrome, certain cancers, and CVD (Kent, 2007) and therefore may impede graft function. It is important to maintain a healthy weight or, if needed, lose weight to prolong graft function and also decrease the risk of morbidity and mortality. Weight should be monitored at every clinic visit, and weight loss should be discussed when necessary by a registered dietitian.

18.6.2.2 Posttransplant Diabetes

Posttransplant patients are at a higher risk for developing diabetes, which is associated with both poor graft function and patient survival. Diabetes can also exacerbate the increased risk of CVD in these patients (Gourishanka et al., 2004). Because transplant recipients must take antirejection medications for the duration of the graft, they are at a higher risk for developing diabetes. It is important to maintain euglycemia and to monitor blood glucose levels at least weekly and then monthly for the first couple of months following the transplant (Gourishanka et al., 2004). If needed, the patient must adhere to a diabetic diet to optimize glycemic control and may be prescribed oral or injection medication as needed to maintain euglycemia.

18.6.2.3 HTN, Dyslipidemia, and CVD

Many RTRs develop cardiac complications such as dyslipidemia and HTN. Those complications, coupled with an increased risk of hyperglycemia and weight gain and/or obesity increase the likelihood of developing metabolic syndrome, which can lead to an increase in morbidity and mortality (Zelle et al., 2010). It is a necessity to monitor blood pressure and pulses at each clinic visit and to monitor lipid profile for 2–3 months following the transplant, and then annually. The patient should follow a cardiac or heart-healthy diet postoperatively with emphasis on whole grains, adequate fruit and vegetable intake, lean protein, low-fat or fat-free dairy products, and the use of fats and oils sparingly. Pending the level of CVD, it may be pertinent to have a registered dietitian educate the patient regarding therapeutic lifestyles changes (Kasiske et al., 2004). It is also imperative to discuss alcohol habits and discourage tobacco use. See Table 18.3 for guidelines and recommendations.

18.6.2.4 Bone Mineral Density

The kidney transplant recipient is at risk for bone loss after transplantation, which leads to the high prevalence of bone fracture. Factors contributing to bone loss include glucocorticoid steroids, calcineurin inhibitors (cyclosporine), persistent hyperparathyroidism, and immobility. It may be necessary to intervene with mediations to prevent bone loss in the first 3 months following the transplant (Kovac et al., 2001).

TABLE 18.3
Therapeutic Lifestyle Changes for Adult Kidney Transplant Recipients

Modification Needed	Goal
Reducing fat	Total fat: 25%–35% of total calories Saturated fat: <7% of total calories Polyunsaturated fat: up to 10% of total calories Monounsaturated fat: up to 20% of total calories
Cholesterol	<200 mg/day
Carbohydrate	50%–60% of total calories; improve glycemic control
Fiber	20–30 g/day of which 5–10 g soluble fiber per day
Plant stanols/sterols	2 g/day
Calories	Match intake to output of energy, attain or maintain standard body weight
Waist circumference	Men: <40 in. (102 cm) Women: <35 in. (88 cm)
Waist to hip ratio	Men: <1.0 Women: <0.8
Physical activity	20–30 min periods of activity 3–4 times per week of planned moderate physical activity including a 5 min warm up and cool down resistance exercise training
Habits	Smoking cessation Alcohol: limit one drink per day with approval of physician

18.6.2.5 Infection and Malignancy

This patient population is also at risk for opportunistic infections. It is standard practice to screen, vaccinate, and/or use prophylaxis to prevent posttransplant viruses (Bia et al., 2010). Posttransplant patients are also at a greater risk for developing malignancy compared to the general public. Age-specific screening for malignancy should be incorporated into care (Bia et al., 2010). And, it is important to maintain a healthy weight as obesity is linked to esophageal adenocarcinoma, endometrial, colorectal, postmenopausal breast, prostate, and renal cancers (Roberts et al., 2010).

18.7 ANTIREJECTION MEDICATIONS—USES, NUTRITION-RELATED SIDE EFFECTS, AND NUTRITIONAL MANAGEMENT

Immunosuppressive medications reduce the incidence and severity of acute rejection considerably, thus improving patient and graft survival. Patients are prescribed immunosuppressive medications immediately following the transplant. Patients may also require induction therapy which generally describes monoclonal or polyclonal antibodies administered via the parenteral route for a short course during transplantation or immediately posttransplant, which is used to prevent or delay acute rejection. Induction therapy is also used to provide immunosuppression, which permits immediate and permanent elimination of one or more of the maintenance medications required after the transplant. It also has an effect of inducing the host's immunological tolerance to the alloantigen. All patients are prescribed maintenance immunosuppressive agents for the life of the transplanted organ and usually include a multimedication regime consisting of corticosteroids, calcineurin inhibitors, antiproliferative agents, and/or mammalian target of rapamycin (mTOR) inhibitors.

Corticosteroids (prednisone, prednisolone, methylprednisone, Solu-Medrol, and Solu-Cortef) are believed to impede the cell cycle of T and B cells by inhibiting cytokine gene transcription and secretion (Czock et al., 2005). They also suppress the production of inflammatory mediators by suppressing prostaglandin synthesis (Granger et al., 2004). Nutrition-related side effects of corticosteroids include hyperglycemia and/or the development of diabetes, hyperphagia, osteoporosis,

HTN, hyperlipidemia, protein catabolism, peptic ulcer disease, fluid retention, and electrolyte disturbances, including hypokalemia and hyponatremia. Corticosteroids may impair wound healing and can increase the risk of infection. Monitoring of blood glucose levels is imperative as well as possibly following a diabetic diet in the event of persistent hyperglycemia. The patient may also be advised to follow a low-sodium diet and maintain a healthy weight, which may include losing weight after graft function has been declared. The patient must consume adequate protein as determined by a registered dietitian, as well as calcium and vitamin D.

Calcineurin inhibitors (cyclosporine, Neoral®, Novartis Pharmaceuticals East Hanover, NJ; Sandimmune®, Novartis Pharmaceuticals, Gengraf, Abbott, Abbott Park, IL; and tacrolimus, Prograf/FK506®, AstellasPharmaUS, Deerfield, IL) limit the lymphocyte proliferation by binding to their respective intracellular binding proteins thus inhibiting phosphatase activity of calcineurin and decrease interleukin-2 transcription (Granger et al., 2004; Lin and Cosgrove, 2006). Nutrition-related concerns are hyperkalemia, hyperglycemia, HTN, hyperlipidemia, hypomagnesemia, hypophosphatemia, and abdominal distress including nausea, vomiting, and diarrhea. The patient may need to follow a low-potassium, low-sodium, low-fat and/or low-carbohydrate diet, and may need magnesium supplementation. The patient may need an antiemetic agent to prevent nausea and/or vomiting.

Antiproliferative agents (azathioprine, Imuran®, Prometheus Laboratories, San Diego, CA; mycophenolatemofetil, CellCept®, Roche Laboratories, Nutley, NJ; mycophenolate sodium, Myfortic®; Novartis Pharmaceuticals, Inc.) also referred to as antimetabolites, suppress the expression of the immune response by inhibiting the proliferation of lymphocytes after they encounter the antigen (Granger et al., 2004). They can cause nausea, vomiting, diarrhea, sore throat, and altered taste acuity. Nutrition therapy includes antiemetic agents as needed and adequate fluid intake to replace losses.

The medication class of mTOR inhibitors (sirolimus, Rapamycin/Rapamune®, Wyeth Pharmaceuticals, Madison, NJ) prevents the regulatory kinase enzyme in the process of cell division (Granger et al., 2004). It is used as part of a maintenance regime and can cause hypertriglyceridemia, hypercholesterolemia, HTN, thrombocytopenia, anemia, diarrhea, acne, rashes, mouth sores, and delayed wound healing. The patient may need to follow a low-fat and low-sodium diet and maintain a healthy weight.

18.8 FOOD SAFETY AND SANITATION

According to the Centers for Disease Control and Prevention (CDC), even though the food supply in the United States is among the safest in the world, each year approximately 76 million illnesses occur including 300,000 hospitalizations and nearly 5000 deaths from foodborne illnesses (CDC, 2010). Because transplant patients are immunocompromised, this patient population may be more vulnerable to foodborne illnesses. One must be attentive when handling, preparing, and consuming foods and knowledgeable about the signs and symptoms of foodborne illness.

18.8.1 Simple Rule of Thumb: When in Doubt Throw It Out

Bacteria can spread throughout the kitchen via food, human contact, counter tops, cutting boards, and utensils. The first line of defense in reducing the risk of foodborne illness is appropriate cleanliness, including proper hand washing, rinsing fresh fruits and vegetables, and finally, washing work surfaces and areas. The patient must wash his/her hands in warm soapy water for at least 20 s before and after handling food (cooked and/or raw food), after using the restroom, changing diapers, and handling garbage or pets. All fresh fruits and vegetables, even those with skins or rinds that are not eaten (melon, oranges, etc.) should be rinsed under running tap water. The lids of canned goods should be cleaned to eliminate the possibility of consuming any debris or microorganisms. All cutting boards, utensils, dishes, and counter tops must be cleaned after preparing food items and before going onto the next food, especially if it is a raw or uncooked protein. One must be mindful of cross contamination that can occur when bacteria spread from one food product to another, especially with raw meat, seafood, poultry, eggs, and milk.

Foods should be cooked and chilled to the proper temperatures to ensure food safety. A food thermometer should be used to determine proper cooking temperatures. Beef and egg dishes should be cooked throughout or to 160°F. Poultry and ham should be cooked to a temperature of 165°F is reached. Seafood should be cooked to 145°F; shrimp, lobster, and crab should be cooked until they turn red and the flesh is opaque; clams, mussels, and oysters should be cooked until the shells open. If the shells do not open, they should be discarded. Foods not consumed at a particular meal should be chilled within 2 h of cooking as a means to reduce the risk of bacterial growth. The refrigerator temperature should be kept at 39°F or below, and the freezer temperature should be kept at 0°F or below.

Foodborne illness unfortunately resembles symptoms of the influenza virus and can sometimes be mistaken for it. The symptoms include nausea, vomiting, diarrhea, fever, chills, and sweating. All transplant recipients on immunosuppressive medications are at an increased risk for severe infection. If there is suspicion of foodborne illness (or the influenza virus), the patient should contact his/her physician or heath care provider immediately. The food thought to be the culprit of causing a foodborne illness should also be preserved in an airtight bag or plastic container and stored in the freezer clearly marked. The packaging material should also be preserved and should include information about the food or beverage item, the date and time it was consumed, and when the symptoms occurred. One should contact the local health department if the food was from a restaurant of other food establishment.

18.9 DIETARY SUPPLEMENTS

Presently, no specific guidelines or recommendations exist regarding vitamin and mineral supplementation in kidney transplant candidates or recipients. Nutrient losses in dialysis patients may be significantly increased with the use of the modern and more efficient dialyzers. Many clinicians will agree that these patients may benefit from supplementation but the question remains: what vitamins and minerals should be supplemented in pre- and posttransplant patients? The Dialysis Outcomes and Practice Patterns Study studied 16,345 hemodialysis patients in the United States, Japan, France, Germany, Italy, Spain, and the United Kingdom and found that patients taking water-soluble vitamins (cobalamin, pyridoxine, ascorbic acid, and folate) had a 16% lower mortality risk compared to those not taking any vitamins (Buchholz, 2006).

Patients with CKD on dialysis often have poor overall intake and thus decreased intake of vitamins and minerals related to anorexia secondary to uremia and to the many dietary restrictions imposed on this patient population. The status of vitamins, especially the B-vitamins, is affected by the dialysis process itself. Increased losses through dialysis and poor intakes have led to routine supplementation of B-vitamins in the adult and pediatric populations. K/DOQI guidelines suggest that children on dialysis necessitate vitamin-B supplementation but the data on which these recommendations are based are limited and extrapolated from adult populations (Don et al., 2010).

Vitamin and mineral supplementation following transplantation is usually not necessary if patients have a good appetite and consume a varied diet. Every patient should be evaluated on an individual basis and recommendations made based on clinical condition and serum laboratory values. For example, calcium and vitamin D supplementation may be needed in those patients with inadequate intakes and/or dislike/intolerance of calcium- and/or vitamin D-rich foods. RTRs are at increased risk for developing bone disease due to the side effects of steroid medications (Connolly, 2002).

Dietary supplements are very popular in Europe, Asia, and the United States. Spanner and Duncan (2005) conducted a cross-sectional survey of 100 adult patients with chronic renal insufficiency to determine the prevalence of dietary supplement use. The investigators found that 45%

of subjects took dietary supplements and that supplement users were more concerned about their health than nonusers. Study subjects took 1–5 or more supplements per day, and dietary supplement was defined as any product containing vitamins, minerals, herbals/botanicals, amino acids, metabolites, and extracts. Another study with a slightly larger sample size of 164 patients was conducted in Germany by Nowack et al. (2009) and described the use of complementary and alternative medicine (CAM) in renal patients treated with dialysis or kidney transplantation. Popularity of CAM in this population was high with 57% of dialysis patients and 49% of transplant patients taking CAM. Transplant patients consumed anywhere from 2 to 12 different CAMs. Study researchers identified 41 different types of CAM products used by patients, of which 22% were not safe for renal patients. Some of these unsafe CAM products included chamomile tea, fruit teas (unspecified), grapefruit juice, vitamins A and E, and St. John's Wort (SJW). These products are thought to either accumulate in renal patients or cause supplement–medication interactions (Nowack et al., 2009).

While patients may report the use of vitamin and mineral supplements to their medical doctor, the use of herbal products and botanicals is often undisclosed. There may be several reasons for not admitting to using herbals. Patients may believe that herbals are safe because they are natural and thus may not consider them a medication. Patients may fail to report the use of herbal products and botanicals for fear of being discouraged from taking them. Unlike over-the-counter and prescription drugs, dietary supplements are not regulated by the Food and Drug Administration. The content and purity of dietary supplements are questionable. They may be contaminated with heavy metals (mercury, lead, arsenic, pesticides) or even certain prescription drugs (steroids, diuretics, anti-inflammatory drugs) making them dangerous to patients with multiple medical conditions who take myriad medications (Allen and Bell, 2002; Foote and Cohen, 1998). Data are lacking on the safety of herbal supplements because little is known about the excretion of botanicals and the ability of the active compounds of herbals to be dialyzed. Cooke et al. (2004) identified popular herbal supplements that may be damaging to the kidneys and are not recommended for use by CKD patients. Selected herbals and renal concerns are listed in Table 18.4.

The use of herbals and botanicals is not recommended in immunosuppressed patients. There have been several case reports confirming episodes of acute rejection in patients taking a popular dietary supplement, SJW. Therapeutic levels of calcineurin inhibitors are significantly lowered

TABLE 18.4
Selected Herbal Supplements Not Recommended for CKD/Kidney Transplant Patients

Herbal Supplement	Effects on the Kidney/Possible Interactions
Rhubarb	High oxalate content of rhubarb may damage the kidneys if used chronically
Juniper berries	This plant can irritate the renal epithelial tissue and increase diuresis
Laxatives such as aloe, senna, cascara	These plants may cause electrolyte imbalance
Echinacea	May interact with antirejection medications
Evening primrose oil	May increase bleeding time
Licorice	May cause hypokalemia, hypocalcemia, hyperphosphatemia; may cause sodium and fluid retention and raise blood pressure
Noni juice	Causes hyperkalemia
Saw Palmetto	May cause hypertension, urine retention
Stevia	May cause hypoglycemia; nephrotoxic in animals
Spirulina (blue-green algae)	May increase serum calcium, serum alkaline phosphatase. This supplement is rich in iron, vitamin A, and mercury—may cause potential vitamin and metal toxicity
Milk thistle	May increase phosphorus absorption
Ginseng (Panax)	Increases blood pressure, anxiety. Causes hypoglycemia, insomnia, and headaches

when SJW is used concurrently with antirejection medications (Allen and Bell, 2002). Barone et al. (2001) described two cases of RTRs who self-medicated with SJW and developed acute graft rejection because of low cyclosporine (CSA) levels. CSA and SJW compete for absorption by using the same mechanisms (P-450 3A4 and/or P-glycoprotein) for metabolism (Radler, 2008). After stopping SJW, both patients' CSA concentrations returned to therapeutic levels. Kidney transplant patients are often prescribed anticoagulants and aspirin; if common herbals such as garlic, ginkgo, and ginseng are taken concomitantly, increased bleeding may occur (Barone et al., 2001). Cardiovascular problems with the use of Ma huang (ephedra) and hypoglycemic episodes with the use of ginseng have also been documented (Allen and Bell, 2002).

Healthcare providers are urged to obtain a detailed history of dietary supplement use from their patients. Ideally, the patient should be asked to bring all of his or her prescribed medications, over-the-counter drugs, and other supplements to the doctor for review (Allen and Bell, 2002).

18.10 PA GUIDELINES, RESTRICTIONS, AND RECOMMENDATIONS

It is well known that regular PA has a significant impact on an individual's health. Many of its benefits are especially important for RTRs, who often suffer from pre-existing HTN, diabetes, overweight/obesity, depression, and osteopenia. Engaging in regular exercise decreases the risk of CVD, reduces blood pressure, improves mood, and helps maintain a healthy body weight and thus better control diabetes. PA also improves and maintains muscle strength. It has been documented that patients have low exercise capacity due to uremic symptoms and the dialysis treatment but that exercise capacity improves significantly following transplantation. Painter et al. (2002) conducted a prospective, randomized clinical trial to study the effects of exercise on peak oxygen uptake, muscle strength, body composition, and quality of life in 97 patients following renal transplantation. The investigators randomized patients into two study groups: exercise intervention (EX) and usual care (UC). Baseline testing was conducted at 1 month after renal transplant with repeat testing completed at 6 and 12 months. Although the peak VO_2 (peak oxygen uptake) increased in both groups from baseline, the EX group continued to have significantly greater gains in oxygen uptake ($p = .01$) at 12 months, which was not true for the UC group. Similarly, muscle strength increased in both groups from baseline but continued to climb in the exercise group compared to the UC group ($p = 0.05$). There was a trend toward higher self-reported physical functioning in the EX group compared to the UC group ($p = .06$). No differences were found in body composition changes between the two groups.

PA is important for organ transplant recipients for the many health benefits mentioned earlier but also for reasons specific to this patient population. For example, CVD is one of the most common causes of death in RTRs. Research has concentrated on reducing certain risk factors for CVD such as HTN and obesity, but little attention has been paid to low exercise capacity in transplant population. HTN and obesity can be improved by regular PA in healthy subjects. The same is true for kidney transplant recipients. Long-term use of corticosteroid medications produces unfavorable side effects such as abnormal glucose levels, weight gain, muscle wasting, and osteopenia/osteoporosis. Exercise can protect against the development of these complications (Gordon et al., 2005; Sethna et al., 2009). Orazio et al. (2009) conducted a cross-sectional study to describe glucose tolerance in 82 RTRs and to identify risk factors associated with abnormal glucose tolerance (AGT). Thirty-five patients were found to have normal glucose tolerance (NGT) and 47 had AGT. Patients with AGT had significantly lower levels of PA compared to RTRs with NGT ($p = .03$). Higher amounts of PA were associated with lower possibility of AGT and PA was found to be an independent predictor of AGT in this patient population (Orazio et al., 2009).

Low levels of PA have been reported in patients with CKD and in patients following kidney transplantation. Hamiwka et al. (2009) studied 20 pediatric RTRs to determine their PA levels and health-related quality of life (HRQOL). Pediatric transplant recipients were compared to age- and gender-matched healthy children. The investigators found that the transplanted children spent significantly less time exercising compared to their healthy counterparts ($p = 0.005$). Similarly, the HRQOL scores were lower in transplant patients than in control subjects ($p = 0.001$), but interestingly, higher HRQOL scores were associated with a higher level of PA in both groups. This validates the need for emphasizing and promoting regular PA for children following renal transplantation (Hamiwka et al., 2009).

Another study of pediatric RTRs by Sethna et al. evaluated aerobic capacity measured by VO_{2max} and compared it to healthy children. Researchers reported 13% lower VO_{2max} in transplant patients compared to their healthy counterparts. Lower hemoglobin levels and use of sirolimus in kidney transplant subjects were found to be risk factors for lower VO_{2max} (Sethna et al., 2009).

Development of exercise regimens specifically tailored to an individual patient based on clinical status and exercise capacity is urgently needed. Healthcare professionals are urged to counsel transplant recipients on health benefits of regular PA and refer them to exercise facilities and physical therapists. Counseling patients on PA should become a routine part of transplant recipient's care (Gordon et al., 2005).

Although no standardized guidelines exist for exercise, the majority of transplant programs around the world recommend that patients engage in at least 15–30 min of PA on most days of the week. Aerobic exercises (walking, hiking, jogging, running, gardening, dancing, bicycling, swimming), strength and resistance training (lifting weights, riding a stationary bike), and stretching exercises (yoga, pilates) are encouraged (ITNS, 2010). Generally, transplant recipients are asked to refrain from heavy lifting and such activities as shoveling, mowing, and raking for 4–6 weeks following surgery (Cleveland Clinic, 2010; Gheith et al., 2008). The best time to begin an exercise program posttransplant is determined by the transplant team and is dependent on a patient's recovery (ITNS.org).

REFERENCES

Allen, D. and Bell, J. 2002. Herbal medicine and the transplant patient. *Nephrol Nurs J* 29(3):269–274.

Barone, G., Gurley, B., Ketel, B., et al. 2001. Herbal supplements: A potential for drug interactions in transplant recipients. *Transplantation* 71:239–241.

Beto, J. and Bansal, V. 2004. Medical nutrition therapy in chronic kidney failure: Integrating clinical practice guidelines. *J Am Dietetic Assoc* 104:404–409.

Bia, M., Adey, D., Bloom, R., et al. 2010. KDOQI US Commentary on the 2009 KDIGO practice guideline for the care of kidney transplant recipients. *Am J Kidney Dis* 56:189–218.

Blue, L. 1992. Nutrition considerations in kidney transplantation. *Top Clin Nutr* 7(3):17–23.

Blue, L. 2002. Adult kidney transplantation. In J. M. Hasse and L. S. Blue eds., *Comprehensive Guide to Transplant Nutrition.* Chicago, IL: American Dietetic Association, 44–57.

Brown, R., Compher, C., and the American Society for Parenteral and Enteral Nutrition (A.S.P.E.N.) Board of Directors. 2010. A.S.P.E.N. clinical guidelines: Adult renal failure. *J Parenter Enteral Nutr* 34:366–377.

Buchholz, P. 2006. Renal vitamins. *J Renal Nutr* 16(2):e1–e6.

Cano, N., Aparicio, M., Brunori, G, et al. 2009. E.S.P.E.N. guidelines on parenteral nutrition: Adult renal failure. *Clin Nutr* 28:401–414.

Cano, N., Fiaccadori, E., Tesinsky, P., et al. 2006. E.S.P.E.N. guidelines on enteral nutrition: Adult renal failure. *Clin Nutr* 25:295–310.

CDC. Centers for Disease Control and Prevention. 2010. Available at:http://cdc.gov/ (accessed September 9, 2010).

Cleveland Clinic. Exercise guidelines after kidney transplant. Available at: http://my.clevelandclinic.org (accessed July 12, 2010).

Connolly, C. 2002. Pediatric kidney transplantation. In J. M. Hasse and L. S. Blue eds., *Comprehensive Guide to Transplant Nutrition.* Chicago, IL: American Dietetic Association, 172–181.

Cooke, J. 2004. Practical aspects of herbal supplement use in chronic kidney disease. *J Renal Nutr* 14(1):e1–e4.

Cupples, S. and Ohler, L. 2003. *Solid Organ Transplantation.* New York: Springer.

Czock, D., Keller, F., Rasche, F., et al. 2005. Pharmacokinetics and pharmacodynamics of systemically administered glucocorticoids. *Clin Pharmacokinet.* 44:61–98.

Don, T., Friedlander, S., and Wong, W. 2010. Dietary intakes and biochemical status of B vitamins in a group of children receiving dialysis. *J Renal Nutr* 20(1):23–28.

Foote, J. and Cohen, B. 1998. Medicinal herb use and the renal patient. *J Renal Nutr* 8(1):40–42.

Gheith, O., El-Saadany, S., Donia, S., et al. 2008. Compliance with recommended life style behaviors in kidney transplant recipients: Does it matter in living donor kidney transplant? *Iranian J Kidney Dis* 2(4):218–226.

Gordon, E., Prohaska, T., Siminoff, L., et al. 2005. Needed: Tailored exercise regimens for kidney transplant recipients. *Am J Kidney Dis* 45(4):769–774.

Gourishanka, S., Jhangri, G., Tonelli, M., et al. 2004. Development of diabetes mellitus following kidney transplantation: A Canadian experience. *Am J Transplant* 4:1876–1882.

Granger, D., Domenick, M., and Ildstad, S. 2004. Transplantation immunology and immunosuppression. In C. M. Townsend, R. Beauchamp, B. Evers, and K. Mattox, eds., *Sabiston Textbook of Surgery: The Biological Basis of Modern Surgical Practice*, 17th edition. Philadelphia, PA: Saunder, 665–697.

Hamiwka, L., Cantell, M., Crawford, S., et al. 2009. Physical activity and health related quality of life in children following kidney transplantation. *Pediatr Transplant* 13:861–867.

International Transplant Nurses Society (ITNS). *What You Should Know: Diet and Exercise after Transplant.* Available at: http://www.itns.org (accessed July 12, 2010).

Kasiske, B., Cosio, F., Beto, J., et al. 2004. Clinical practice guidelines for managing dyslipidemias in kidney transplant patients: A report from the managing dyslipidemias in chronic kidney disease work group of the national kidney foundation kidney disease outcomes quality initiative. *Am J Transplant* 4 (Suppl. 7):13–53.

Kent, P. 2007. Issues of obesity in kidney transplant. *J Renal Nutr* 17:107–113.

Kent, P. 2008. Transplantation. In L. Byham-Gray, J. Burrowes, and G. Chertow, eds., *Nutrition and Health: Nutrition in Kidney Disease*. Totowa, NJ: Humana Press, 263–286.

Kopple, J. 2001. The National Kidney Foundation K/DOQI clinical practice guidelines for dietary protein intake for chronic dialysis patients. *Am J Kidney Dis* 38:S68–S73.

Kovac, D., Lindic, J., Kandus, A., et al. 2001. Bone mineral density in kidney transplant recipients. *Transplant Proc* 33:3668–3669.

Lentine, K., Rocca Rey, L., and Bacchi, G., et al. 2008. Obesity and cardiac risk after kidney transplantation: Experience at one center and comprehensive literature review. *Transplantation* 86:303–312.

Lin, S. and Cosgrove, C. 2006. Perioperative management of immunosuppression. *Surg Clin N Am* 86:1167–1183.

Linden, P. 2009. History of solid organ transplantation and organ donation. *Crit Care Clin* 25:165–184.

Martins, C., Pecoits-Filho, R., and Riella, M. 2004. Nutrition for the post-renal transplant recipients. *Transplant Proc* 36:1650–1654.

Meier-Krieshe, H., Vaghela, M. and Thambuganipalle, R., et al. 1999. The effect of body mass index on long term renal allograft survival. *Transplantation* 68:1294–1297.

National Kidney Foundation. 2009. KDOQI™ (Kidney Dialysis Outcomes Quality Initiate) Clinical practice guideline for nutrition in children with CKD: 2008 Update. *Am J Kidney Dis* 52:S1–S124.

Nowack, R., Ballé, C., Birnkammer, F., et al. 2009. Complementary and alternative medications consumed by renal patients in southern Germany. *J Renal Nutr* 19(3):211–219.

Orazio, L., Hickman, I., Armstrong, K., et al. 2009. Higher levels of physical activity are associated with a lower risk of abnormal glucose tolerance in renal transplant recipients. *J Renal Nutr* 19(4):304–313.

Organ Procurement and Transplantation Network (OPTN). 2010. Available at: http://optn.transplant.hrsa.gov (accessed July 12, 2010).

Painter, P., Hector, L., Ray, K., et al. 2002.A randomized trial of exercise training after renal transplantation. *Transplantation* 74:42–48.

Pham, P-T., Pham, P-C., and Danovitch, M. 2010. The acute care of the transplant recipient. In D. McKay and S. Steinberg, eds., *Kidney Transplantation: A Guide to the Care of Kidney Transplant Recipients.* Springer Science + Business Media, LLC, 207–235.

Radler, D. 2008. Dietary supplements. In L. Byham-Gray, J. Burrowes, and G. Chertow, eds., *Nutrition and Health: Nutrition in Kidney Disease*. Totowa, NJ: Humana Press, 531–541.

Roberts, D., Dive, C., and Renehan, A. 2010. Biological mechanisms linking obesity and cancer risk: New perspectives. *Ann Rev Med* 61:301–316.

Sethna, C., Salerno, A., McBride, M., et al. 2009. Cardiorespiratory fitness in pediatric renal transplant recipients. *Transplantation* 88:395–401.

Singh, D., Lawen, J., and Alkhadair, W. 2005. Does pretransplant obesity affect the outcome in kidney transplant recipients? *Transplantation Proc* 37:717–720.

Spanner, E. and Duncan, A. 2005. Prevalence of dietary supplement use in adults with chronic renal insufficiency. *J Renal Nutr* 15(2):204–210.

St. Luke's Episcopal Hospital. Texas Medical Center. 2009. *A Guide to Living Kidney Donation*. Available at: www.stlukeshouston.com (accessed July 12, 2010).

Teplan, V., Valkovsky, I., Teplan, Jr., V., et al. 2009 Nutritional consequences of renal transplantation. *J Renal Nutr* 19(1):95–100.

USRDS. 2010. *United States Renal Data System*. Available at: http://www.usrds.org/ (accessed September 9, 2010).

Zelle, D., Corpeleijin, E., van Ree, R., et al. 2010. Markers of the hepatic component of the metabolic syndrome as predictors of mortality in renal transplant recipients. *Am J Transplant* 10:106–114.

19 Establishing Quality Improvement Parameters

Lynn K. Thomas
University of South Carolina School of Medicine

CONTENTS

19.1 INTRODUCTION

> We know nothing of the principle of health, the positive of which pathology is the negative, except from observation and experience. And nothing but observation and experience will teach us the ways to maintain or to bring back the state of health.
>
> **(Nightingale, 1860)**

Florence Nightingale (Figure 19.1), in mid-nineteenth century, was one of the first health care practitioners to collect and analyze data to be used as the basis for improving patient outcomes. Years later, Ernest Codman, founder of the American College of Surgeons (ACS), took on the task of recording outcomes, but in his zeal for "documenting end results" and for publicly insulting his colleagues, he was ostracized and forced to resign from the organization he had created (Neuhauser, 2002). In 1917, the ACS finally established a hospital standardization program. The standards focused on care within hospitals and had clinical review as one of the five minimum standards (Roberts et al., 1987). Once the minimum standards were in place, the ACS began surveying health care organizations to determine their suitability to become accredited. After a few years, the minimum standards were expanded and more rigorous criteria were put in place (Luce et al., 1994). The ACS also united with the American College of Physicians, the American Hospital Association, the American Medical Association, and the Canadian Medical Association to form the Joint Commission on Accreditation of Hospitals Organization (JCAHO). In 1975, the JCAHO expanded to include ambulatory care

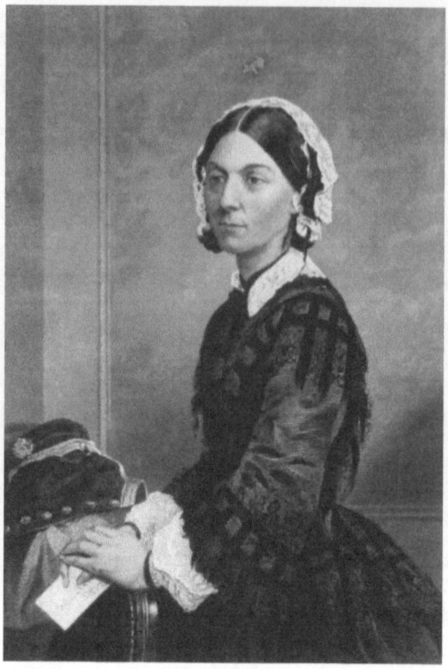

FIGURE 19.1 Florence Nightingale. (Courtesy of the National Library of Medicine.)

centers such as outpatient surgery and dialysis clinics. Today's dialysis centers must be certified by the Centers for Medicare and Medicaid Services (CMS) and receive accreditation through JCAHO or the Accreditation Association for Ambulatory Health Care.

19.2 EVIDENCE-BASED PRACTICE

After World War II, improvements in statistical analysis enabled reliable measurements of new therapeutic and interventional procedures. Data collection increased and produced the framework for systemic data synthesis, meta-analyses, and evidence-driven decision making. This framework ultimately led to the use of clinical practice guidelines that focused on the process of care delivery (Eknoyan, 2010).

The process of health care delivery includes the interactions among physicians, health care providers, facility personnel, and patients. At the patient level, services include diagnosis, treatment, management, and recovery. By observing the different services provided in the delivery of health care, an evaluation of the process can be made. Outcome data are also used to determine whether the goals of patient treatment have been achieved. Disease progression statistics and patient reports of health status and quality of life are used to determine any additional sets of quality improvement indicators.

The increasing use of electronic health records gives timely access to many new streams of data. Using multiple methods for data collection, a robust inventory of variations and complications can be documented. The combined information can be used to improve efficiency, increase patient safety, and generally advance health care delivery through the development of evidence-based clinical practice guidelines and quality improvement indicators (Steinwachs and Hughes, 2008).

Currently, clinical practice guidelines are grounded in research and defined through evidence-based practice. In some settings, the term "evidence-based guidelines" is used. These guidelines generally start with a literature search and end with graded recommendations. The National Kidney Foundation delineates the ideal grading system as having certain characteristics: (1) it offers support to help the user make informed decisions; (2) it provides simple, clear, and consistent grading

TABLE 19.1
Evidence-Based Guideline Resources

American Dietetic Association	www.adaevidencelibrary.com
Centre for Evidence-Based Medicine	www.cebm.net
Clinical Evidence	www.clinicalevidence.bmj.com
Cochrane Library	www.thecochranelibrary.com
Essential Evidence Plus	www.essentialevidenceplus.com
Health Sciences Research	www.nlm.nih.gov/hsrinfo/datasites.html
National Guidelines Clearinghouse	www.guideline.gov
University of York Centre for Reviews and Dissemination	www.crd.york.ac.uk/CMS2web

TABLE 19.2
Total Weighted Performance Score

Hgb < 10 g/dL:50%	Use 10 points for each measure
Hgb > 12 g/dL:25%	Subtract 2 points for every 1.0% below the performance standard
Urea reduction ratio > 65%:25%	Sum to create total performance score
	Performance scores are posted at Dialysis Compare Website www.medicare.gov/dialysis

among specialties; (3) it is a comprehensive evaluation of the overall quality of evidence; (4) it provides evaluation of important clinical outcomes; (5) it contains a risk benefit analysis; and (6) it is applicable to a wide range of clinical questions. The National Kidney Foundation's Kidney Disease Outcomes Qualifications Initiative (NKF KDOQI, 2002) guidelines for grading a study's quality use an ABC approach: **A** = least bias, **B** = susceptible to some bias, and **C** = significant bias. Guidelines are extremely useful in assisting the decision-making process in specific clinical circumstances. It offers basic recommendations that are supported by review of the current literature. Overall, the clinical expertise of the practitioner remains crucial (Roberts and Reed, 2009; Uhlig et al., 2006). A list of evidence-based guideline resources can be found in Table 19.1.

19.3 QUALITY IMPROVEMENT

In chronic kidney disease (CKD), quality improvement serves to both prolong the time before a patient needs dialysis and increase the quality of care after dialysis begins. The CKD community now relies on 13 standardized sets of criteria developed by the National Kidney Foundation, the NKF KDOQI. In 1997, the first two guidelines addressed vascular access and adequacies of dialysis, both hemodialysis and peritoneal (National Kidney Foundation, 1997a and 1997b). A new worldwide endeavor, which began in 2003, called Kidney Disease: Improving Global Outcomes (KDIGO™) is building on the KDOQI guidelines.

In addition to the NKF KDOQI guidelines, the new End-Stage Renal Disease Quality Improvement Program from the CMS, measures three core indicators: two on anemia management and one on hemodialysis adequacy. These measures are weighted and summed to make the total performance score (Table 19.2). As this bundled program is implemented, additional quality improvement indicators are being considered: bone mineral metabolism and dialysis adequacy calculated by Kt/V (dialyzer clearance of urea × dialysis time/volume of urea distribution) in addition or instead of urea reduction ratio (CMS, 2011). Dialysis entities and state agencies also assign patient outcome indicators that incorporate outcome objectives specific to the patient populations of each unit. These indicators must be met within specific ranges for centers to maintain accreditation/certification (Table 19.3).

TABLE 19.3
Measures Assessment Tool from the Centers for Medicare and Medicaid Services

Tag	Condition/Standard	Measure	Values	References	Source
494.40 Water and dialysate quality:					
V196	Water quality	Maximum chloramine (must determine)	≤0.1 mg/L daily/shift	AAMI RD52	Records
V196	Use max. chloramine value if only one test is performed	Maximum total chlorine (may determine)	≤0.5 mg/L daily/shift		
V178		Action/maximum bacteria—product water/dialysate	50 CFU/mL/<200 CFU/mL		
V180		Action/maximum endotoxin—product water/ dialysate	1 EU/mL/<2 EU/mL (endotoxin units)		
494.50 Reuse of hemodialyzers and blood lines (only applies to facilities that reuse dialyzers and/or bloodlines)					
V336	Dialyzer effectiveness	Total cell volume (hollow fiber dialyzers)	Measure original volume	KDOQI HD Adequacy 2006;	Records
			Discard if after reuse <80% of original	AAMI RD47	Interview
494.80 Patient assessment: The interdisciplinary team (IDT), patient/designee, RN, MSW, RD, physician must provide each patient with an individualized and comprehensive assessment of needs					
V502	Health status/comorbidities	Medical/nursing history, physical exam findings	Refer to Plan of care & QAPI sections (below) for values	Conditions for Coverage	Chart
V503	Dialysis prescription	Evaluate: HD every month; PD first month & q 4 months		KDOQI Guidelines (see POC)	
V504	BP and fluid management	Interdialytic BP and weight gain, target weight, symptoms			
V505	Lab profile	Monitor labs monthly and as needed			
V506	Immunization and medical history	Pneumococcal, hepatitis, influenza; med allergies			
V507	Anemia (Hgb, Hct, iron stores, ESA need)	Volume, bleeding, infection, ESA hypo-response			
V508	Renal bone disease	Calcium, phosphorus, PTH, and medications			
V509	Nutritional status	Multiple elements listed			
V510	Psychosocial needs	Multiple elements listed			
V511	Dialysis access type and maintenance	Access efficacy, fistula candidacy			

V512	Abilities, interests, preferences, goals, desired participation in care, preferred modality and setting, expectations for outcomes	Reason why patient does not participate in care, reason why patient is not a home dialysis candidate			
V513	Suitability for transplant referral	Reason why patient is not a transplant candidate			
V514	Family and other support systems	Composition, history, availability, level of support			
V515	Current physical activity level and referral to vocational & physical rehabilitation	Abilities and barriers to independent living; achieving physical activity, education and work goals			
494.90 Plan of care: The IDT must develop and implement a written, individualized comprehensive plan of care that specifies the services necessary to address the patient's needs as identified by the comprehensive assessment and changes in the patient's condition, and must include measurable and expected outcomes and estimated timetables to achieve outcomes. Outcome goals must be consistent with current professionally accepted clinical practice standards.					
V543	(1) Dose of dialysis/volume status	Management of volume status	Euvolemic and BP 130/80 (adult); lower of 90% of normal for age/height/weight or 130/80 (pediatric)	KDOQI HD Adequacy 2006	Chart
	Monitor each treatment			KDDOQI Hypertension 2004	
V544	(1) Dose of dialysis (HD adequacy)	Adult HD < 5 h 3×/week, minimum spKt/V	≥1.2; min. 3 h/tx if RKF < 2 mL/min	KDOQI HD Adequacy 2006	DFR
	Monitor adequacy monthly	Adult HD 2×/week, RKF < 2 mL/min	Inadequate treatment frequency		
		HD 4–6×/week, minimum spKt/V	≥2.0/week		
V544	(1) Dose of dialysis (PD adequacy—adult)	Minimum delivered Kt/V_{urea}	≥1.7/week	KDOQI PD Adequacy 2006	Chart
	Monitor 1st month and every 4 months				
V544	(1) Dose of dialysis (PD adequacy—pediatric) Monitor 1st month and every 6 months	Minimum delivered KtA/V_{urea}	≥1.8/week	KDOQI PD Adequacy 2006	Chart
V545	(2) Nutritional status—Monitor albumin and body weight monthly; other parameters at V509, monitor as needed for impact on nutrition	Albumin	≥4.0 g/dL BCG preferred; if BCP: lab normal % usual wt, % standard wt, BMI, est. % body fat	KDOQI Nutrition 2000	Chart
		Body weight and other parameters listed at V509	KDOQI CKD 2002		

(*Continued*)

TABLE 19.3 (Continued)
Measures Assessment Tool from the Centers for Medicare and Medicaid Services

Tag	Condition/Standard	Measure	Values	References	Source
V546	(2) Nutritional status (pediatric) monitor monthly	Length/height, weight, BMI, nPCR	Normalized nPCR for HD teen, nPCR N/A younger	KDOQI Pediatric Nutrition 2008	Chart
V546	(3) Mineral metabolism and renal bone disease	Calcium corrected for albumin (BCG)	Normal for lab; preferred upper level <10/mg/dL	KDOQI Bone Metabolism and	Chart
	Monitor calcium and phosphorus monthly	Phosphorus	All: 3.5–5.5 mg/dL	Disease 2003	
	Monitor intact PTH every 3 months	Intact PTH	Adult: 150–300 pg/mL; Pediatric: 200–300 pg/mL		
V547	(4) Anemia—Hgb non-ESA—monitor monthly	Hemoglobin (Adult and pediatric)	>10.0 g/dL	KDOQI Anemia 2006	DFR
V547	(4) Anemia—Hgb on ESA—monitor monthly	Hemoglobin (Adult and pediatric)	<12.0 g/dL[a]	DFR	
V548		Hemoglobin (Adult and pediatric)	10–12.0 g/dL[b]		
		Hemoglobin (Adult and pediatric)	11–12.0 g/dL, ≤13.0 g/dL[c]		
V549	(4) Anemia—Monitor iron stores routinely	Adult and pediatric: transferrin saturation	>20% (HD, PD), or CHr > 29 pg/cell	KDOQI Anemia 2006	DFR
		Adult and pediatric: serum ferritin	HD: >200 ng/mL; PD: >100 ng/mL HD/PD: <500 ng/mL or evaluate if indicated		
V550	(5) Vascular access	Fistula	Preferred[d,e]		DFR
V551		Graft	Acceptable if fistula not possible[d,e]	2006	Interview
		Central venous catheter	Avoid, unless bridge to fistula/graft or to PD, if transplant soon, or in small adult/peds pt[d]	CW	
V552	(6) Psychosocial status	Survey physical and mental functioning annually	Achieve and sustain (case-mix adjusted) scores of average or above, with no declines of ≥10 points	Conditions for Coverage	Chart Interview
		KDQOL-36 survey annually or more often as needed		CMS CPM 4/1/08; DOPPS	

V553	(7) Modality	Home dialysis referral	Candidacy or reason for non-referral	Conditions for Coverage	Chart
V554		Transplantation referral			Interview
V555	(8) Rehabilitation status	Productive activity desired by patient	Achieve and sustain appropriate level, unspecified	Conditions for Coverage	Chart
		Pediatric: Formal education needs met			Interview
		Vocational and physical rehab referrals as indicated			
V562	(d) Patient education and training	Dialysis experience, treatment options, self-care, QOL, infection prevention, rehabilitation	Documentation of education in record	Conditions for Coverage	Records
				CMS CPM 4/1/2008	Interview
494.110 Quality assessment and performance improvement (QAPI): The dialysis facility must develop, implement, maintain, and evaluate an effective, data-driven QAPI program with participation by the professional members of the IDT. The program must reflect the complexity of the organization and services (including those under arrangement), and must focus on indicators related to improved health outcomes and the prevention and reduction of medical errors. The dialysis facility must maintain and demonstrate evidence of its QAPI program including continuous monitoring for CMS review. Refer to your ESRD Network's goals for targets for aggregate patient outcomes.					
V627	Health outcomes: Physical and mental functioning	Survey adult/pediatric patients	Achieve and sustain appropriate status	Conditions for Coverage	Records
		KDQOL-36 survey annually or more often as needed	↑ % completing survey	CMS CPM 4/1/2008	
V627	Health outcomes: Patient hospitalization	Standardized hospitalization ratio (1.0 is average, >1.0 is worse than average, <1.0 is better than average)	↓ hospitalizations	Conditions for Coverage	DFR
V627	Health outcomes: Patient survival	Standardized mortality ratio (1.0 is average, >1.0 is worse than average, <1.0 is better than average)	↓ mortality	Conditions for Coverage	DFR
				CMS CPM 4/1/08	
V629	(i) HD adequacy (monthly)	HD: Adult (patient with ESRD >3 months)	↑ % with spKt/V ≥1.2 or URR ≥65% if 3 times/week dialysis; spKt/V >2.0 if 5–6 times/week dialysis	Conditions for Coverage	DFR
				CMS CPM 4/1/2008, MIPPA	Records

(*Continued*)

TABLE 19.3 (Continued)
Measures Assessment Tool from the Centers for Medicare and Medicaid Services

Tag	Condition/Standard	Measure	Values	References	Source
V629	(i) PD adequacy (rolling average, each patient tested ≤4 months)	PD: Adult	↑ % with weekly Kt/V_{urea} ≥1.7 (dialysis + RKF)	Conditions for Coverage	DFR
				CMS CPM 4/1/2008	Records
V630	(ii) Nutritional status	Facility set goals; refer to parameters listed in V509	↑ % of patients within target range on albumin and other nutritional parameters set by the facility	Conditions for Coverage	Records
V631	(iii) Mineral metabolism/renal bone disease	Calcium, phosphorus, and PTH	↑ % in target range monthly	Conditions for Coverage CMS CPM 4/1/2008	Records
V632	(iv) Anemia management	Mean hemoglobin (patient with ESRD at 3 months)	↑ % with mean 10–12 g/dL	Conditions for Coverage	DFR
	Patients taking ESAs and/or patients not taking ESAs	Mean hematocrit	↑ % with mean 30%–36%	CMS CPM 4/1/2008, MIPPA	Records
		Serum ferritin and transferrin saturation or CHr	Evaluate if indicated		
V633	(v) Vascular access (VA)	Cuffed catheters > 90 days	↓ to<10%[f]		DFR
	Evaluation of VA problems, causes, solutions	AV fistulas for dialysis using two needles	↑ to ≥65%[f] or ≥66%[g]		Records
		Thrombosis episodes	↓ to <0.25/pt-year for fistulas; 0.50/pt-year for (grafts	CMS CPM 4/1/2008	CW 2/09
		Infections per use-life of access	↓ to <1% (fistula); <10% (graft)		
		VA patency	↑ % with fistula >3 years and graft >2 years		
V634	(vi) Medical injuries and medical errors identification	Medical injuries and medical errors reporting	↓ frequency through prevention, early identification and root cause analysis	Conditions for Coverage	Records
V635	(vii) Reuse	Evaluation of reuse program including evaluation and reporting of adverse outcomes	↓ adverse outcomes	Conditions for Coverage	DFR Records

V636	(viii) Patient satisfaction and grievances	Report and analyze grievances for trends	Prompt resolution of patient grievances	Conditions for Coverage	Records
		CAHPS In-Center Hemodialysis Survey or any patient satisfaction survey	↑ % of patients satisfied with care	CMS CPM 4/1/2008	Interview
V637	(ix) Infection control	Analyze and document incidence for baselines and trends	Minimize infections and transmission of same	Conditions for Coverage	DFR
			Promote immunizations		Records
V637	Vaccinations	Hepatitis B, influenza, and pneumococcal vaccines	Documentation of education in record	Conditions for Coverage	Records
		Influenza vaccination by facility or other provider	↑ % of patients vaccinated on schedule	CMS CPM 4/1/2008	
			↑ % of patients receiving flu shots 10/1–3/31		

Abbreviations: BP, blood pressure; BCG/BCP, bromcresol green/purple; BMI, body mass index; CAHPS, consumer assessment of healthcare providers and services; CFU, colony-forming units; CHr, reticulocyte hemoglobin; DOPPS, Dialysis Outcomes and Practice Patterns Study; ESA, erythropoiesis stimulating agent; KDOQI, Kidney Disease Outcomes Qualifications Initiative; MIPPA, Miedicare Improvements for Patients and Providers Act of 2008; nPCR, normalized protein catabolic rate; PTH, parathyroid hormone; RKF, residual kidney function; spKt/V = single-pool Kt/V; QoL, quality of life.

Note: *DFR* = Dialysis Facility Reports; *CW* = CROWNWeb; *Chart* = Patient Chart; *Records* = Facility Records; *Interview* = Patient/Staff Interview.

[a] FDA “box” warning.
[b] Medicare reimbursement.
[c] KDOQI Anemia CKD 2007.
[d] KDOQI Vascular Access.
[e] Fistula First.
[f] KDOQI 2006.
[g] Fistula First.

The newest initiatives involve patients in the development of clinical practice guidelines. Patients provide feedback on their health care experiences and then collaborate with researchers to define objectives and indicators (Díaz Del Campo et al., 2011).

19.4 DEVELOPMENT OF PROTOCOLS

Many quality improvement indicators are grouped into practice protocols or criteria. Numerous protocols have already been established by the NKF and the CMS. It is well known that these guidelines can result in improved patient outcomes and provide the structure for systematic patient care reviews. Protocol development should advance according to center needs and resources (Fetter, 2003; Figure 19.2).

The CKD dialysis clinic environment, with its interdisciplinary structure, is ideal for the development of locally needed patient-care-focused protocols (Roberts, 2008). A possible development schematic for nutrition counseling is found in Figure 19.1.

An example of a focus area is patients who are gaining excessive weight between dialysis treatments. Data for this focus area would be collected from the current literature and from the information on patient treatment sheets.

The pilot study:

> All patients with inter-dialytic weight gains more than 5% of dry weight will trigger patient counseling. As a sub-study, try different approaches to patient education. A new idea to consider is cohesive counseling in order to send the same message throughout differing disciplines. Example: If a patient arrives with excessive fluid gains, the diet technician or nurse should be ask the patient to use a check list to identify foods and fluids consumed since the last treatment. Once the list is completed, the staff has the option to refer to the dietitian (if available) or pick from a list of appropriate counseling messages. If the fluid gains are from too much liquid, then pathway one. If the fluid gains are from too many salty foods,

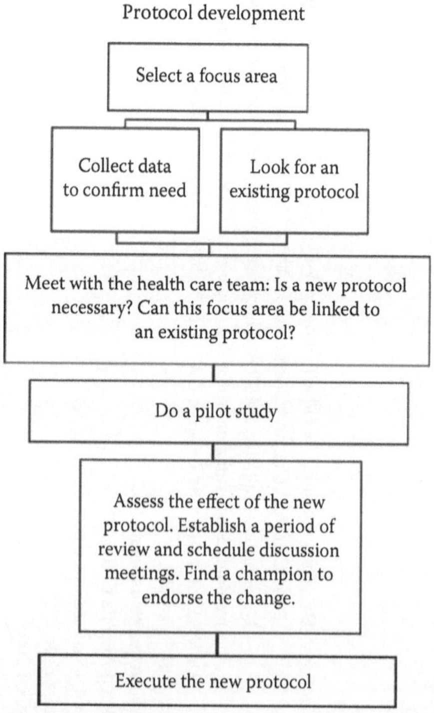

FIGURE 19.2 Protocol development.

then pathway two. Using this approach eliminates the "cut back on all fluids approach." No one wants to advise limiting the nutritional supplement or a fortified juice, along with the ice chips. Salty snack foods might be really be the culprit.

Now, assess the effect of the new protocol. Did the number of excessive inter-dialytic weight gains among the patients improve? Was the staff time adequate to educate the patient? How much additional training was required? Was the ebb and flow of patient care interrupted by this protocol? When the new protocol is executed, always add a date for review or renewal. As needed, collect outcome data to provide justification for new staffing or equipment or materials.

19.4.1 Resistance to Change

Protocols and guidelines implementation can be hindered by resistance to change. Guideline developers must be aware of how presentation will affect the successful execution of new standards. Barriers should be discussed and enablers identified. There is an additive effect on individual guidelines when seen in the context of multiple factors. Resource constraints, workloads, complexity of guidelines, and protocols must be considered when the clinician is looking for ways to break down resistance by changing attitudes. Successful strategies include having open discussions, spelling out the whys of a new standard, having agreement among stakeholders, and scheduling education and training. The application of new guidelines or protocols should be as seamless as possible and should not disrupt the daily routine (Jones et al., 2007).

19.5 STAGES OF CKD

A 2000 NKF KDOQI working group was the first to develop a system of defining CKD and classifying the different stages of disease progression. The overarching goal was to create a method for early identification and treatment of kidney disease. Chronic kidney disease is defined as persistent kidney damage for 3 months. It is associated with a decreased glomerular filtration rate (GFR) in most cases, although disease can also be confirmed by biopsy or other markers (Kent, 2005). The classification stages (Table 19.4), published in 2002, are based on laboratory indicators for severity of disease, the level of complications associated with each stage, risks for loss of kidney function, and the development of cardiovascular comorbidity (National Kidney Foundation, 2002). Diminishing GFR not only impacts general nutritional status but also changes electrolyte balance and mineral metabolism. Most clinical practice guidelines and the development of quality improvement indicators are usually concentrated in Stage 5. This is when the CKD health care teams have the most contact and follow-up opportunities with the patient.

TABLE 19.4
Stages of Chronic Kidney Disease

Stage	Glomerular Filtration	GFR (mL/min/1.73 m^2)
1	Normal rate[a]	≥90
2	Mildly deficient	60–89
3	Moderately deficient	30–59
4	Severely deficient	15–29
5	Failure	≤15 or dialysis

Abbreviation: GFR, glomerular filtration rate.

[a] Certain kidney damage can abnormalities in blood, urine, or be apparent on imaging before changes in GFR are noted.

19.6 CLINICAL PRACTICE GUIDELINES FOR STAGE 1–3 CKD PATIENTS

Typically, CKD patients in stages 1–3 have not been referred to a nephrologist, nor do they see a renal dietitian (RD) for dietary management. If a dietitian is not available, established valid and reliable nutrition screening tools should be used by other health care professionals who have been trained to employ the instrument. Most screening tools take 10–15 min to complete. Good examples are the Mini-Nutritional Assessment, short form (see Chapter 7), the Malnutrition Universal Screening Tool, and the Malnutrition Screening Tool.

The causes of CKD are many and most often are secondary to another illness such as diabetes mellitus, hypertension, and vascular disease. In an outpatient setting, quality improvement indicators for nutrition should focus on the management of the primary disease, weight control, and exercise. Examples might be serum glucose maintained within acceptable standards, improvement in choosing healthy foods, weight loss as appropriate, and establishment of an exercise routine. The patient should always be involved in deciding goal focus areas. Written or online educational materials; frequent follow-up in the office, on the Internet, by mail, or by phone; assignments such as food and/or exercise diaries; and counseling groups can help to increase success for the patient. The U.S. Department of Agriculture (2011) has developed various educational tools for healthy eating. In particular, its Choose My Plate site (http://www.choosemyplate.gov) offers multiple educational materials. Many other organizations have disease-specific nutritional resources. The physician or other health care practitioners should always be aware of the possible progression of renal disease and be alert to evidence of malnutrition (ADA Evidence Based Library, 2011).

Quality improvement opportunities also exist with the hospitalized CKD patient. A recent study (Campos Gutiérrez et al., 2011) suggests that deterioration of kidney function could be identified earlier with the implementation and dissemination of a clinical protocol. This might involve charting creatinine changes or sudden weight fluctuations during hospitalization. Longitudinal electronic health records will one day make this approach very effective in identifying early CKD by combining outpatient data with inpatient data.

19.7 CLINICAL PRACTICE GUIDELINES FOR STAGE 4 CKD PATIENTS

In stage 4 CKD, dietary interventions play an important part in delaying the decline of kidney function (Levey et al., 2006). NKF KDOQI guideline number 24 suggests that a lower protein diet should be one of the first dietary modifications considered. The Nurse's Health study and the Third National Health and Nutrition Examination Survey (NHANESIII) found that there was a relationship between higher protein consumption and indicators of decreased kidney function (Knight et al., 2003; Wrone et al., 2003). A meta-analysis that included more than 2000 patients showed that a reduced-protein diet helped to slow the rate of renal impairment (Fouque and Laville, 2009). A lower protein diet hinders the generation of nitrogenous metabolites and delays the development of uremia. Following a lower protein diet is not without risk, however. At least 50% of the total daily dietary protein should be of high biologic value. Clinical practice guidelines should advise the monitoring of not only protein intake but also energy consumption. Adequate caloric intake will allow protein to be metabolized appropriately. NKF KDOQI guideline number 25 recommends a daily energy intake range of 30–35 cal/kg for most nondialyzed adults. Meeting energy needs can be challenging because appetite is reduced in advancing kidney disease.

Food-frequency questionnaires, 3-day dietary intake reports, and dietary interviews can be used to monitor adequacy of both protein and energy consumption. Objective data should also be monitored. KDOQI recommends serum albumin and actual/standard body weight be measured every 1–3 months. Other laboratory values, such as potassium, calcium, and phosphorus, should also be monitored for changes. If qualitative assessment of protein intake is not available, then normalized protein nitrogen appearance (nPNA) should be calculated every 3–4 months. A subjective global assessment is also recommended quarterly, as are dietary counseling sessions (National Kidney Foundation, 2000). The subjective global assessment focuses on nutrient intake and body composition (McCann, 1996). Nutritional status should be assessed more frequently if there is evidence that there is inadequate food intake, protein-energy malnutrition, or the presence of a comorbidity that worsens baseline nutrition status.

Quality improvement indicators can be constructed around laboratory reports with the goal of all values being within expected parameters. Quantitative indicators should be driven by changes in weight, food intake, gastrointestinal function, activities of daily living, comorbidities, and physical signs of malnutrition. Measurement of these factors is very important since poor nutritional status predicts poor outcome and the development of protein-energy malnutrition (National Kidney Foundation, 2000).

19.8 CLINICAL PRACTICE GUIDELINES FOR STAGE 5 CKD PATIENTS

Once a patient begins dialysis, extensive nutritional assessment is provided by a skilled RD. The 2008 CMS Conditions for Coverage make these statements:

1. Patients have the right of access to a qualified renal dietitian who will provide a comprehensive nutrition assessment and counseling for nutritional needs. The dietitian will also assist with a plan of care and a quality assessment and performance improvement program. Patients will have the opportunity to participate in their care plan.
2. The renal dietitian will be registered with the American Dietetic Association and have at least one year of professional work experience as an RD in a clinical setting. The dietitian will be able to independently perform the duties of nutrition assessment, evaluation of laboratory values, and provide assistance to an interdisciplinary team in terms of management of anemia, bone mineral disorders, and kinetic modeling.

19.8.1 Frequency and Minimum Criteria for Nutritional Assessments

In its Conditions for Coverage (CMS, 2008), the CMS mandates that a new dialysis patient receive an initial nutritional assessment within 3 months of beginning treatment. Afterward, an annual follow-up assessment is required, at minimum, on all stable patients. Unstable patients need to be reassessed monthly.

Every patient is reviewed monthly for changes in weight, albumin, and dialysis adequacy parameters. Quarterly reviews include, but are not limited to, metabolic and glycemic control, cardiovascular health, anthropometric data, self-management skills, and motivation to make changes. A plan of care with established monitoring goals for monitoring laboratories and weight changes is also reviewed monthly (short term) and annually (long term).

An implementation plan must be completed or updated within 15 days of any assessment. It should include active problems, desired outcomes, and planned or completed interventions. Professionally accepted clinical practice standards and CMS clinical performance measures must be used to derive outcome expectations.

19.8.2 Serum Albumin and Other Measures of Nutritional Status

Serum albumin is a widely used marker of visceral protein stores in dialysis patients. It is easily available and highly predictive of mortality risk (Lowrie et al., 1995). NKF KDOQI guideline 3 states that serum albumin is a valid and clinically useful measure of protein-energy malnutrition in dialysis patients (National Kidney Foundation, 2000). The CMS clinical performance measures also suggest using serum albumin as the main indicator of nutritional status (CMS, 2008).

The recommendation to use serum albumin as the sole performance measure comes with cautions. Serum albumin, although recommended by the NKF KDOQI and CMS guidelines, has not been shown to be a reliable measure of nutrition status (de Mutsert et al., 2009). Levels are extremely susceptible to different influences such as inflammation, infection, decreased synthesis from liver disease, acute stress, chronic stress, gastrointestinal loss, tissue injury, and volume overload. Levels are best interpreted over time by using multiple serum albumin values or by pairing serum albumin with other markers (Ikizler, 2009). A composite approach more fully reflects the complicated nature of the complete nutrition assessment. Serum albumin should be partnered with a measurement such as change in dry weight or nPNA and at least one other reliable indicator of possible malnutrition.

According to NKF KDOQI guideline 4, serum pre-albumin is also a valid and clinically useful measure of protein and energy malnutrition. Unfortunately, the same limitations apply to its use as an indicator of malnutrition. The C-reactive protein test can be used in conjunction with serum albumin to evaluate inflammation as the reason for a subnormal value. A very low serum cholesterol reading is also an indicator of acute infection or starvation. Markers for iron deficiency, such as total iron binding capacity (TIBC), transferrin, transferrin saturation, or mean corpuscular volume, can be used to provide clues to the cause of a low serum albumin. Other tests might include total protein, lymphocyte count, alpha-1 acid glycoprotein, creatinine, magnesium, zinc, and potassium (National Kidney Foundation, 2000; Thompson, 2003; Tsirpanlis, 2005). An example of a composite measure of performance might be to pair serum albumin and serum creatinine since a relationship has been established by reports in the literature (Segall et al., 2008).

Other measures of nutritional status can be derived from monitoring such items as change in usual dry weight over time or in the findings from repetitive anthropometric assessment. Significant variations in weight may be overlooked in the presence of pretreatment fluid gains, so it is important to access changes on a monthly basis. Anthropometric assessments should be completed at least every 6 months. Indicators should address the interventions that are put in place once change is noted. The effectiveness of the intervention should be compared to baseline. No single indicator provides a comprehensive assessment of a patient's nutritional health.

19.9 PATIENT-CENTERED CONCEPTS

Often patients are excluded from the development of quality improvement indicators. Patient consultations in the form of focus groups and surveys can be conducted in order to identify patient care areas that should be targets for possible clinical practice guidelines. Targets suggested by patients include care provided by various health care professionals, patient education and training, treatment choices and effectiveness, and health outcomes (Díaz Del Campo et al., 2011; Rubin et al., 1997).

19.10 WHAT DOES KDIGO MEAN?

The incident of CKD is increasing worldwide. For the last 7 years, the KDIGO endeavor has been trying to broaden the scope of current guidelines to reduce the variability of care and improve patient outcomes worldwide. A major focus of the initiative is to translate evidence-based research into well-defined statements that which can be incorporated into clinical practice.

A secondary goal is to establish a more consistent approach to the development of guidelines. The complications from kidney disease are universal. The grading system used to rate the strength of recommendations and quality of the supporting evidence is variable in the extreme. A global public health approach could improve the pace of development, widen the area of dissemination, and increase implementation of evidence-based clinical practice guidelines (Eknoyan et al., 2004; Uhlig et al., 2006).

At this time, KDIGO has published three guidelines: care of the transplant recipient, mineral and bone disorders, and hepatitis C in CKD. Others are planned, including acute kidney injury and care of lipid disorders.

19.11 SUMMARY

Quality improvement indicators or clinical practice guidelines are important to facilitate the excellence in care that every patient deserves. Clinicians should be careful to find the correct balance of national and local guidelines. The guidelines should be valid, appropriate, and easily incorporated into the daily routine. They should be grounded in evidence-based research. A system of indicators/guidelines reviews should be in place in each clinic and for every area of practice. Implementation of guidelines requires the input of all practitioners so obstacles can be identified and corrected.

REFERENCES

American Dietetic Association (ADA) Evidence Based Library. 2011. *Nutrition Screening*. Available at: www.adaevidencelibrary.com/topic.cfm?cat=3584 (accessed August 2011).

Campos Gutiérrez, B., Lou Arnal, L., Gimeno Orna, J., et al. 2011. Undiagnosed kidney disease in hospitalized patients: An opportunity for improvement. *Nefrologia* 31(1):70–75.

Centers for Medicare and Medicaid Services Conditions for Coverage (CMS). 2008. Available at: http://www.cms.gov/CFCsAndCoPs/downloads/ESRDfinalrule0415.pdf (accessed April 12, 2011).

Centers for Medicare and Medicaid Services (CMS). (2011) Available at: https://www.cms.gov/ESRDQualityImproveInit/downloads/QIPODF09212010.pdf (accessed April 10, 2011).

de Mutsert, R., Grootendorst, D., Indemans, F., et al. 2009. Association between serum albumin and mortality in dialysis patients is partly explained by inflammation, and not by malnutrition. *J Renal Nutr.* 19(2):127–135.

Díaz Del Campo, P., Gracia, J., Blasco, J., et al. 2011. A strategy for patient involvement in clinical practice guidelines: Methodological approaches. *BMJ Qual Saf.* Published Online First: April 2, 2011. doi: 10.1136/bmjqs.2010.049031

Eknoyan, G. 2010. Why we need clinical practice guidelines in chronic kidney disease. *J Renal Nutr.* 20(5):S127–S130.

Eknoyan, G., Lameire, N., Baroum, R., et al. 2004. The burden of kidney disease: Improving global outcomes. *Kidney Int.* 66:1310–1314.

Fetter, M. 2003. Geriatric assessment and management protocols. *J Infusion Nurs.* 26:153–160.

Fouque, D. and Laville, M. 2009. Low protein diets for chronic kidney disease in non-diabetic adults. *Cochrane Database Syst Rev.* 3:CD001892.

Ikizler, T. 2009. Nutritional requirements in hemodialysis patients. In Mitch, W. and Ikizler, T. eds. *Handbook of Nutrition and the Kidney*, 6th edition. Philadelphia, PA: Lippincott Williams & Wilkins, 177–195.

Jones, N., Suurdt, J., Ouelette-Kuntz, H., et al. 2007. Implementation of the Canadian clinical practice guidelines for nutrition support: A multiple case study of barriers and enablers. *Nutr Clin Pract.* 22:449–457.

Kent, P. 2005. Integrating clinical nutrition practice guidelines in chronic kidney disease. *Nutr Clin Pract.* 20(2):213–217.

Knight, E., Stampfer, M., Hankinson, S., et al. 2003. The impact of protein intake on renal function decline in women with normal renal function or mild renal insufficiency. *Ann Intern Med.* 138:460–467.

Levey, A., Greene, T., Samak, M., et al. 2006. Effect of dietary protein restriction on the progression of kidney disease: Long-term follow-up of the modification of diet in renal disease study. *Am J Kidney Dis.* 48(6):879–888.

Lowrie, E., Huang, W., and Lew N. 1995. Death risk predictors among peritoneal dialysis and hemodialysis patients. *Am J Kidney Dis.* 26:220–228.

Luce, J., Bindman, A., and Lee, P. 1994. A brief history of health care quality assessment and improvement in the United States. *West J Med.* 160(3):263–268.

McCann, L. 1996. Subjective global assessment as it pertains to nutrition status. *Dialysis Transplant.* 25(4):190.

National Kidney Foundation. 1997a. DOQI clinical practice guidelines for hemodialysis and peritoneal adequacy. *Am J Kidney Dis.* 30:Suppl 3.

National Kidney Foundation. 1997b. DOQI clinical practice guidelines for vascular access. *Am J Kidney Dis.* 30:S150–S191.

National Kidney Foundation. 2000. KDOQI nutrition in chronic renal failure. *Am J Kidney Dis.* 35(6) Suppl 2:S1–S141.

National Kidney Foundation. 2002. KDOQI clinical practice guidelines for chronic kidney disease: evaluation, classification, and stratification. Available at: www.kidney.org (accessed April 6, 2011).

Neuhauser, D. 2002. Ernest Amory Codman, MD. *Qual Saf Health Care.* 11(2):104–105.

Nightingale, F. 1860. *Notes on Nursing*. New York: Appleton and Company, 129.

Roberts, J., Coale, J., and Redman, R. 1987. A history of the joint commission on accreditation of hospitals. *JAMA* 258:936–940.

Roberts, S. 2008. Evidence based protocols: Why protocols are beneficial and considerations for implementation. *Support Line* 30(2):23–26.

Roberts, S. and Reed, L. 2009. Understanding and applying evidence based guidelines in clinical practice. *Support Line* 3192:16–21.

Rubin, H., Jenckes, M., Fink, N., et al. 1997. Patient's view of dialysis care: Development of a taxonomy and rating of importance of different aspects of care. CHOICE study. *Am J Kidney Dis.* 30(6):793–801.

Segall, L., Covic, A., Mardare, N., et al. 2008. Nutritional status evaluation in maintenance hemodialysis patients. *Rev Med Chir Soc Med Nat Iasi.* 112(2):343–350.

Steinwachs, D. and Hughes, R. 2008. Health services research: Scope and significance. In: Hughes, R., ed., *Patient Safety and Quality: An Evidence-Based Handbook for Nurses*. Books and Documents. Available at: www.ncbi.nlm.nih.gov/pubmed/21328761

Thompson, C. 2003. Laboratory assessment. In Charney, P. and Malone, A., eds., *ADA Pocket Guide to Nutrition Assessment.* Chicago, IL: American Dietetic Association, 63–141.

Tsirpanlis, G. 2005. The pattern of inflammation and a potential new clinical meaning and usefulness of C-reactive protein in end-stage renal failure patients. *Kidney Blood Press Res.* 28(1):55–61.

Uhlig, K., MacLeod, A., Craig, J., et al. 2006. Grading evidence and recommendations for clinical practice guidelines in nephrology. *Kidney Int.* 70:2058–2065.

U.S. Department of Agriculture. 2011. Choose my plate. Available at: www.choosemyplate.gov (accessed August 2011).

Wrone, E., Carnethon, M., Palaniappan, L., et al. 2003. Association of dietary intake and microalbuminuria in healthy adults: Third national health and nutrition examination survey. *Am J Kidney Dis.* 41(3):580–587.

20 Counseling Strategies

Matthew Orr
University of South Carolina School of Medicine

CONTENTS

20.1 GRABBING THE LOW-HANGING FRUIT: SOLUTION-FOCUSED INTERVENTIONS FOR BRIEF COUNSELING

One of the most challenging tasks for patients with chronic health conditions is to navigate all the lifestyle modifications their health care providers tell them they must make. Some may argue that this is never any truer than it is for patients with chronic kidney disease (CKD), who are often expected to adapt to highly restrictive diets as well as modify other health behaviors, such as physical activity, smoking cessation, and medication adherence. This chapter provides a practical patient-centered approach to counseling patients who have difficulty making these changes. Although the focus of this book is dietetics, most health care providers will no doubt find themselves counseling patients with CKD on these other health behaviors as well.

20.2 DEVELOPING A SOLUTION FOCUS

20.2.1 Solution-Focused Therapy

Solution-focused therapy (SFT) is based on the belief that people are experts about their own lives, that they already possess the resources necessary to solve their problems, and that change occurs more readily when the focus is on their strengths and past successes rather than their weaknesses and failures (Berg, 1994; de Shazer, 1988). This approach not only empowers patients to manage their lives but also fits well into busy health care practices when time is at a premium. The application of SFT to primary medical care has been proposed and described by others for more than a decade (Cheng, 2007; Giorlando and Rae, 1997; Greenberg et al., 2001; Poon, 1997).

People so often focus on their problems or what is not going well in their lives. This is especially true of people living with chronic illness for whom treatment (i.e., lifestyle modifications) can be as inconveniencing or unbearable as the illness itself, if not more so from the perspective of patients, such as those with CKD, who must live with these modifications daily, even though they may not experience their symptoms every day. People in this situation often present as overwhelmed, discouraged, and seeking relief, but they dread hearing the next generic or cumbersome instruction or recommendation offered by yet another health care clinician. They often welcome a solution-based approach because it helps them identify and tap into their own resources and repertoire of successful experiences, whether now or in the past, and it does so in a simple fashion. Walter and Peller (1992) summarize the core elements of constructing solutions as follows:

> *One*, define what the client wants rather than what he or she does not; *two*, look for what is working and do more of it; *three*, if what the client is doing is not working, then have him or her do something different. (p. 6)

These basic tenets of solution building are embodied in the techniques described in this chapter; each technique contains some element of both exploring what has gone well in the past and discovering what is going well right now and what the patient thinks will go well in the future. As these techniques are applied, the conversation between the clinician and the patient becomes less problem oriented and more solution focused (e.g., taking into account what patient wants vs. what he or she does not want), and there is a shift of viewpoint from what holds the patient back to what propels him or her forward. The idea is not to suggest that there is a behavioral intervention that will "cure" chronic illness; rather, the idea is to promote methods that empower people to improve their quality of life and perhaps influence the course of their illness. This approach encourages patients to grab the low-hanging fruit on the tree, so to speak, rather than to simply diagnose what they are doing wrong and then construct interventions to correct those deficits. This latter approach is akin to asking the patient to navigate a winding, obstacle-filled path to the top of the tree, where the fruit is no healthier or tastier.

20.2.2 Circular Questions

The framework and techniques described here are also informed by the circular-questioning methods of brief systemic family therapy (Fleuridas et al., 1986). The circular-questioning interview style focuses on illuminating the connections and distinctions between people and their behavior; it is in contrast to a linear approach, which typically only captures disparate pieces of information that have diagnostic but little interventional value. Central to this approach is the idea that "developing an awareness of the reciprocal interrelatedness of behaviors may, in and of itself, promote spontaneous change" (Fleuridas et al., 1986, p. 113). While this approach originally focused on family relationship processes, it can be extremely useful in health behavior counseling because it helps individuals and families become more aware of the role of behavior in the disease process and its management. For example, instead of the clinician asking the patient, "What is difficult about following the diet?" a circular style will sound as follows:

"Tell me about a time when you were able to follow one of the food recommendations?"
"Where were you?"
"Who was there?"
"What was going on?"
"What did you do?"
"What did (they) do?"
"What happened next?"
"And then what happened?"
"How often does it go this way?"
"What is different about when it does go this way?"

Instead of focusing on *why* patients have not been able to follow their diets, for example, this approach aims to help patients discover, in their own words, the specific factors or resources (i.e., people, places, actions, and abilities) that have contributed to successful decision making and behavior, such as following a dietary recommendation in the above example. Each response to a question about past successes represents another possible solution in the here and now. If a patient identifies that her last dietary success was that she ordered a salad for lunch, that her best friend was with her and ordered the same thing, and that she was motivated by knowing that she would be eating an early dinner, she has just verbalized several supportive psychosocial factors on which the clinician and patient can construct future solutions, namely, building in more social supports and modifying her eating schedule. While this focus on social supports and daily schedules is nothing new to health counseling, the advantage of SFT methods and using a circular questioning style is that it is the patient who generates these ideas, and what is more, her responses reveal what has worked for her.

Indeed, questions are key to collecting information and getting to know patients. However, a circular question in and of itself can serve as a potent intervention technique (McGee et al., 2005). For example, "What has been going well with your food choices?" is more effective than asking "How is your diet going?" The value of the former question is much more than the difference between open-ended and closed-ended questions. The value is that the patient has to stop and think about what *specifically* has been going well, which raises his or her level of insight into and awareness of the particular circumstances of the situation and highlights possible solutions.

20.2.3 "Tell Me ..."

One of the most fruitful single-item interventions for moving a patient's cognitive process is actually a statement rather than a question: "Tell me (more) about ..." This has been called a "curious command" (Mitchell, 2005), and while there are others, such as "Please share with me ... ," "Describe to me ... ," and so on, there seems to be no more gentle, yet effective, patient-centered prompt than "Tell me ..." because it (1) expresses empathy and genuine interest and concern for the patient; (2) asserts that there is not necessarily one all-encompassing explanation but a variety of possible explanations for the patient's situation; and (3), perhaps most importantly, declares that the patient is capable of being in control of his or her life, at least enough to identify and discuss these possibilities.

20.3 TECHNIQUES

20.3.1 Exceptions to the Problem

Central to the concept of constructing solutions is identifying *exceptions to the problem* (Berg, 1994; de Shazer, 1988). This technique encourages patients to explore the times when they have not been mired in their current problem. The intent of this intervention is to determine what has worked in the past for the patient in order to promote doing more of it in the here and now. Consider the following excerpt from an interview between a clinician and a patient, Sue, whose current distress is her uncontrolled diabetes and concomitant fatigue and low mood:

Clinician: Tell me about the last time your blood sugar was under control.
Sue: It's been a while since it was really down. It's always so up and down.
Clinician: It sounds like you've been dealing with a lot (*expressing empathy*). How about just tell me about the last time you felt better than you do now. (*Clarifying and simplifying the request out of respect for her condition – fatigue and possible poor concentration*)
Sue: Oh I guess it was a month ago .... Yeah, it was definitely last month.
Clinician: What was different about last month?
Sue: I was going on my walks, eating pretty good food, and I was spending more time reading my Bible. I let myself get away from that. Yeah, that's it exactly! My daughter and her kids moved back in with me and she's had all of this trouble with money and I've had to help her carry the kids to school and around town because she works at night. I love them, but I'd just like some time to myself again.

Highlighting exceptions to the problem is a solution-focused application of circular techniques and helps to illuminate the relationship between the times when patients have lived well with their illness and the behaviors that contributed to that success. When we ask people about their problems, they tell us about their problems. When we ask them about their prior successes, they will tell us about what has worked for them in the past, and this may offer possible solutions for their present distress.

Clinician: My goodness. It sounds like you know how to take care of yourself! How did you make all of that happen ... the walking and eating and the Bible study?
Sue: Oh, well, I used to be pretty active and fit when I was young, but then had kids and let myself go. I've been battling weight problems for about twenty years, and then I found out I had diabetes. I decided I had to take care of myself and I was doing really well until this last year and then I've been up and down ... lots of stress you know?
Clinician: Wow, you are a determined person. You take care of yourself and then you take care of your daughter and grandkids. ... You're not going to let anything happen to them it sounds like. I wonder if it is a matter of finding ways to do both at the same time.
Sue: I think that is very true.
Clinician: Something tells me you will find a way to make it happen. In the meantime, I would be happy to help you sort out how you might do it when you feel up to it.

20.3.2 Compliments

In the preceding exchange the clinician punctuates Sue's comments about her behavior in the past with *compliments*. Giving compliments (Berg, 1994; de Shazer, 1988) is another solution-focused and circular interviewing method that helps bring to light people's strengths and resources. The clinician refrains from focusing on "why" having her daughter and grandchildren living her causes her stress and how she might cope with it. Instead, the clinician compliments her determination and her ability to take care of herself and suggests that she had simply transferred that determination and care from herself to them. This is inherently more empowering than suggesting that she is not coping well enough.

There is always something for which patients can be complimented—the fact that they managed to make it to their appointment that day or that they have made it through adversity to get to their current point in the life are examples. One can wonder aloud: "How did you manage to make that happen?" or "Where or from whom did you learn to make it happen?" Patients living with chronic and potentially debilitating illnesses can feel patronized and dismissed if clinicians move directly into teaching cognitive and behavioral coping skills because this sends the message that what they have been doing is wrong and that they must learn something new in order to succeed. By focusing on a patient's indisputable accomplishments, such as making his or her appointment or keeping his or her diabetes under control for 6 months prior to a current symptomatic episode, clinicians can help to establish that the evidence demonstrates that the patient possesses the necessary resources to succeed in his or her own way.

20.3.3 Miracle Question

Synonymous with SFT is the *miracle question* (Berg, 1994; de Shazer, 1988). The purpose of this technique is to help patients identify what they would like to be different about themselves or situations, rather than thinking only about what they do not like about their lives. This focus on something positive that they would like to see happen is, in essence, setting a goal for behavior change. To apply this technique, the clinician instructs:

> Suppose this evening you get tired and go to sleep … , and in the middle of the night, when you are fast asleep, a miracle happens and something changes that makes things better for you. … But because you were asleep you did not know it had happened. … When you wake up the next morning, what do you notice that tells you a miracle happened? What has changed/improved? What else do you notice? What else?

This can be highly effective at identifying specific behaviors that are amenable to change; however, the clinician may need to help move the patient through this exercise. It is common for patients to respond, "I would be rich" or "I would have a million dollars." A solution-focused response to this would be, "Sounds like that might make a difference. Now let's think about something a bit more reasonable, something a bit more likely to happen soon." People also often answer this question with a negative that states the opposite of the problem. For example, "I wouldn't have kidney disease" or "My husband would listen to me more" or "My son would stop asking me for money." These are not issues people can resolve or change overnight because they cannot change the fact that they have a disease or immediately change another person's behavior. But these wishes are not necessarily impossible and focusing on them provides an excellent opportunity to highlight the roles people play in their own frustrations and promotes a sense of control and influence over these problems by asking: "If that happened what would you notice was different about yourself?"

This helps people focus on themselves and on the behaviors or characteristics that are more likely under their immediate control and influence as well as emphasizes beginning with small, manageable changes. With just this one question, people often shift from an external focus on what other people are doing wrong to being quite specific about what they themselves can do to improve their situation. Clinicians may also hear common responses such as, "I would pray first thing when I woke up" or "I would get up and make my own breakfast" or "I would ask my husband to help me make breakfast."

Such responses indicate that the patients are intentionally thinking about what actions they could take to improve their situations. The question-response exchange also suggests that the possibility of change is within the patient's reach and that the patient is capable of making these changes. Therefore, it is not necessary to follow up with a plan to implement these changes; the patient's realization of these possibilities is intervention enough since it is up to each patient to decide how and when to put them into action. Of course, clinicians may wish to pursue this discussion further.

20.4 ONE THING TECHNIQUE

20.4.1 One Thing

The *one thing* technique can be used to build upon the miracle question or can stand on its own as an intervention. Like the miracle question, it helps bring into focus what the patient would like be different about his or her situation and leads the way toward identifying concrete ways to achieve a goal. It begins:

> Tell me just one thing that you would like to see be different about yourself or your situation?

The patient's response is followed by:

> What is one thing that you could do to make this happen?

An alternative to this question in situations where there is a premium on decreasing the pressure the patient is feeling and increasing manageability of the problem, is as follows:

> What is one thing that *could change or improve about you or your situation* that will make it *more likely* that will happen?

The idea is to use as many follow-up questions as necessary to "peel the layers of the onion" and arrive at a concrete, manageable action the patient can take. The following is an example of such a conversation between a primary care physician and Linda, a 52-year-old female patient with CKD who had not experienced many symptoms before a recent bout of persistent fatigue, swollen ankles, and changes in her urination, which frightened her and led to her lamenting her struggle to stick to her diet and nutrition plan:

Dr: Tell me just one thing that you would like to see be different about yourself or your situation?

Linda: If I could stick to the diet plan that would help, of course.

Dr.: What is something that you could do to make this happen?

Linda: It is so hard, this diet is so blah! If there was some way to stick to it I would do it.

Dr: It does sound like a tremendous challenge! What is just one thing that could change or be different about you or your situation will make it just a little more likely that will happen?"

Linda: I don't know .... I guess it would be being able to fix my own food and not worry about having to cook or eat with the rest of my family. If I don't to take care of my husband and my son and grandchildren, no one will, and we eat a lot of big family dinners every week with my sisters and their families and I cook for everyone. I can't expect them to eat stuff from my boring diet and it's hard to turn down that tasty food when it's right there. Yeah, I suppose that would be it ... things would be easier if I only had to cook for myself.

This exchange could stop here and still be productive since the patient has now acknowledged a potential solution, and it would be appropriate to emphasize her autonomous decision making by letting her sit with this thought. However, the physician decides it would be more helpful to peel the layers of the onion to identify solutions that depend less on the cooperation of others:

Dr.: What would have to happen to make it a little more likely you will cook for yourself?

Linda: (chuckling) Oh, I'd have to move out.

Dr.: That doesn't sound like an option at this point, does it? Short of moving out, what's one thing that will make it a bit easier to get a meal or two to yourself?

Linda: That's funny, you say a meal or two and I'm always thinking that I have to eat right [at] every meal or what's the use. I can probably shoot for a meal or two each week when it's just me and my husband if you think that might help.

Dr.: It sounds like a great start. When you get to the point where you are ready to make this adjustment, what do you think it will be that makes it happen the first time?

Linda: I guess it will be that I tell my husband and son that this is something I have to do. They were pretty concerned when they saw my ankles all swollen. And then buy the right things at the grocery store.

The physician could continue by exploring what it will take for Linda to follow through on her decision to tell her husband and to actually make the right purchases at the grocery store, and so on. However, Linda's physician is determined that she had come a long way during this visit. He did not want to frustrate her and also wanted to support her sense of autonomy and choice in deciding how she would put these possibilities into action.

20.4.2 Scaling Questions

Another method for exploring possibilities and setting goals is the use of *scaling questions* (Berg, 1994). These serve a variety of purposes and can be applied to any situation, such as gauging patients' level of interest in change, determining their readiness to change, helping them to see their problem in terms of establishing small and manageable goals, and supporting their progress toward behavior change. These are just some examples related to behavioral health counseling, and the wording of the questions can be adapted to fit any focus. The intervention can be thought of as having two stages: (1) introduction of the scale and (2) and following up and concretizing goals and hypothetical solutions.

20.4.2.1 Introduction of the Scale

In gauging the patient's *readiness to change*, the following is a versatile template for staging the question:

> On a scale from 1 to 10, with 1 being the least ready you have been and 10 being the most ready you can imagine being, how ready would you say you are today to try this eating plan?

For gauging the patient's *willingness to explore change* (i.e., gauging the level of interest), the word "ready" would be replaced by "willing," and the question would be modified as follows:

> ... How willing would you say you are today to think about the information I am giving you?

This can also be done for the patient's *confidence* that he or she can follow through on a plan:

> ... How confident are you today that you will be able to stick to your plan?

For *happiness, satisfaction, motivation, health, support from family, and so on*:

> ... Where would you say your level of happiness (satisfaction, motivation, health, support from family) is today?

20.4.2.2 Following Up and Concretizing Goals and Hypothetical Solutions

Initially, patients often struggle to assign a number to their responses. They seem to feel compelled to talk more about what is not going well in their lives. When this happens it is important for the clinician to stick to the question and help guide the patient back to a specific answer. The following question usually helps patients get their bearings and offer a rating on the scale:

> Okay, so where does that put you on the scale right now? ... What number would you give that?

The next step is critical to helping the patient identify a concrete goal and think about possible behavioral solutions toward that goal. Let us assume that a patient is asked how hopeful he is about his situation and that he has responded that he is at 6. Then the clinician asks:

> What would be different about you or your life that would move you to 6 ½?

This is also an opportunity to use the one thing intervention to increase specificity and focus:

What is one thing that could change or improve about you or your situation that would push you to a 6 ½?

The emphasis here is on asking the patient to consider a hypothetical question: what would have to happen to move his or her rating to the positive side of the scale. Framing the question in this way and stressing just a half-point movement decreases the pressure many patients feel to change everything all at once because it essentially gives them permission to consider small, reasonable goals and manageable steps toward achieving those goals in the form of hypothetical possibilities.

20.4.3 From Scaling Questions to the One Thing

For instance, consider Charles, a patient with CKD, who displays low mood and says that he is discouraged about not being able to control his diabetes or hypertension. Charles has previously dismissed recommendations to quit smoking and change his diet. But when asked how confident he is that he can improve these conditions without changing his smoking or diet, he now rates himself 4 on the 1–10 scale.

Clinician: What would be different about you or your life that would move you to 4 ½?
Charles: If I could control my sugar and blood pressure without giving things up.
Clinician: What might be one thing that could change or improve about you or your situation that would push you up just that half a point?"
Charles: A 4 ½ eh? I guess if it didn't cost so much to eat healthy! That's a big deal when you live on a fixed income!

There are two essential points in this exchange that exemplify the nature of a solution-focused approach. First, it would not be surprising if some clinicians decided to point out to Charles the discrepancy between his refusal to quit smoking or change his diet and his "4" confidence rating that he can become healthier without doing so. This may be useful in increasing his motivation to change. However, such discrepancies are often obvious to patients, and pointing them out may only increase the pressure they feel. Typically, the issue is that they do not know how to resolve the discrepancies and feel stuck rather than being unaware of them. Second, Charles' final response demonstrates the importance of continuing to peel the layers of the onion. Given his previous response, some clinicians may simply assume that Charles will say that not having to give anything up would make things better; however, clinicians often find that asking that next question, along the same line, often yields tangible results. While the clinician and patient still have work to do to move toward solutions, the door to solution room has been opened because his response indicates he might prefer to discuss dietary changes than his smoking and, most importantly, that he has at least explored the possibility of making changes to his diet in the past.

Clinician: Sometimes when folks are dealing with so much the littlest of changes don't seem to count for much, but they really do make a difference in the long run. I wonder what could be the smallest change you could make and still be on a fixed income even if it didn't seem like it would make a difference.
Charles: Small change .... Hmmm ... well, my wife has been on me about my potato chips. I suppose I could cut back on those. (Chuckling) I don't know if that would make much of a difference!

Charles has just asserted that change, no matter how small, is still a possibility, and that he is capable of making it when he is ready. Restraining the size of the proposed change reduces the pressure of the change process from being like a tidal wave over which the patient feels no control to a cup of water over which the patient has control and can sip from when he chooses. Since this is a statement rather than a question, it does not require a definitive response about his plan or purchasing food; instead, it promotes imagination and hypothetical solutions regarding existing food choices and options.

Clinician: Wow! Potato chips huh? So using that same scale of 1–10, how likely are you to cut back on your chips for just two days this next week if you pick the days?

Charles: Scale of 1–10. … (Laughing) Probably a 2 on that! … Nah, I'm probably at a 6, especially if I can pick the days. It'll have to be the weekdays because I like to have chips while I'm watching football and basketball on TV.

Clinician: Okay, I'm impressed. What would it take to push you to a 6.5 for those two days?

Charles: I usually take the whole bag of chips and just keep eating them. I guess I could just put some in a bowl and just eat those.

Clinician: Great idea! I wonder if there is something else that you could have on hand for when you get to the bottom of the bowl in case you still have a hankering for the chips.

Charles: To be honest, yeah, well they're still like chips, but my wife got some unsalted pretzels and I ate those a couple of times. She really wanted me to eat celery sticks like it said in that pamphlet. I guess I could do that once or twice too.

Clinician: It sounds like you may have some options. Now what else can we bug you about, or is that enough for today?

This dialogue illustrates how the conversation cycles back to a scaling question to concretize small, manageable goals and hypothetical possibilities. The clinician does not impose a set requirement or recommendations on the patient; instead, he or she poses his suggestions as "I wonder what would happen if" questions that the patient can do with what he chooses. Fortunately for the change process, framing issues in this hypothetical way reduces the pressure on the patient and opens up a discussion of possibilities. Here, Charles comes up with several possibilities on his own, and the clinician does not try to dictate how or when Charles should implement them. The visit finishes with an affirmation that Charles has options, which he himself generated. The clinician pairs this with a playful question intended to bring the visit to a close, but that, most importantly, acknowledges both the challenges of trying to change and how much work the patient did during that visit.

20.5 REFRAMING

A *reframe* redefines the problem as something inherently more positive. Because reframing makes the problem seem more amenable to change, it can be a useful and empowering technique when the patient seems to resist making changes. It is usually the case that the more complex is the problem, the harder it is to change, and the more resistant the patient seems. So methods that diminish the perceived potency of problems typically allow the patient to feel more hopeful and optimistic about change.

For example, it is common for patients being counseled about smoking cessation to counter the clinician's comments with an emphatic I'm-not-interested-in-changing-anything type of response, such as the following:

> My father smoked all of his life, and he lived to be … 85 years old.

This closes the door on productive health behavior counseling for clinicians who tend to get revved up at this type of response and who want to probe for evidence that the father actually experienced low quality of life and that smoking ultimately led to his death. This is often a fruitless approach because there is no guarantee that the father's perceived quality of life suffered and, more importantly, it turns the conversation into a power struggle. It can be much more fruitful to respond to the patient by saying:

> So, smoking was a part of your father's health care plan; what other things did your father do to live to be 85 years old?

This statement and the question together reframe the father's behavior (smoking) as normal for him and turn the focus to other, less emotionally laden discussions of health behaviors, which the clinician and patient can explore together. Many patients will respond as this patient did, by saying:

> That's a good question. Well, actually he did quit smoking—when he was 75—and walked two miles almost every day at the mall with a friend of his.

Discussing a patient's father rather than the patient himself can help loosen his defensiveness about his own decisions and behavior enough to consider alternative points of view. Even if the patient does not acknowledge the smoking, discussing other behaviors, such as physical activity and eating, can suggest the possibility of making smaller changes that from the patient's perspective seem more manageable. For example, about the "other things his father did" the patient responds:

> Oh, well he always said putting extra salt on your food was bad for you. And he worked every day on his farm until he was 70 and then worked a large garden when the farm work was too much.

This response opens the doors for the clinician to explore what the patient feels were the motivation behind these behaviors; highlight them as health behaviors (i.e., diet and physical activity) and then amplify them toward the patient by asking as follows:

> What are your healthy habits when it comes to eating? What serves as your farm for physical activity like your father had?

20.5.1 Life Lessons: Reframing

It can be particularly useful with behaviors that are highly resistant to change, such as diet and physical activity, to reframe them as lessons the patient is teaching to others rather than emphasizing them as problems. Consider the following questions:

> What is it that you try to teach your children about how to handle adversity such as this?
> What is it that you'd like your children (others) to learn from you about handling illness and pain?
> If you look down the road five years, what do you want to be able to say your children learned from you about the way you handled your situation?

Many patients will respond, "Hmmm … I hadn't really thought about it like that before." The potency of reframing questions is that they emphasize relationships with loved ones, especially children, and this tends to increase patients' self-awareness about the stakes of their behavior and makes the discussion of that behavior, as well as the potential behavior change, more meaningful. In essence, reframing the behavior as a life lesson takes the covert, private worry people may have about the impact of their behavior on their loved ones and makes it an overt, public reality that cannot be as easily suppressed.

For those patients without children or dependents, an alternative reframing question can be asked that creates the same frame of thought:

> When you get to that point in your life when you are looking back on what you have accomplished and what your legacy has been, what do you want people to be able to say about you?

20.6 CRYSTAL BALL

Crystal ball interventions are simply solution-focused, circular questions that help the patient focus on the future and articulate short- and long-term goals. Crystal ball questions are largely self-explanatory and elaborate on the other techniques discussed in this chapter. They can help further illuminate and concretize goals and solutions when used to follow up those other interventions. Also, clinical experience suggests that the more complex a problem is and the more resistant the patient is to engage in the change process, the more useful will a future focus and these crystal ball techniques become. Some examples of crystal ball questions are as follows:

Where would you like to be in six months? A year? ... Five years?
What will you be doing?
Who will be there?
What things that you are doing now put you closer to that vision?
Let's pretend that/when you wake up one day and your symptoms are controlled, people are off your back, you've only gone to your doctor for regular visits, etc. What would you guess would be one thing that you would look back and say you did to make that more likely to happen?
Six months (or one year) from now what do you want to be able to look back and say you accomplished between now and then?
What will you notice is different about yourself at the time you are ready to make a change?
What will be a sign that something different needs to happen or that you need to make a change?

20.7 CONCLUSION

This chapter has elucidated a framework of solution-focused counseling strategies for health behavior change, in general, and for diet counseling, in particular. These techniques are versatile and can be adapted to a variety of behavior change issues, as well as to various interpersonal styles. It is certainly not a comprehensive review of SFT or of the circular questioning interviewing style. It provides a practical explanation of several valuable techniques for initiating and supporting the behavior change process. The intention is to introduce readers to the potential clinical utility of a solution-focused approach as an alternative to or in addition to other established and promising models of dietary health behavior counseling (Spahn et al., 2010).

REFERENCES

Berg, I. 1994. *Family Based Services: A Solution Focused Approach*. New York: WW Norton.

Cheng, M. 2007. New approaches for creating the therapeutic alliance: Solution-focused interviewing, motivational interviewing, and the medication interest model. *Psychiatr Clin North Am*. 30:157–166.

deShazer, S. 1988. *Investigating Solutions in Brief Therapy*. New York: WW Norton

Fleuridas, C., Nelson, T., and Rosenthal, D. 1986. The evolution of circular questions: Training family therapists. *J Marital Fam Ther*. 12:113–127.

Giorlando, M. and Rae, J. 1997. On becoming a solution-focused physician: The MED-STAT acronym. *Fam Syst Health*. 15:361–373.

Greenberg, G., Ganshorn, K., and Danilkewich, A. 2001. Solution-focused therapy. Counseling model for busy family physicians. *Can Fam Phys*. 47:2289–2295.

McGee, D., Del Vento, A., and Beavin Bavelas, J. (2005). An interactional model of questions as therapeutic interventions. *J Marital Fam Ther*. 31:371–384.

Mitchell, C. 2005. *Effective Techniques for Dealing with Highly Resistant Clients*. Johnson City, TN: Clifton W. Mitchell Publishing.

Poon, V. 1997. Short counseling techniques for busy family doctors. *Can Fam Phys*. 43:705–713.

Spahn, J., Reeves, R., Keim, K., et al. 2010. State of the evidence regarding behavior change theories and strategies in nutrition counseling to facilitate health and food behavior change. *J Am Diet Assoc*. 110:879–891.

Walter, J. and Peller, J. 1992. *Becoming Solution-Focused in Brief Therapy*. New York: Brunner/Mazel.

Index

G

H

K

L

M

N